Trauma Emergencies

Editors

CHRISTOPHER HICKS
KIMBERLY A. BOSWELL

EMERGENCY MEDICINE CLINICS OF NORTH AMERICA

www.emed.theclinics.com

Consulting Editor
AMAL MATTU

February 2023 • Volume 41 • Number 1

ELSEVIER

1600 John F. Kennedy Boulevard • Suite 1800 • Philadelphia, Pennsylvania, 19103-2899

http://www.theclinics.com

EMERGENCY MEDICINE CLINICS OF NORTH AMERICA Volume 41, Number 1
February 2023 ISSN 0733-8627, ISBN-13: 978-0-323-93969-0

Editor: Joanna Gascoine

Developmental Editor: Axell Ivan Jade Purificacion

Emergency Medicine Clinics of North America (ISSN 0733-8627) is published quarterly by Elsevier Inc., 360 Park Avenue South, New York, NY, 10010-1710. Months of issue are February, May, August, and November. Business and Editorial Offices: 1600 John F. Kennedy Boulevard, Suite 1800, Philadelphia, PA 19103-2899. Customer Service Office: 6277 Sea Harbor Drive, Orlando, FL 32887-4800. Periodicals postage paid at New York, NY, and additional mailing offices. Subscription prices are $100.00 per year (US students), $381.00 per year (US individuals), $778.00 per year (US institutions), $220.00 per year (international students), $490.00 per year (international individuals), $958.00 per year (international institutions), $100.00 per year (Canadian students), $449.00 per year (Canadian individuals), and $958.00 per year (Canadian institutions). International air speed delivery is included in all *Clinics'* subscription prices. All prices are subject to change without notice. **POSTMASTER:** Send address changes to *Emergency Medicine Clinics of North America*, Elsevier Periodicals Customer Service, 11830 Westline Industrial Drive, St. Louis, MO 63146. Customer Service (orders, claims, online, change of address): Elsevier Periodicals **Customer Service, 11830 Westline Industrial Drive, St. Louis, MO 63146. Tel: 1-800-654-2452 (U.S. and Canada); 314-453-7041 (outside U.S. and Canada). Fax: 314-453-5170. E-mail: journalscustomerservice-usa@elsevier.com (for print support); journalsonlinesupport-usa@elsevier.com (for online support)**.

Reprints. For copies of 100 or more of articles in this publication, please contact the Commercial Reprints Department, Elsevier Inc., 360 Park Avenue South, New York, NY 10010-1710. Tel.: 212-633-3874; Fax: 212-633-3820; E-mail: reprints@elsevier.com.

Emergency Medicine Clinics of North America is covered in *MEDLINE/PubMed (Index Medicus), Current Contents/Clinical Medicine, EMBASE/Excerpta Medica, BIOSIS, SciSearch, CINAHL, ISI/BIOMED,* and *Research Alert.*

Contributors

CONSULTING EDITOR

AMAL MATTU, MD, FAAEM, FACEP
Professor and Vice Chair, Department of Emergency Medicine, University of Maryland School of Medicine, Baltimore, Maryland

EDITORS

KIMBERLY A. BOSWELL, MD, FACEP
Assistant Professor, Department of Emergency Medicine, University of Maryland School of Medicine, R. Adams Cowley Shock Trauma Center, University of Maryland Medical Center, Baltimore, Maryland, USA

CHRISTOPHER HICKS, MD, MEd, FRCPC
Department of Emergency Medicine, St. Michael's Hospital, Toronto, Ontario, Canada

AUTHORS

HENRY AJZENBERG, MD
Division of Emergency Medicine, University of Toronto, Toronto, Ontario, Canada

SAMUEL AUSTIN, DO
Fellow, Trauma and Surgical Critical Care, R Adams Cowley Shock Trauma Center, Baltimore, Maryland, USA

JEANNIE CALLUM, MD, FRCPC
Queen's University, Kingston, Ontario, Canada

WAN-TSU W. CHANG, MD
Associate Professor, Departments of Emergency Medicine and Neurology, Program in Trauma, University of Maryland School of Medicine, Baltimore, Maryland, USA

TIM CHAPLIN, MD
Department of Emergency Medicine, Queen's University, Kingston, Ontario, Canada

LUIS TEODORO DA LUZ, MD, MSc
Sunnybrook Health Sciences Centre, Toronto, Ontario, Canada

SAGAR B. DAVE, DO
Assistant Professor, Departments of Emergency Medicine and Anesthesiology, Emory University School of Medicine, Emory Critical Care Center, Emory University, Atlanta, Georgia, USA

JULIANNA DEUTSCHER, MD, PGY-5, FRCP-EM
Department of Medicine, Faculty of Medicine, University of Toronto, Toronto, Ontario, Canada

EMMA DUCHESNE, MD, PGY-4, FRCP-EM
Department of Emergency Medicine, Kingston Health Sciences Centre, Queen's University, Kingston, Ontario, Canada

CHRIS EVANS, MD
Trauma Services, Department of Emergency Medicine, Kingston General Hospital, Queen's University, Kingston, Ontario, Canada

JENNIFER GUYTHER, MD
Assistant Professor, Departments of Emergency Medicine and Pediatrics, University of Maryland School of Medicine, Baltimore, Maryland, USA

BARBARA HAAS, MD, PhD, FRCSC
Assistant Professor, Department of Surgery and Interdepartmental Division of Critical Care Medicine, University of Toronto, Sunnybrook Health Sciences Centre, Toronto, Ontario, Canada

DANIEL HAASE, MD, RDMS, RDCS
Assistant Professor, Departments of Emergency Medicine and Surgery, R Adams Cowley Shock Trauma Center, Baltimore, Maryland, USA

JOSEPH HAMERA, MD
Visiting Clinical Instructor, Department of Emergency Medicine, Fellow, Critical Care, R Adams Cowley Shock Trauma Center, University of Maryland School of Medicine, Baltimore Maryland, USA

JULIE LA, MD, MESc
Division of General Surgery, Queen's University, Kingston, Ontario, Canada

LORRAINE LAU, MScA, MD, FRCPC
Department of Emergency Medicine, McGill University Health Centre, Montreal, Quebec, Canada

CAROLINE LEECH, MBChB, FRCEM, FIMC RCSEd, FEWM
University Hospitals Coventry and Warwickshire NHS Trust, The Air Ambulance Service, United Kingdom

ASHLEY MENNE, MD
Assistant Professor, Department of Emergency Medicine, R Adams Cowley Shock Trauma Center, University of Maryland School of Medicine, Baltimore Maryland, USA

KATERINA PAVENSKI, MD, FRCPC
Department of Laboratory Medicine, St. Michael's Hospital, Toronto, Ontario, Canada

ANDREW PETROSONIAK, MD, MSc, FRCPC
Department of Emergency Medicine, St. Michael's Hospital, Toronto, Ontario, Canada

MATT PIASECZNY, MD, MSc
Department of Emergency Medicine, Queen's University, Kingston, Ontario, Canada

ZAFFER QASIM, MD, FRCEM, EDIC
Assistant Professor of Emergency Medicine and Critical Care, Department of Emergency Medicine, Perelman School of Medicine, University of Pennsylvania, Philadelphia, Pennsylvania, USA

VANESSA R. SALASKY, MD
Clinical Fellow, Department of Neurology, Section of Neurocritical Care and Emergency Neurology, University of Maryland Medical Center, Baltimore, Maryland, USA

KARI SAMPSEL, MD, MSc, FRCP
Emergency Physician, Medical Director, Sexual Assault and Partner Abuse Care Program, The Ottawa Hospital, University of Ottawa, Ottawa, Ontario, Canada

JESSE SHRIKI, DO, MS
Associate Professor, Department of Critical Care, Banner-University Medical Center, Phoenix, Arizona, USA

REUBEN J. STRAYER, MD
Maimonides Medical Center, Brooklyn, New York, USA

JAKE TURNER, BMEDSCI, BMBS, FRCA, FIMC RCSEd
The Air Ambulance Service, United Kingdom; Anaesthetic Department, Nottingham University Hospitals NHS Trust, Nottingham, United Kingdom; Lincolnshire and Nottinghamshire Air Ambulance, United Kingdom

RACHEL WILTJER, DO
Resident, PGY-5, Combined Emergency Medicine and Pediatrics Residency, University of Maryland Medical Center, Baltimore, Maryland, USA

CAMILLA L. WONG, MHSc, MD, FRCPC
Associate Professor, Division of Geriatric Medicine, St. Michael's Hospital, Toronto, Ontario, Canada

Contents

Shock is a life-threatening condition of circulatory failure leading to inadequate organ perfusion and tissue oxygenation. In a trauma patient, shock may be due to hypovolemia, cardiogenic, obstructive or distributive causes individually or in combination. The physiological response to major hemorrhage is dependent on a variety of autonomic reflexes, mechanism of injury, bleeding source, and baseline physiology of the patient. This article discusses the common causes of shock and the accompanying physiology, how clinical assessment can support the diagnosis and effective treatment of shock, and the common pitfalls in trauma patients.

Traumatic brain injury (TBI) continues to be a leading cause of morbidity and mortality worldwide with older adults having the highest rate of hospitalizations and deaths. Management in the acute phase is focused on preventing secondary neurologic injury from hypoxia, hypocapnia, hypotension, and elevated intracranial pressure. Recent studies on tranexamic acid and continuous hypertonic saline infusion have not found any difference in neurologic outcomes. Care must be taken in prognosticating TBI outcomes, as recovery of consciousness and orientation has been observed up to 12 months after injury.

Blunt and penetrating vascular injuries to the neck represent a significant burden of mortality and disability among trauma patients. Blunt cerebrovascular injury can present with signs of stroke either immediately or in a delayed fashion. Most injuries are detected with computed tomography angiogram and managed by antiplatelet agents or unfractionated heparin. In contrast, for patients presenting with penetrating neck injuries, assessment for hard signs of vascular and aerodigestive injury should be done and prompt emergent surgical consultation if present. Overall management priorities for penetrating neck injuries focus on airway management, hemorrhage control, and damage control resuscitation before definitive surgical repair.

Damage-control resuscitation is the standard of care for the hemorrhaging trauma patient. This approach combines rapid hemostasis and early-ratio-based blood product administration. These patients often require initiation of a massive hemorrhage protocol to support the systematic and coordinated delivery of care during this critical phase of resuscitation. Emerging evidence supports that this includes more than blood product administration alone but rather a comprehensive suite of treatments. In this article, we review the existing evidence and provide a pragmatic framework, the 7 Ts of massive hemorrhage protocol, to guide the care of patients with life-threatening traumatic hemorrhage.

Hemorrhage, in particular, noncompressible torso hemorrhage, remains a significant contributor to mortality in trauma cases. Despite many advances in resuscitation, noncompressible sites of bleeding have presented a particular challenge. Resuscitative endovascular balloon occlusion of the aorta (REBOA) is one technique that can be used to temporarily stop hemorrhage from these sites to allow transfer to definitive care. Although the technique is relatively straight-forward, it carries significant risk, in particular, from ischemia due to aortic occlusion. This article describes the role and considerations for the use of REBOA in the critically injured patient.

The utilization of extracorporeal membrane oxygenation (ECMO) in trauma mirrors wider trends toward increased utilization of ECMO throughout various forms of critical illness. ECMO can safely be performed on trauma patients with or without anticoagulation. Most of the trauma ECMO cases are for the management of post-traumatic respiratory failure, but they can be used for certain cases of circulatory failure as well. Cannulation of patients for ECMO is technically feasible in the hands of surgeons and intensivists involved in the care of trauma patients. A sound understanding of the ECMO circuit components can help troubleshoot system malfunctions. Emerging technologies may combine extracorporeal circulatory support with endovascular hemorrhage control to prolong the viable survival of exsanguinating patients.

Intimate partner violence and human trafficking commonly affect patients presenting to the emergency department including the trauma bay. Although these forms of violence and exploitation are not always the underlying cause of that particular emergency department encounter, screening is important regardless of the presenting condition because this presentation may be the only opportunity to receive help and ultimately plants the seed for future access to help regardless of what a patient chooses to do following this first encounter. There are important medical care considerations in these patients beyond trauma bay procedures that can make the difference in saving a life.

Polytrauma patients often require medications to treat pain, treat agitation, and facilitate painful procedures. Though analgesia will be deferred in obtunded patients in profound shock, reduced-dose opioids or ketamine should be administered to unstable patients with severe pain with good mental status. Agitation commonly complicates polytrauma presentations, and is treated according to the danger it presents to patient and staff. Severe agitation can be effectively managed with dissociative-dose ketamine, which facilitates ongoing resuscitation, including CT. Severely painful procedures can be effectively facilitated by propofol or dissociative-dose ketamine, with continuous attention to ventilation and application of a step-by-step response to hypoventilation.

Bedside ultrasound assessment has become a routine aspect of care in trauma resuscitation and the critical care setting. Although early research was focused on its role in blunt trauma, it has shown utility in the assessment of penetrating trauma by rapidly identifying hemopericardium and facilitating appropriate intraoperative management. In addition, ultrasound is a reliable test in identifying hemopneumothorax or diaphragmatic injuries. The Rapid Ultrasound in Shock and Hypotension and the Focused Rapid Echocardiographic Examination can diagnose etiologies of shock and guide resuscitation in the critically ill patient. Finally, the role of transesophageal echocardiography is expanding in the trauma setting as more research emerges.

Procedures such as central access and tube thoracostomy are integral in the care of the injured patient. However, both increasing life span and patient complexity of comorbidities can hinder procedural success. Careful forethought should be completed before, simply, charging ahead with a procedure. This article covers the details needed to be successful in carrying out these 2 procedural "staples" in trauma. From anatomy to pain control to postprocedural management, this article will be the building block for technical success. Understanding what you are doing and careful planning ahead are now more than ever crucial to patient care.

Although resuscitation in trauma requires a multidisciplinary and multifaceted approach, one of the "Big Five" procedures may need to be performed as lifesaving and improving intervention. Understanding, timing, and techniques of these elusive and difficult-to-master procedures can be the difference between life and death. This article focuses on and reviews these five critical procedures: cricothyroidotomy, burr hole craniotomy, resuscitative thoracotomy, emergent hysterotomy, and lateral canthotomy. Prepare the team, system, and yourself when performing any of these procedures. It is important to be facile with your equipment and familiar with the steps to maximize success.

The relative proportion of trauma patients who are older adults continues to rise as the population ages. Older adults who experience trauma have unique needs compared with their younger counterparts. There are specific considerations that must take into account. Treating older adults with traumatic injuries requires specific skills, knowledge, and specialized protocols to optimize outcomes. This article reviews the most important aspects of geriatric trauma care. We focus on presentation and initial resuscitation, triage guidelines and the issue of undertriage, the importance of multidisciplinary and specialized geriatric care, and common injuries and their management.

Emergency department response to the pediatric trauma patient starts with the basics–ABCDE. Certain important differences in pediatric patients, such as airway physiology and drug dosing, must be considered but standardized resources are available. Pediatric blunt and penetrating trauma treatment also have mechanisms and nuances that distinguish them from adult cases. Pediatric literature is slowly growing which can shape evidence-based practice for care including blood transfusions, medications, and procedures.

EMERGENCY MEDICINE
CLINICS OF NORTH AMERICA

SERIES OF RELATED INTEREST

Critical Care Clinics
https://www.criticalcare.theclinics.com/

THE CLINICS ARE NOW AVAILABLE ONLINE!
Access your subscription at:
www.theclinics.com

EMERGENCY MEDICINE
CLINICS OF NORTH AMERICA

FORTHCOMING ISSUES

May 2023
Updates in Obstetric and Gynecologic Emergencies
Sarah B. Dubbs and Brittany Guest, Editors

August 2023
Cardiac Arrest
William J. Brady and Amandeep Singh, Editors

November 2023
Endocrine and Metabolic Emergencies
George Willis and Bennett A. Myers, Editors

RECENT ISSUES

November 2022
Cardiovascular Emergencies
Jeremy S. Boemen and Leen Alblaihed, Editors

August 2022
Respiratory and Airway Emergencies
Haney Mallemat and Terren Trott, Editors

May 2022
Toxicology Emergencies
Christopher P. Holstege and Joshua D. King, Editors

SERIES OF RELATED INTEREST

Critical Care Clinics
https://www.criticalcare.theclinics.com/

Foreword

Trauma Emergencies

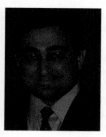

Amal Mattu, MD
Consulting Editor

One of the defining features of a good emergency physician is one's ability to provide initial resuscitation to any type of patient that shows up in the emergency department (ED)...adult and pediatric, medical, trauma, minor or major illness or injury. Over the years, however, emergency medicine in many settings has become very "compartmentalized." In many locales, we find dedicated pediatric hospitals, heart centers, cardiac arrest centers, stroke centers, and trauma centers. The compartmentalization occurs even within individual hospitals...separate adult versus pediatric versus trauma EDs. When an emergency physician works in one of these settings, it becomes very easy to ignore the necessity of maintaining a broad range of knowledge and skills. For example, I work in a large academic medical center with a separate adult ED, pediatric ED, and trauma receiving unit. It certainly is tempting to ignore the need to maintain pediatric and trauma skills in my practice.

On a regular basis, however, I am reminded of the need to maintain a sound knowledge of resuscitation of pediatric and trauma patients when those patients show up in the *adult* ED unexpectedly. I was often reminded of this when I worked in a community hospital ED as well. Specifically with regards to trauma, it was, and still is, not uncommon for victims of penetrating or blunt trauma to be brought to our "nontrauma ED" by the patient's friends or family or by prehospital personnel. Whether the dedicated trauma team was upstairs or across town, it was *our* responsibility in the "nontrauma ED" to initiate the resuscitation and oftentimes perform life-saving interventions. *If you call yourself an emergency physician, you must know how to manage victims of trauma no matter where you work.*

With this tenet in mind, we present to you our latest issue of *Emergency Medicine Clinics of North America*, an issue dedicated to maintaining and raising your knowledge and skills in emergency trauma care. Our Guest Editors are both emergency physicians who have exceptional knowledge in caring for the trauma patient, and they both are outstanding educators. Dr Kimberly Boswell is an emergency physician with

Emerg Med Clin N Am 41 (2023) xiii–xiv
https://doi.org/10.1016/j.emc.2022.10.003
0733-8627/23/© 2022 Published by Elsevier Inc.

emed.theclinics.com

fellowship training in trauma and critical care from the Maryland Shock Trauma Center, where she still works. Dr Christopher Hicks is an emergency physician and internationally recognized expert in trauma care who works at the busiest trauma center in Toronto, St. Michael's Hospital. Dr Boswell and Dr Hicks have brought together an outstanding group of colleagues from the United States and Canada to provide some of the latest advances in trauma care for emergency physicians. They address basic resuscitation as well as advanced concepts, such as extracorporeal life support; imaging techniques; special patient populations; and an assortment of critical trauma procedures.

This issue of *Emergency Medicine Clinics of North America* represents an important addition to the emergency medicine literature, and it also nicely exemplifies how far our specialty has progressed in trauma care beyond the basics of "A-B-C." I would again emphatically argue that if you call yourself an emergency physician, you must maintain your knowledge and skills in managing patients with trauma regardless of your practice setting. Mastering the concepts that these editors and authors provide within the following pages will do just that. Kudos to the contributors for an outstanding issue!

Amal Mattu, MD
Department of Emergency Medicine
University of Maryland School of Medicine
Baltimore, MD 21201, USA

E-mail address:
amattu@som.umaryland.edu

Preface

Inside and Out: Trauma Resuscitation at the Speed of Light

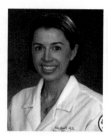 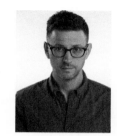

Kimberly A. Boswell, MD, FACEP   Christopher Hicks, MD, MEd, FRCPC
Editors

Trauma is changing. True, the force of gravity is constant, cars still hurt, and humanity's thirst for violence runs deep beyond reckoning. But how we respond to injury, and the science and innovation that support our practice scarcely resemble trauma care from even a decade ago. Gone are the non-evidence-based peculiarisms of advanced trauma life support (ATLS): the savage fluid boluses, the primacy of the trauma surgeon, the mechanistic thoughtlessness of an algorithmic approach to everything. We know more now than we ever did, about managing neurotrauma, understanding shock (goodbye and good riddance, 3-to-1 rule), executing life-saving procedures, and attending to pain and agitation in ways we once ignored. We continue to push the boundaries of what new technology can do for meaningful survival, from advanced ultrasound to resuscitative endovascular occlusion of the aorta (REBOA) and ECMO (extracorporeal membrane oxygenation). Most poignantly, we are no longer looking away from difficult issues in trauma, from injuries in the aging population to intimate partner violence and human trafficking. These very real issues speak to the integral role that emergency medicine plays in patient safety and advocacy. Once preached to, emergency medicine is now comfortably leading this drive to advance and excel.

If this seems like a lot, that's by design. We encourage starting with the 2018 *Emergency Medicine Clinics of North America* trauma issue[1] to set the stage for understanding this quantum leap in care that we are currently living through. The current issue pushes our understanding even further. In that respect, we are grateful to the

Emerg Med Clin N Am 41 (2023) xv–xvi
https://doi.org/10.1016/j.emc.2022.10.002
0733-8627/23/© 2022 Published by Elsevier Inc.

authors for assembling such outstanding and boundary-pushing work. Buckle up and enjoy the ride.

Kimberly A. Boswell, MD, FACEP
Department of Emergency Medicine
University of Maryland School of Medicine
R. Adams Cowley Shock Trauma Center
University of Maryland Medical Center
22 South Greene Street, P1G01
Baltimore, MD 21202, USA

Christopher Hicks, MD, MEd, FRCPC
Department of Emergency Medicine
St. Michael's Hospital, 30 Bond Street
Toronto, ON M5B 1W8, Canada

E-mail addresses:
kboswell@som.umaryland.edu (K.A. Boswell)
chrismikehicks@gmail.com (C. Hicks)

REFERENCE

1. Hicks CM, Petrosoniak A. Damage control: advances in trauma resuscitation. Emerg Med Clin N Am 2018.

Shock in Trauma

Caroline Leech, MBChB, FRCEM, FIMC RCSEd, FEWM[a,b,]*,
Jake Turner, BMedSci, BMBS, FRCA, FIMC RCSEd[b,c,d]

KEYWORDS

- Shock • Trauma • Hypovolemia • Physiology • Resuscitation

KEY POINTS

- Understanding the cardiovascular responses to hemorrhage and injury aids interpretation of the vital signs following trauma.
- Hypotension following injury can be caused by several conditions other than, or in addition to, hypovolemia.
- There are several clinical pitfalls if clinicians use only pulse and blood pressure to assess the severity of hypovolemia.

INTRODUCTION

Shock is a life-threatening condition of circulatory failure leading to inadequate organ perfusion and inadequate tissue oxygenation. Left untreated, poor perfusion leads to anaerobic metabolism, lactic acidosis, and progressive cellular and organ dysfunction resulting in irreversible multiorgan failure and death.

Inadequate perfusion may result from failure of the pump (the heart), inadequate circulating blood volume (absolute or relative), or obstruction to the flow of blood through the circulatory system. Traditionally, shock has been subdivided into 4 main subtypes (**Fig. 1**). In practice, there is often considerable overlap, with different types of shock coexisting in the same patient. In trauma patients, this includes patients with more than one system injury (eg, traumatic brain injury [TBI], hypovolemia) or medical events (eg, sepsis, cardiac, neurological) contributing to the mechanism of injury resulting in a mixed picture of shock.

In healthy, uninjured patients, oxygen consumption (Vo_2) is closely regulated and serves as a carbon acceptor in the generation of ATP by mitochondria. In shock states when oxygen delivery decreases, reducing Vo_2 below a critical level to maintain cellular metabolic demands, mitochondrial aerobic function is impaired. This results

[a] University Hospitals Coventry & Warwickshire NHS Trust, Coventry CV2 2DX, UK; [b] The Air Ambulance Service, Blue Skies House, Butlers Leap, Rugby, Warwickshire, CV21 3RQ. UK; [c] Anaesthetic Department, Nottingham University Hospitals NHS Trust, Derby Road, Nottingham NG7 2UH, UK; [d] Lincs & Notts Air Ambulance Headquarters, HEMS Way, Lincoln LN4 2GW, UK
* Corresponding author. Emergency Department, University Hospitals Coventry & Warwickshire NHS Trust, Walsgrave, Coventry CV2 2DX, UK.
E-mail address: Caroline.Leech@uhcw.nhs.uk

Emerg Med Clin N Am 41 (2023) 1–17
https://doi.org/10.1016/j.emc.2022.09.007
emed.theclinics.com
0733-8627/23/© 2022 Elsevier Inc. All rights reserved.

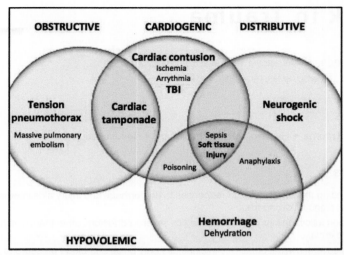

Fig. 1. Venn diagram showing the different subtypes of shock. TBI, traumatic brain injury.

in a cellular oxygen debt and accumulation of metabolic acids generated by anaerobic processes.[1] As oxygen debt progresses, the likelihood of cellular injury increases with a reduction in cellular membrane integrity, osmosis, and swelling. Intracellular organelles become damaged, cellular synthetic mechanisms cease, and lysosomes are activated resulting in cellular necrosis and death. Tissues with the greatest basal metabolic oxidative requirements (brain, myocardium, liver, kidneys) are particularly vulnerable, and depending on the extent and severity of cellular injury, can develop multiorgan dysfunction and failure.[2]

Hypovolemic shock results from inadequate circulating blood volume secondary to hemorrhage or excessive fluid loss. In the context of major trauma, hypovolemic shock secondary to uncontrolled hemorrhage is the most common cause of death in the military setting,[3] and the second most common cause of death (after TBI) in the civilian setting.[4] Bleeding may occur from damaged veins, arteries, solid organ parenchyma, and/or fractured bones. The rate of hemorrhage, presenting physiology, and trajectory of deterioration will depend on the anatomy of injury, source of bleeding, and patient factors (age, comorbidities, polypharmacy). Alternative or coexisting causes of shock in trauma often complicate the clinical assessment and management of these patients and are discussed in more detail later.

CASE SCENARIOS
Case 1: Incisional Torso Hemorrhage

A 25-year-old male patient has sustained an incisional wound to the left chest in the anterior axillary line 7th intercostal space. On arrival to the resus room, the patient is agitated, diaphoretic with no palpable radial pulses, BP 180/154, and a thready slow carotid pulse (HR 50). The patient has unrecordable peripheral oxygen saturations and looks centrally pale (lips, tongue, and conjunctivae). The prehospital team has placed an intravenous cannula and administered tranexamic acid.

The trauma team leader (TTL) tasks the anesthetic team to prepare for a rapid sequence intubation to facilitate ongoing management and resuscitation of the patient, but not to undertake this intervention until appropriate volume resuscitation has been undertaken. The TTL confirms with the team that this patient is most likely critically hypovolemic and to disregard the spurious blood pressure. The anesthetic team sedates the patient with judicious doses of ketamine and full monitoring and oxygen is applied.

The trauma team fully exposes the patient (to exclude additional incisional wounds) and undertakes a primary survey. There is reduced air entry on the left side and absence of pleural sliding on ultrasound. There is no emphysema or active bleeding from the wound. An extended FAST scan excludes any significant pericardial tamponade but does identify free fluid within the left splenorenal fossa. Bilateral wide bore intravenous access is obtained and warmed blood products are started as there is no recordable blood pressure. A left-sided thoracostomy is performed (lung down, comes up, no blood) with insertion of a chest drain. Invasive blood pressure monitoring confirms that the patient is a transient responder to volume resuscitation with an opening BP of 40/30, improving to 75/52. The patient's heart rate improves from an initial 42 beats per minute, to 118 with volume resuscitation as the underfilled left ventricular C-fiber–mediated bradycardia resolves.

The TTL, in collaboration with the consultant surgeon, agrees that the patient should be taken directly to theater for a trauma laparotomy for hemorrhage control.

Case 2: Blunt Polytrauma

A 67-year-old male patient has been run over by a heavy goods vehicle and sustained lower abdominal, pelvic, and bilateral femoral injuries. On arrival, the patient is confused, has palpable radial pulses and a NIBP of 100/40 with a heart rate of 75. The pulse oximetry trace is poor, but intermittently reading 94% on 15L oxygen. The prehospital team stated that the patient was initially unconscious but has become confused en route to hospital. Drug history includes bisoprolol, amlodipine, ramipril, aspirin, and furosemide.

Primary survey identifies bilateral rib fractures, no surgical emphysema, lower abdominal contusions and tenderness, pelvic tenderness with a pelvic binder that is correctly positioned over the greater trochanters, bilateral closed femoral fractures splinted with traction devices, and left frontotemporal bruising with bilaterally reactive pupils. The patient has a Glasgow Coma Score (GCS) of 13 (M5, V4, E4), is cool peripherally, and has palpable radial pulses with a consistent BP of 98/45 and HR of 70. A venous blood gas confirms a normal baseline hemoglobin, but with deranged acid-base status (pH 7.18, BE -8.2, Lac 3.4) consistent with a shock state.

The TTL summarizes to the team the current injuries and main issues: this is an older patient with clinical signs of significant hypovolemia for his baseline physiology. Plan is for careful volume resuscitation to a MAP 80 to 90, and when able, a whole-body CT due to the high blunt-mechanism injury burden. The anesthetic team is asked to place a radial arterial line to help guide ongoing volume resuscitation and blood products are commenced. The patient responds to 2 units of blood and is transferred to CT, which demonstrates the femoral fractures, complex pelvic fractures, bilateral rib fractures, and pulmonary contusions but with no active bleeding.

PHYSIOLOGY OF HYPOVOLEMIA
Shock Classification

The traditional ATLS classification of hypovolemic shock with 4 classes defined by % blood loss, heart rate, blood pressure, respiratory rate, and GCS has been shown to overestimate the degree of tachycardia and hypotension associated with increasing blood loss.[5] The physiological response to bleeding in trauma is complex, variable, and dependent on both injury and patient-related factors.[6,7]

Hemodynamic Reflexes to Hypovolemia

There are 3 main compensating reflexes that need to be understood when considering the physiological response to acute hypovolemia: the arterial baroreceptor reflex, the reflex elicited by activation of the cardiac C-fiber afferents, and the arterial chemoreceptor reflex (**Table 1**). Only a proportion of patients with hypovolemia will present with hypotension and tachycardia.

Simple hemorrhage without significant soft tissue injury (eg, *penetrating trauma*) is often biphasic with an initial baroreceptor-mediated reflex tachycardia and peripheral vasoconstriction. As hemorrhage progresses, there is a subsequent vagally mediated depressor response resulting in bradycardia and peripheral vasodilation. This is referred to as a biphasic response and may be secondary to cardiac C-fiber–mediated reflexes (**Fig. 2**).[8] This second reflex may confer some degree of protection with the bradycardia supporting diastolic filling, increasing stroke volume, and improving coronary perfusion.[7]

With tissue injury and ischemia in *blunt trauma*, it is the baroreceptor-mediated tachycardia and peripheral vasoconstriction response which predominates. This intense vasoconstriction redistributes blood flow and oxygen delivery from metabolically active organs such as the gastrointestinal tract, increasing oxygen debt, and promoting subsequent multiorgan dysfunction.[7]

In military battlefield casualties, explosions and *blast injury* are currently the primary mechanism of trauma.[9] Casualties are likely to have extensive tissue damage with severe blood loss from a combination of blunt and penetrating trauma, with a minority having hypoxia secondary to blast lung. The cardiorespiratory response to blast lung causes a characteristic triad of bradycardia, prolonged hypotension, and apnea followed by rapid shallow breathing.[10] This reflex will augment any biphasic response to severe hemorrhage as a consequence of secondary blast injury.

Administration of *opioids* for analgesia may have a deleterious impact on hemodynamic stability in the context of hypovolemia. In simple hemorrhage, morphine may

Table 1
Hemodynamic reflexes

Reflex	% Blood Loss	Receptor Location	Mechanism	Effects	Clinical Signs
Arterial baroreceptor	10-15%	Carotid sinus, aortic arch	As pulse pressure decreases, activity decreases	↓ Vagal activity = predominant sympathetic activity	Tachycardia ↑ SVR
Cardiac C-fibers	> 20%	Left ventricular myocardium	Contracting around empty chamber	↑ Vagal activity	Bradycardia
Arterial chemoreceptor	> 20%	Carotid and aortic bodies	Hypoxia, hypercarbia, acidosis	↑ vagal & slight ↑ sympathetic activity	↑ SVRBradycardia ↑ SVR

Abbreviations: RR, respiratory rate; SVR, systemic vascular resistance.

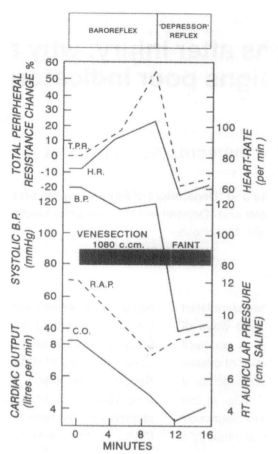

Fig. 2. Changes in HR, systolic arterial blood pressure, cardiac output, peripheral resistance, and right atrial pressure during controlled hemorrhage in male human volunteer.[6]

attenuate (reduce) the biphasic response (autonomic mediated bradycardia and vasodilation), which is protective for end-organ and coronary perfusion. Even hemodynamically stable opioids such as fentanyl can precipitate hemodynamic collapse in patients with propound hypovolemia and should be used judiciously.[11]

Arterial Injury Shock

Arterial injury shock is the physiologic response to a major arterial vascular injury whereby elastic arterial diastolic recoil is impaired across the entire arterial system. This results in immediate and profound hemodynamic instability with a disproportionate loss of diastolic pressure and subsequent reduction in left ventricular coronary perfusion. Characteristically there is minimal or no response to volume resuscitation, as the underlying shock etiology is one of diastolic recoil failure, rather than hypovolemia.

Patients with significant defects to large arterial structures are at risk of this phenomenon. It tends to occur more frequently in penetrating trauma as elastic arterial structures are more resistant to the shear forces of blunt trauma. Arterial injury shock will lead to a very rapid and profound hemodynamic decompensation, often resulting in cardiac arrest within minutes of injury, unless early prehospital vascular control can be achieved. In comparison, exsanguinating small arterial, venous, solid organ, or bony bleeding often results in a slower physiologic deterioration, with either complete or transient response to volume resuscitation.

Clinical Assessment

A thorough assessment of the primary survey, prodromal events, mechanism/kinematics of injury, and familiarity with bleeding mimics are essential in identifying the etiology of shock in the trauma patient.

The 'hateful eight' of hypovolemia

Compensatory mechanisms, biphasic autonomic responses to hypovolemia, and unreliability of noninvasive blood pressure (NIBP) contribute to the challenges of shock assessment. A broader clinical assessment of the patient, in correlation to the mechanism of injury is key. This clinical assessment is sometimes referred to as the 'hateful eight' and can be used to identify patients with life-threatening hemorrhagic shock (**Box 1**).

Compensated shock

Hypovolemic, cardiogenic, and obstructive shock states are all characterized by a reduced cardiac output. To offset this reduction in stroke volume and maintain cardiac output, the sympathetic nervous system increases the heart rate and stimulates peripheral vasoconstriction diverting blood centrally to restore preload. This is recognized by pale and sweaty skin, prolonged capillary refill time, reduced pulse pressure, and acidosis-driven increased minute ventilation. In these early stages, cardiac output and blood pressure are maintained. Although the blood pressure is maintained, perfusion of peripheral tissues is impaired, and an oxygen debt accumulates.

Distributive shock states may not present with the classic skin changes or tachycardia described earlier. Pathological vasodilatation may prevent compensatory vasoconstriction, resulting in flushed warm peripheries in the early stages. Tachycardia may also be absent in neurogenic shock with high cord lesions, due to unopposed vagal tone.

Decompensated shock

When compensatory mechanisms fail, perfusion to the vital organs becomes compromised and decompensation occurs. The brain relies on a constant blood flow to

| Box 1 | | |
Clinical signs of hypovolemia		
Air hunger		
Low end-tidal CO_2		
Sweaty/clammy		
Pallor (lips, tongue, palms, soles)		
Venous collapse		
Abnormal pulse (brady or tachycardia)		
Hypotension		
Altered mental status (agitated, unconscious)		

maintain function and as blood flow decreases, cognition is impaired, resulting in confusion/agitation. The presence of peripheral pulses and NIBP measurements are unreliable indicators for decompensated shock.

The speed at which decompensation occurs will depend partly on the physiological reserve of the patient and the cause of the shock state. Patients in cardiogenic and distributive shock states have a limited ability to compensate and therefore are liable to decompensate rapidly. Other confounding factors can affect the patient's response to shock (**Table 2**), and a high index of suspicion is essential in these patient groups if shock is to be identified.

'Low flow' or 'no flow' states

Patients with ongoing hemorrhage will deteriorate from decompensated shock into cardiac arrest with no palpable central pulse. During the early stages of hypovolemic cardiac arrest, the patient will be in a low output state, and may have a rapid or normal rate narrow complex pulseless electrical activity. Cardiac activity may still be present on ultrasound and this finding can prioritize management away from chest compressions (which will impede right ventricular filling[13]) and toward volume replacement with blood products. As the patient further declines, the electrocardiographic complexes will widen, slow, and decline into asystole with no cardiac activity on ultrasound (**Fig. 3**): this requires chest compressions. End-tidal CO_2 should be monitored throughout as a surrogate for right ventricular stroke volume and return of spontaneous circulation. Hemorrhage control, oxygenation, and volume resuscitation is the priority for these patients.

Clinical Pitfalls

Palpable pulses. Traditionally, palpation of the carotid, femoral, and radial pulse has been used to estimate the blood pressure and perfusion of trauma patients. A loss

Table 2	
Factors affecting the physiologic response to shock	
Confounders	**Changes in Response to Hypovolemia**
Advancing age	Older patients have less physiological reserve and can decompensate earlier. Resting blood pressure is higher and hypotension may be present at systolic blood pressures <110 mm Hg.[12]
Comorbidities	Major cardiovascular, renal, hepatic, and endocrine disorders may tolerate shock states poorly, rapidly accumulating a critical oxygen debt with an increase of risk end-organ injury, dysfunction, and failure.
Medications	Medicines that slow the heart rate and block the sympathoadrenal axis can mask early signs of hemorrhagic shock by preventing a compensatory tachycardia and peripheral vasoconstriction.
Pacemaker	A pacemaker with a fixed rate will limit the ability of the patient to mount a compensatory tachycardia and lead to earlier decompensation.
Younger patients/athletes	The resting heart rate may be in the region of 50 bpm. This should be taken into account when assessing for relative tachycardia.
Pregnancy	Blood may be shunted from the uterine and placental circulation into the maternal circulation to the detriment of the fetus. Significant hypovolemia may occur before signs of shock are evident.
Hypothermia	Hypothermia can reduce RR, HR, and BP independent of hypovolemia.

Low Output State in Trauma (LOST)

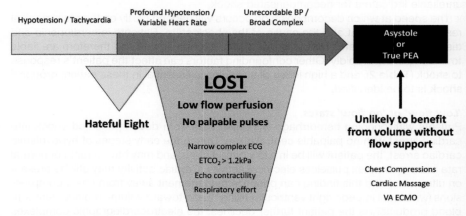

Fig. 3. The physiological spectrum of a low output state due to hypovolemia. PEA, pulseless electrical activity.

of the radial pulse is used as a surrogate marker for the need for fluid replacement in many trauma protocols. However, in some patients, a radial pulse may only become absent when the systolic blood pressure is below 60 mm Hg and therefore this clinical sign may underestimate the degree of shock.[14]

Noninvasive blood pressure. NIBP is standard monitoring for all patients but is prone to several pitfalls. An accurate measurement depends on cuff size and fit and no vascular limb injury. In low output states, an erroneous reading is common (eg, 200/180). Studies demonstrate that it is imprecise when compared to invasive blood pressure monitoring.[15] Interpretation relies on a trend rather than an individual reading and mean blood pressure measured noninvasively is more accurate than systolic blood pressure. The reference ranges for different ages of children need to be available and consideration that older patients have higher baseline blood pressures when well. Pulse pressure is the difference between systolic and diastolic blood pressures. In trauma patients with a blood pressure in the normal range, a narrow pulse pressure is an independent early predictor of active hemorrhage requiring blood product transfusion and surgical intervention for hemorrhage control.[16,17]

Shock index (SI). SI is the heart rate divided by the systolic blood pressure. A SI greater than one is considered to be abnormal. SI performs better than hypotension alone for triaging patients with critical bleeding and need for emergent injury. However, it includes the pitfalls of noninvasive blood measurement and undertriages patients who have a bradycardic response to shock.

Permissive Hypotension

The underlying principles for resuscitation of the shocked patient focus on restoring perfusion and eliminating oxygen debt. However, for patients with active noncompressible torso hemorrhage, contemporary management advocates damage control resuscitation, until definitive hemorrhage control can be achieved.[18] Permissive hypotension is a key component of this approach and describes the permissive acceptance of adequate, but suboptimal blood pressure and end-organ perfusion.

The role of permissive hypotension (palpable central pulse or SBP 80–90 mm Hg) in the management of the actively bleeding trauma patient has become widespread, and is supported by several national guidelines such as the European Guideline on Management of Major Bleeding and Coagulopathy Following Trauma[19] and the National Institute for Health and Care Excellence (NICE) Guidelines for the Management of Bleeding Trauma Patients.[20] Despite this, permissive hypotension remains contentious, with risks when applied generically to trauma patients, especially in the context of TBI.[21]

The NICE guidelines[20] advocate a restrictive approach to volume resuscitation until early definite control of bleeding, titrating volume resuscitation to a palpable central pulse. However, in patients with concurrent TBI, the guidance advocates a restrictive approach if bleeding is the predominant factor, and a less restrictive approach if TBI is the predominant condition. These challenges are compounded by the fact that physiological parameters are of limited diagnostic value in assessing the severity of major hemorrhage[22] and that up to 45% of UK trauma patients with TBI are intoxicated, making pre-CT exclusion of significant brain injury challenging.[23] We also know that hypotension in TBI increases mortality,[24,25] and both the Brain Trauma Foundation (SBP >110 mm Hg) and Association of Anaesthetists (MAP 80 mm Hg) advocate normal hemodynamic targets to maintain penumbral cerebral perfusion and minimize secondary brain injury.[26,27]

A 2014 Cochrane meta-analysis examining the timing and volume of fluid administration in hemorrhage concluded there was 'no evidence for or against the use of early or larger volume intravenous fluid administration in uncontrolled haemorrhage.'[28] There are several relevant limitations for the studies included within this Cochrane review; exclusion of TBI, utilization of large volumes of cold crystalloid fluids as the comparator group, predominantly younger patients with a high incidence of penetrating trauma, immortality bias, and exclusion of patients with comorbidities.[21] The vast majority of UK trauma is multisystem and blunt in nature (penetrating trauma accounting for <3% of cases),[29] making the extrapolation of data supporting permissive hypotension for penetrating trauma challenging.[30] The studies analyzed by the Cochrane meta-analysis also do not reflect modern trauma care with early access to balanced blood product resuscitation, a high incidence of concurrent TBI, and an aging trauma population with increasing comorbidities tolerating periods of hypoperfusion poorly.

Hypotension should be recognized as the decompensation of a bleeding trauma patient, often requiring immediate blood product resuscitation to maintain adequate cerebral and end-organ perfusion. We need to consider patient factors (age, comorbidities), injury factors (type and severity), and duration of shock when providing individualized modern trauma care. The remaining components of damage control resuscitation should be aggressively pursued with the normalization of coagulopathy, avoidance of hypothermia/hypocalcemia/hyperkalemia, and rapid surgical or interventional radiologically achieved hemorrhage control.

BLEEDING MIMICS
Prodrome and Comorbidities

Prodromal events such as ingestion of illicit substances, exertion, fear, and severe anxiety can all precipitate a sympathomimetic response to injury, mimicking early shock physiology. These mimics are short-lived and readily managed with reassurance, time, and judicious doses of analgesics.

Incisional trauma, breach of pleural and peritoneal membranes, and blood irritation of thoracic and abdominal cavities can precipitate a profound vagal reflex mimicking a biphasic C-fiber–mediated response to major hemorrhage. As with prodromal mimics, vagal reflexes may resolve with reassurance, time, and analgesia.

Cardiogenic Shock

Cardiogenic shock occurs when there is myocardial dysfunction in the presence of adequate left ventricular filling pressures, resulting in inadequate end-organ oxygen delivery. Without intervention, cardiogenic failure will result in reduced cardiac output, impaired coronary perfusion, and a spiral of worsening myocardial function (**Fig. 4**).

Myocardial dysfunction may be preexisting (ischemic heart disease, cardiomyopathy, heart failure), but in the context of major trauma can be secondary to a variety of factors; commotio cordis, cardiac contusion, myocardial injury, coronary injury, valvular disruption, and cardiomyopathy.

Commotio cordis
Commotio cordis or 'concussion of the heart' is caused by a blunt impact to the chest wall over the heart during the vulnerable phase of the cardiac cycle.[31] This can result in an electrophysiological R-on-T phenomenon causing ventricular fibrillation. There is no mechanical damage to the myocardium or surrounding organs, and cardiac arrest should be managed as per advanced life support guidance.

Cardiac injury
High-energy blunt trauma to the thorax can result in myocardial contusion, valvular disruption, coronary dissection, and rib fracture-associated penetrating trauma to the heart and pericardium. Myocardial contusions may impair contraction, and in severe cases result in cardiogenic shock. The right ventricle is most commonly injured in blunt trauma because of its position behind the sternum. Diagnosis includes ECG,

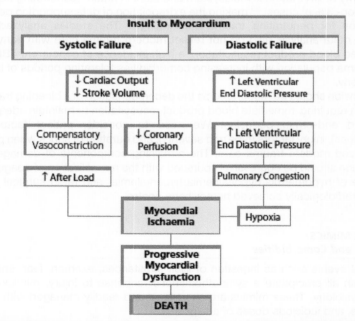

Fig. 4. Cardiogenic shock. Tim Nutbeam, Matthew Boylan, ABC of Prehospital Emergency Medicine, Wiley, 2013.

cardiac troponins, and echocardiography. ECG changes include nonspecific ST-segment and T-wave changes, conduction delays, dysrhythmias, and sinus tachy-cardia.[32] Cardiac troponins are highly sensitive for myocardial injury, but may also be raised due to hypoperfusion from hypovolemia or other causes of hypotension.[32] A normal 12-lead ECG and troponin blood test excludes cardiac contusion. Echocardiography is a useful screening tool for patients who develop cardiac complications or unresponsive hypotension after blunt chest wall trauma. Segmental wall motion abnormalities representing regional hypokinesia and RV dilatation are characteristic findings in severe cardiac contusion. Echo is also helpful to diagnose valvular disruption or pericardial effusions in the context of coronary lesions and myocardial lacerations.[32]

Penetrating trauma to the thorax may cause a pericardial effusion, but can also cause coronary disruption, valvular/papillary injury, and damage to the conduction system of the heart. The assessment and clinical management of penetrating trauma to the chest remains unchanged (see below for more detail in the obstructive shock section), but in patients with refractory shock states and conduction abnormalities, direct cardiac injury should be considered.

Cardiomyopathy

Cardiomyopathy is defined as a disease of the myocardium that impairs its ability to contract due to dilation, thickening, or stiffening. Although patients may have preexisting cardiomyopathy, this condition can also occur acutely in the context of major trauma, complicating the clinical assessment and management of patients with shock in trauma.

Following a TBI or multisystem trauma with a high tissue-injury burden, excess catecholamines are released, depleting the myocardium of energy stores **(Fig. 5)**,[33] impairing contractility and resulting in a stunned myocardium with regional wall motion abnormalities in the basal and midventricular regions. This pattern of myocardial impairment is referred to as a Takotsubo cardiomyopathy.[34–37] Concurrent hypoxia

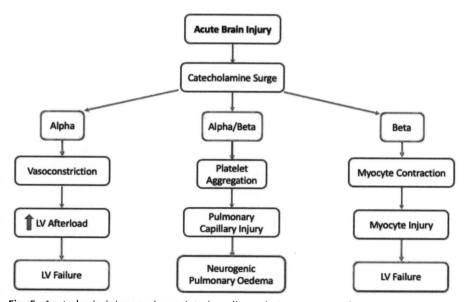

Fig. 5. Acute brain injury and associated cardiorespiratory compromise.

and hypercarbia from concussive injury to the brain, resulting in abnormal ventilation or apnea, can compound this catecholamine-driven myocardial injury.[38] Recognition of a stunned myocardium/cardiomyopathy can be challenging, and a thorough clinical examination, assessment of the patient's physiology, and correlation with echocardiography may guide diagnosis. Management requires judicious volume resuscitation and inotropic support as required.

Patients with sustained or profound myocardial hypoperfusion due to prolonged hypovolemia, particularly on a background of preexisting ischemic heart disease, may sustain irreversible myocyte injury. This can result in delayed (24–48 hours) cardiac failure and multiorgan dysfunction despite aggressive and early resuscitative efforts.

Obstructive Shock

Extracardiac obstruction to blood flow can cause impaired ventricular diastolic filling or excessive right ventricular afterload, impairing cardiac output and resulting in end-organ oxygen debt. Causes include cardiac tamponade, tension pneumothorax, and pulmonary embolism.

Cardiac tamponade is most commonly caused by incisional trauma to the torso including the supraclavicular region, lower neck, thorax, or epigastrium. There have also been case reports of pericardial effusion and tamponade caused by blunt trauma, either due to rib fractures and bone-fragment injury, or due to blunt cardiac chamber lacerations or coronary vessel disruption.[39] Cardiac tamponade must be a differential diagnosis for all patients with decompensated shock in the context of penetrating trauma. Signs of cardiac tamponade include tachypnea, cardiovascular compromise, electrical alternans (alternating height of consecutive QRS complexes), pulsus paradoxus (fall of systolic blood pressure of >10 mm Hg during the inspiratory phase of respiration), muffled heart sounds, and distended neck veins (absent if concurrent hypovolemia). In patients with compensated shock, further imaging may guide diagnosis: CT or bedside transthoracic echocardiography with visualized effusion and right atrial/ventricular collapse have a high specificity.[40] For patients who are periarrest or in cardiac arrest, immediate resuscitative thoracotomy is indicated within 15 minutes of loss of vital signs.[41] Note that a proportion of neurologically intact survivors from pre-hospital thoracotomy have a presenting rhythm of asystole, and therefore this should not be used as a prognostic determinant for this cohort of patient.[42]

Tension pneumothorax in the spontaneously ventilating patient has a very different pathophysiology to the positive pressure ventilated patient.[43] In spontaneous ventilation, a one-way pleural defect is required for gas accumulation in the intrapleural space, and progressive tachypnea, dyspnea, pleuritic chest pain, and hypoxia (masked by high-flow oxygen) are the presenting features. Hemodynamic compromise only occurs at the point of hypoxic cardiac arrest and concurrent hypovolemia should always be considered in spontaneously ventilating patients with a tension pneumothorax and cardiovascular collapse. In positive pressure ventilated patients, a nonvalved pleural defect will suffice for gas accumulation in the intrapleural space, increasing the incidence of tension physiology. This will result in rapid hemodynamic compromise, high ventilatory pressures, decreased oxygen saturations, and subsequent cardiovascular collapse. Both distended neck veins and a deviated trachea are unreliable and rarely identified signs of a tension pneumothorax.[44] The acuity of cardiovascular collapse is also related to the volume status of the patient, with concurrent hypovolemia decreasing this threshold in patients with a tension pneumothorax when positive pressure ventilated.

Dynamic hyperinflation (gas trapping) due to excessive positive pressure ventilation in patients with severe bronchospasm may also reduce venous return sufficient to cause an obstructive shock state, particularly in the presence of hypovolemia. Consideration of mechanical ventilatory strategies and gentle bag-valve ventilation of hypovolemic patients can minimize hemodynamic compromise by reducing the inspiratory pressure.

Distributive Shock

A reduction in peripheral vascular resistance can unmask compensated hypovolemia, or in the context of profound vasodilation/vasoplegia will decrease right ventricular preload, resulting in reduced cardiac output and subsequent end-organ oxygen debt. Septic, anaphylactic, and neurogenic shock are the most common subtypes of distributive shock.

Neurogenic shock occurs secondary to damage to the spinal cord above the level of T10, with loss of sympathetic outflow leading to unopposed peripheral vasodilatation. Injuries to the spinal cord above T6 may also damage the cardioaccelerators and result in bradycardia, compounding this vasoplegic-mediated neurogenic shock. Clinical suspicion of spinal cord injury with neurogenic shock is supported by spinal pain/tenderness, limb paralysis and paresthesia, flaccid areflexia, diaphragmatic breathing, flushed warm skin despite hypotension, and priapism. The timing of onset of neurogenic shock can vary considerably (minutes to hours post injury) and can also develop in patients with anatomical injuries below T5.[45] The whole length of the sympathetic cord supplies innervation to the vasculature and therefore interruption at any level has the capacity to produce the vasoplegic shock independent of heart involvement. Log-rolling or repositioning may precipitate vasovagal stimulation. In the early phases of neurogenic shock, there may be tachyarrhythmias making it hard to differentiate from hypovolemic shock.[46] The hypotension that characterizes neurogenic shock may lead to hypoperfusion of the spinal cord with subsequent ischemia and secondary injury. Treatment after exclusion of hypovolemia on imaging and fluid resuscitation

Table 3	
Summary of trauma shock etiologies, and diagnostic features	
Etiology of Shock	**Clinical Diagnosis**
Tension pneumothorax	Respiratory compromise Chest ultrasound, chest x-ray, or thoracostomy
Hypovolemia	Hateful eight signs Blood gas Hb (very late sign) eFAST, chest x-ray/pelvic x-ray
Cardiac tamponade	Mechanism Distended neck veins Cardiac ultrasound
Cardiac contusion	Mechanism Abnormal ECG, troponin T, echo
Neurogenic shock	Clinical signs of spinal cord injury – motor and sensory deficit Vasodilatation – warm peripheries, distended peripheral veins, priapism Bradycardia with hypotension
Traumatic brain injury	External signs of head injury, prehospital low GCS Alternating bradyarrhythmia and tachyarrhythmia
Soft tissue injury	Mechanism, signs of limb injury Unresponsive tachycardia

to maintain blood volume, includes preventing fluid overload, monitoring urine output/ fluid balance, and judicious use of vasopressors to maintain an MAP of 85 to 90 mm Hg.[47]

Rewarming hypothermic major trauma patients with cutaneous vasoconstriction, or administration of anesthetic agents with vasodilatory profiles can precipitate cardiovascular collapse in patients with compensated hypovolemia. This should be anticipated when rewarming a bleeding polytrauma patient and treated with balanced blood product resuscitation as required. The use of vasopressors to offset this phenomenon should be avoided, as may worsen end-organ microcirculatory perfusion, oxygen delivery, and trauma-induced coagulopathy.

Table 3 summarizes the common causes of shock in trauma patients.

As **Fig. 1** illustrates, there are also several medical conditions that can mimic bleeding and may also account for the primary cause of the injury. Examples include relative hypovolemia from dehydration or sepsis causing collapse, drug use/overdose leading to behavioral disturbance, and cardiac ischemia or arrhythmia leading to syncope. The importance of interpreting the prodromal events, patient comorbidities, physical examination findings, and response to treatment are all crucial in recognizing these trauma mimics and managing them appropriately.

SUMMARY

Shock in trauma is complex and varied in presentation and etiology. The physiological response to major hemorrhage is dependent on a variety of autonomic reflexes, mechanism of injury, bleeding source, and the patient's baseline physiology. A number of bleeding mimics can also result in trauma shock, occurring in isolation or in combination with major hemorrhage. A thorough understanding of how patients respond to bleeding, the differential diagnoses, and recognition of individualized tolerability to shock is essential when assessing and resuscitating major trauma patients.

CLINICS CARE POINTS

- Hypovolemia may induce bradycardia via cardiac C-fiber and arterial chemoreceptor reflexes.
- Penetrating injury without tissue damage may produce a biphasic hemodynamic response.
- Traumatic brain injury or multisystem trauma with a high tissue-injury burden may cause release of excess catecholamines resulting in a stunned myocardium and cardiogenic shock.
- Rewarming hypothermic major trauma patients can precipitate cardiovascular collapse in patients with compensated hypovolemia.

DISCLOSURE

None of the authors have any financial or professional conflicts of interest to declare.

REFERENCES

1. Rixen D, Siegel JH. Bench-to-bedside review: Oxygen debt and its metabolic correlates as quantifiers of the severity of hemorrhagic and post-traumatic shock. Crit Care 2005;9(5):441–53.
2. Cowley RA, Mergner WJ, Fisher RS, et al. The subcellular pathology of shock in trauma patients: studies using the immediate autopsy. Am Surg 1979;45(4): 255–69.

3. Champion HR, Bellamy RF, Roberts CP, et al. A profile of combat injury. J Trauma 2003;54(5 Suppl):S13–9.
4. Sauaia A, Moore FA, Moore EE, et al. Epidemiology of trauma deaths: a reassessment. J Trauma 1995;38(2):185–93.
5. Guly HR, Bouamra O, Spiers M, et al. Vital signs and estimated blood loss in patients with major trauma: testing the validity of the ATLS classification of hypovolaemic shock. Resuscitation 2011;82(5):556–9.
6. Little RA, Kirkman E, Driscoll P, et al. Preventable deaths after injury: why are the traditional 'vital' signs poor indicators of blood loss? J Accid Emerg Med 1995; 12(1):1–14.
7. Kirkman E, Watts S. Haemodynamic changes in trauma. Br J Anaesth 2014; 113(2):266–75.
8. Evans RG, Ventura S, Dampney RA, et al. Neural mechanisms in the cardiovascular responses to acute central hypovolaemia. Clin Exp Pharmacol Physiol 2001; 28(5–6):479–87.
9. Champion HR, Holcomb JB, Young LA. Injuries from explosions: physics, biophysics, pathology, and required research focus. J Trauma 2009;66(5): 1468–77, discussion 1477.
10. Kirkman E, Watts S. Characterization of the response to primary blast injury. Philos Trans R Soc B Biol Sci 2011;366(1562):286–90.
11. Pain in the Polytrauma Patient – painandpsa.org [Internet]. [cited 2022 Jun 6]. Available at: https://painandpsa.org/pain-in-the-poly-trauma-patient/.
12. Eastridge BJ, Salinas J, McManus JG, et al. Hypotension begins at 110 mm Hg: redefining 'hypotension' with data. J Trauma 2007 Aug;63(2):291–7 [discussion: 297-299].
13. Watts S, Smith JE, Gwyther R, et al. Closed chest compressions reduce survival in an animal model of haemorrhage-induced traumatic cardiac arrest. Resuscitation 2019;140:37–42.
14. Deakin CD, Low JL. Accuracy of the advanced trauma life support guidelines for predicting systolic blood pressure using carotid, femoral, and radial pulses: observational study. BMJ 2000;321(7262):673–4.
15. McMahon N, Hogg LA, Corfield AR, et al. Comparison of non-invasive and invasive blood pressure in aeromedical care. Anaesthesia 2012 Dec;67(12):1343–7.
16. Bankhead-Kendall B, Teixeira P, Roward S, et al. Narrow pulse pressure is independently associated with massive transfusion and emergent surgery in hemodynamically stable trauma patients. Am J Surg 2020;220(5):1319–22.
17. Priestley EM, Inaba K, Byerly S, et al. Pulse Pressure as an Early Warning of Hemorrhage in Trauma Patients. J Am Coll Surg 2019 Aug;229(2):184–91.
18. Nevin DG, Brohi K. Permissive hypotension for active haemorrhage in trauma. Anaesthesia 2017;72(12):1443–8.
19. Rossaint R, Bouillon B, Cerny V, et al. The European guideline on management of major bleeding and coagulopathy following trauma: fourth edition. Crit Care Lond Engl 2016;20:100.
20. Glen J, Constanti M, Brohi K, Guideline Development Group. Assessment and initial management of major trauma: summary of NICE guidance. BMJ 2016; 353:i3051.
21. Wiles MD. Blood pressure in trauma resuscitation: 'pop the clot' vs. 'drain the brain. Anaesthesia 2017;72(12):1448–55.
22. Lecky F, Woodford M, Edwards A, et al. Trauma scoring systems and databases. Br J Anaesth 2014;113(2):286–94.

23. Harrison DA, Prabhu G, Grieve R, et al. Risk Adjustment In Neurocritical care (RAIN)–prospective validation of risk prediction models for adult patients with acute traumatic brain injury to use to evaluate the optimum location and comparative costs of neurocritical care: a cohort study. Health Technol Assess Winch Engl 2013;17(23):vii–viii, 1–350.
24. Berry C, Ley EJ, Bukur M, et al. Redefining hypotension in traumatic brain injury. Injury 2012;43(11):1833–7.
25. Chesnut RM, Marshall LF, Klauber MR, et al. The role of secondary brain injury in determining outcome from severe head injury. J Trauma 1993;34(2):216–22.
26. Carney N, Totten AM, O'Reilly C, et al. Guidelines for the Management of Severe Traumatic Brain Injury, Fourth Edition. Neurosurgery 2017;80(1):6–15.
27. Nathanson MH, Andrzejowski J, Dinsmore J, et al. Guidelines for safe transfer of the brain-injured patient: trauma and stroke Guidelines from the Association of Anaesthetists and the Neuro Anaesthesia and Critical Care Society. Anaesthesia 2020;75(2):234–46.
28. Kwan I, Bunn F, Chinnock P, et al. Timing and volume of fluid administration for patients with bleeding. Cochrane Database Syst Rev 2014;(3):CD002245.
29. Whittaker G, Norton J, Densley J, et al. Epidemiology of penetrating injuries in the United Kingdom: A systematic review. Int J Surg Lond Engl 2017;41:65–9.
30. Bickell WH, Wall MJ, Pepe PE, et al. Immediate versus delayed fluid resuscitation for hypotensive patients with penetrating torso injuries. N Engl J Med 1994; 331(17):1105–9.
31. Link MS. Commotio cordis: ventricular fibrillation triggered by chest impact-induced abnormalities in repolarization. Circ Arrhythm Electrophysiol 2012;5(2): 425–32.
32. Kaye P, O'Sullivan L. Myocardial contusion: emergency investigation and diagnosis. Emerg Med J 2002;19(1):8–10.
33. Clifton GL, Robertson CS, Kyper K, et al. Cardiovascular response to severe head injury. J Neurosurg 1983 Sep;59(3):447–54.
34. Prasad Hrishi A, Ruby Lionel K, Prathapadas U. Head Rules Over the Heart: Cardiac Manifestations of Cerebral Disorders. Indian J Crit Care Med 2019;23(7): 329–35.
35. Banki NM, Zaroff JG. Neurogenic Cardiac Injury. Curr Treat Options Cardiovasc Med 2003;5(6):451–8.
36. Kawano H, Okada R, Yano K. Histological study on the distribution of autonomic nerves in the human heart. Heart Vessels 2003;18(1):32–9.
37. Gruhl SL, Su J, Chua WC, et al. Takotsubo cardiomyopathy in post-traumatic brain injury: A systematic review of diagnosis and management. Clin Neurol Neurosurg 2022;213:107119.
38. Wilson MH, Hinds J, Grier G, et al. Impact brain apnoea - A forgotten cause of cardiovascular collapse in trauma. Resuscitation 2016;105:52–8.
39. Almond P, Morton S, OMeara M, et al. A 6-year case series of resuscitative thoracotomies performed by a helicopter emergency medical service in a mixed urban and rural area with a comparison of blunt versus penetrating trauma. Scand J Trauma Resusc Emerg Med 2022;30(1):8.
40. Spodick DH. Acute Cardiac Tamponade. N Engl J Med 2003;349(7):684–90.
41. Lott C, Truhlář A, Alfonzo A, et al. European Resuscitation Council Guidelines 2021: Cardiac arrest in special circumstances. Resuscitation 2021;161:152–219.
42. Davies GE, Lockey DJ. Thirteen survivors of prehospital thoracotomy for penetrating trauma: a prehospital physician-performed resuscitation procedure that can yield good results. J Trauma 2011;70(5):E75–8.

43. Roberts DJ, Leigh-Smith S, Faris PD, et al. Clinical Presentation of Patients With Tension Pneumothorax: A Systematic Review. Ann Surg 2015;261(6):1068–78.
44. Leigh-Smith S, Harris T. Tension pneumothorax—time for a re-think? Emerg Med J 2005;22(1):8–16.
45. Taylor MP, Wrenn P, O'Donnell AD. Presentation of neurogenic shock within the emergency department. Emerg Med J EMJ 2017;34(3):157–62.
46. Gondim FaA, Lopes ACA, Oliveira GR, et al. Cardiovascular control after spinal cord injury. Curr Vasc Pharmacol 2004;2(1):71–9.
47. Walters BC, Hadley MN, Hurlbert RJ, et al. Guidelines for the management of acute cervical spine and spinal cord injuries: 2013 update. Neurosurgery 2013; 60(CN_suppl_1):82–91.

Neurotrauma Update

Vanessa R. Salasky, MD[a], Wan-Tsu W. Chang, MD[b],*

KEYWORDS

- Traumatic brain injury • Intracranial pressure • Coagulopathy • Antifibrinolytic
- Hyperosmolar therapy • Craniectomy • Hypothermia

KEY POINTS

- Although there has been an overall decline in traumatic brain injury (TBI) -related mortality, rates of hospitalization have increased owing to an increase in falls, anticoagulation therapy, and injuries in older adults.
- The risk of hematoma expansion increases from 15.6% to 43% from mild to severe TBI; thus, a follow-up head computed tomographic scan is recommended to evaluate for stability of the hemorrhagic lesion.
- There is mixed evidence for the use of tranexamic acid in isolated TBI. The CRASH-3 trial found a potential mortality benefit with early administration in subgroup analysis of patients with mild and moderate TBI.
- Management of elevated intracranial pressure and herniation syndromes should follow a tiered approach. Hyperventilation should only be used as a temporizing measure and bridge to definitive therapy.
- Decompressive craniectomy and therapeutic hypothermia can be considered as salvage therapy for refractory intracranial hypertension, although studies have not shown any benefit in outcomes.

A CHANGING EPIDEMIOLOGY

Traumatic brain injury (TBI) is the leading cause of morbidity and mortality worldwide. In the United States, 1.7 million people annually are diagnosed with TBI.[1] TBI accounts for 1.4% of emergency department (ED) visits and 4.8% of injuries presenting to the ED.[2] Despite an overall decline in TBI-related mortality, rates of hospitalizations have been on the rise. The National Hospital Discharge Survey demonstrated a 10.6% increase in TBI-related hospitalizations over 1995 to 2010.[1] Likely explanations for this increase in hospitalizations are the concomitant increase in falls as well as increased anticoagulation therapy among older adults.[1,3] Falls now supersede motor

[a] Department of Neurology, Section of Neurocritical Care and Emergency Neurology, University of Maryland Medical Center, 22 South Greene Street, G7K18, Baltimore, MD 21201, USA;
[b] Departments of Emergency Medicine and Neurology, Program in Trauma, University of Maryland School of Medicine, 22 South Greene Street, G7K18, Baltimore, MD 21201, USA
* Corresponding author.
E-mail address: wchang1@som.umaryland.edu

Emerg Med Clin N Am 41 (2023) 19–33
https://doi.org/10.1016/j.emc.2022.09.014
0733-8627/23/© 2022 Elsevier Inc. All rights reserved.
emed.theclinics.com

vehicle accidents as the most common cause for TBI with 61% of TBIs in those age 65 years and older being fall-related. Moreover, adults greater than 75 years of age have the highest rates of TBI-related hospitalizations and deaths.[2]

Pathophysiology

TBI is defined in 2 stages, primary and secondary brain injury. Primary injury refers to the insult that occurs on impact, resulting in hematoma, contusion, vascular injury, swelling, or diffuse axonal injury (DAI). Secondary injury refers to the cascade of cellular and biochemical events occurring as early as minutes to hours after the initial insult, and persisting over days, that contributes to secondary decline. Mechanisms of secondary injury in TBI include glutamate toxicity, blood-brain barrier disruption, free radical formation, oxidative stress, mitochondrial dysfunction, and a maladaptive immune reaction. It is these secondary injuries that promote additional cell death and necrosis, and lead to ischemia, hypoxemia, and edema.[4]

Definitions

TBI is an umbrella term for a heterogenous group of injuries with several classification schemes according to mechanism, primary structural pathologic condition, or clinical severity.

Mechanistic categories include closed head, penetrating, and blast injury. Closed head injuries involve direct impact outside the skull and can result in deceleration/acceleration or rotational forces. Penetrating injuries result from direct penetration of an object into the brain parenchyma, most commonly owing to gunshot wounds or shrapnel. Blast injuries are a newer entity within TBI, most commonly incurred by military personnel from high-grade explosives that cause significant thermal, mechanical, and electromagnetic energy to be transferred to the brain. Blast injuries often cause early and severe cerebral edema, subarachnoid hemorrhage (SAH), and vasospasm.[5]

When defined according to primary pathologic condition, TBI can be thought of as either focal or diffuse (**Table 1**). Focal injuries include cerebral contusions and hematomas: epidural, subdural, subarachnoid, intraparenchymal, or intraventricular. Cerebral contusions result from coup injuries, causing direct injury of underlying brain tissue, or contrecoup injuries, causing injury to the contralateral brain region. Contusions are classically seen in the inferior frontal and anterior-inferior temporal lobes. Subdural hematomas occur from of tearing of bridging veins between the dura and arachnoid space, causing accumulation of blood in a concave pattern that crosses suture lines. Cerebral contusions and subdural hematomas are the most frequently seen abnormalities in severe TBI. In epidural hematoma, injury to the middle meningeal artery or vein causes blood to collect between the skull and dura mater, and because it does not cross suture lines, presents in a classic convex appearance. SAH results from tearing of vessels in the subarachnoid space, and in traumatic SAH, this usually occurs at the site of impact or contralaterally. Intraventricular hemorrhage can be caused by a ruptured subependymal vein, extension from an intraparenchymal hematoma, or redistribution from the subarachnoid space. It is important to note that there is often overlap in presentation with multiple blood patterns present.

Diffuse injuries include DAI, causing damage to white matter tracts and cerebral edema. Patients with DAI often present in coma, do not present with high intracranial pressure (ICP), and have unfavorable outcomes.[5] Cerebral edema results from disruption of cerebral autoregulation or the blood-brain barrier. Both cytotoxic and vasogenic edema can occur and can appear focally or diffusely.

Various vascular injuries can also occur, including dural venous sinus tear or occlusion, arterial dissection, and traumatic aneurysms. These injuries are best identified by

Table 1
Classification of traumatic brain injury by structural pathologic condition

		Pathophysiology	Imaging Characteristics
Focal injuries	Cerebral contusion	Coup/contrecoup injury	Inferior frontal and anterior-inferior temporal lobes
	Subdural hematoma	Bridging vein injury	Concave (crescent shaped)
			Crosses suture lines
	Epidural hematoma	Middle meningeal artery/vein, diploic vein, or dural venous sinus injury	Convex (lens shaped)
			Does not cross suture lines
			Adjacent to skull fractures
	Subarachnoid hemorrhage	Pial vessel injury	Cerebral convexities
			Basal cisterns
	Intraventricular hemorrhage	Subependymal vein injury	Layering within ventricular system
		Extension from intraparenchymal hemorrhage	
		Redistribution from subarachnoid space	
Diffuse injuries	Diffuse axonal injury	Axonal shear injury	Cortical–white matter junction
			Midline white matter structures
	Cerebral edema	Cerebral autoregulation or blood-brain barrier disruption	Cytotoxic or vasogenic edema

computed tomographic venography and computed tomographic arteriography, respectively. Arterial dissection involves a tear in the intimal layer of a blood vessel, which can result in a false lumen, luminal occlusion, or pseudoaneurysm. Luminal occlusion or emboli can subsequently result in ischemia or infarcts, which often occur in a delayed fashion.

The Monro-Kellie doctrine asserts that there is a fixed volume in the intracranial vault, consisting of 3 different compartments: blood, cerebrospinal fluid (CSF), and brain tissue. If there is an increase in the volume of 1 compartment, one or both of the other compartments must decrease in volume in order to maintain constant ICP. There are autoregulatory mechanisms that maintain cerebral perfusion across a range of mean arterial pressure (MAP). However, once these compensatory mechanisms fail, elevated ICP can result in herniation syndromes and cerebral ischemia. In TBI, an increase in volume is usually experienced as hemorrhage or cerebral edema.

EVALUATION

The clinical examination is paramount in the diagnosis of TBI and should be tracked serially over time to detect clinical improvement or decline. Pupillary size, reaction to light, and the motor examination are critical components of the neurologic assessment. Anisocoria is defined as greater than 1-mm difference in pupillary diameter between the eyes and can be an important marker of neurologic decline. Pupillary constriction relies on innervation from parasympathetic fibers carried by cranial nerve 3, the nucleus and exiting fibers of which are located at the level of the midbrain. Transtentorial herniation compressing the ipsilateral oculomotor nerve produces a unilateral dilated and nonreactive pupil, which should prompt empiric treatment for elevated ICP. Traumatic carotid dissection can result in a Horner syndrome whereby sympathetic innervation to the pupil, eyelid, and sweat glands is disrupted, causing ipsilateral miosis, ptosis, and depending on the site of the lesion, anhidrosis.

The Glasgow Coma Score (GCS) is the most common severity assessment score for TBI and should be obtained as part of the primary survey of the traumatically injured patient. It assesses the degree of disordered consciousness, and like the pupillary assessment, should be tracked throughout a patient's course. The GCS consists of 3 components: best eye opening (1–4), verbal (1–5), and motor (1–6) response to stimulation with the sum score ranging from 3 to 15. TBI is commonly defined based on GCS as mild (GCS 13–15), moderate (GCS 9–12), or severe (GCS $\leq$8). It is recommended that all 3 components be reported for an individual patient, (i.e. E1V1M2). Although it is a useful tool with excellent interrater reliability, one should keep in mind that it does not distinguish between primary pathologic conditions for brain injury and can be confounded by other factors like intoxication, sedation, and paralytics.

Clinical signs of increased ICP include asymmetric, dilated, or nonreactive pupils, motor posturing, neurologic decline of greater than 2 GCS points, or Cushing reflex (bradycardia, hypertension). Any signs of increased ICP or herniation should prompt empiric treatment. Interventions include elevation of the head of the bed, maintaining neutral head position, hyperventilation, and osmotic therapy, which are described in more detail in later discussion.

PRINCIPLES OF NEURORESUSCITATION

Appropriate assessment and triage of TBI patients are critical. Like other traumatic injuries, the initial assessment focuses on airway, breathing, and circulation, and in TBI especially, stabilizing the cervical spine. The Brain Trauma Foundation (BTF) further recommends that patients with severe TBI be transported to a facility with a computed tomographic (CT) scanner, neurosurgical care, and ICP monitoring capabilities.[6]

Airway, breathing, and circulation

Intubation should be considered for any comatose patient with severe TBI (GCS <9) or for patients with moderate TBI (GCS 9–12) with significant extracranial injuries, agitation, or declining mental status.[7] Brain-injured patients often have depressed mental status and respiratory drive; thus, securing the airway is necessary to prevent secondary hypoxic injury. Preoxygenation with 100% FiO2 followed by rapid sequence intubation (RSI) with in-line cervical spine stabilization is the preferred method for intubation. The reflex sympathetic response from intubation is of particular concern in this patient population because this can increase ICP. Pretreatment with fentanyl can be considered to blunt the hemodynamic response. Esmolol should be avoided in the patient with multitrauma or hemorrhagic shock given the risk of transient hypotension. Induction agents may include ketamine or etomidate. These are hemodynamically neutral agents, thus may avoid exacerbating brain injury that can occur with hypotension.[8] Previous concerns over ketamine causing increased ICP have since been debunked.[9]

Much attention has been given to prehospital intubation and RSI in patients with severe TBI, especially given the importance of preventing hypoxia in this population. There is limited data from retrospective trials demonstrating worse outcomes in prehospital RSI compared with those intubated in the ED.[10,11] One large study comparing prospectively enrolled patients with severe TBI undergoing paramedic RSI compared with historical controls found increased mortality and worse functional outcomes.[12] A 2009 expert panel assembled by BTF concluded that the existing literature regarding paramedic RSI in patients with severe TBI is inconclusive, and that additional research is needed to identify patients who might benefit from early intubation. This panel also noted that poorer outcomes in these studies may reflect unrecognized oxygen desaturations or hyperventilation, and that the success of paramedic RSI depends on emergency medical services (EMS) characteristics.[13] A randomized controlled trial (RCT) published in 2010 compared paramedic RSI and hospital intubation in 312 patients with severe TBI and showed better outcomes at 6 months in the paramedic intubation group and no differences in in-hospital mortality.[14] Although this remains a controversial topic, current recommendations advise against prehospital RSI in patients who are spontaneously breathing and recommend maintaining an SpO2 greater than 90% on supplemental oxygen.[6]

Both hypotension and hypoxia are associated with worse outcomes and are the main focus of prehospital and ED care. A single episode of hypotension, defined as systolic blood pressure (SBP) <90 mm Hg, occurring from time of injury through resuscitation has been associated with doubled mortality, and patients whose hypotension was not corrected before ED arrival have worse outcomes.[15,16] Hypoxemia has similarly been associated with worse outcomes.[17] The BTF recommends prehospital continuous O2 monitoring, correction of hypoxemia for o_2 saturation goal greater than 90%, and administration of isotonic fluids for goal SBP >90 mm Hg.[6] Hypotonic fluids (D5W or ½ NS) can worsen cerebral edema and should be avoided. Neither hypertonic saline nor albumin has been shown to be an effective resuscitative fluid.[18,19]

Current evidence now supports a target SBP ≥110 mm Hg for patients 15 to 49 years old or older than 70 years old and SBP ≥100 mm Hg for patients 50 to 69 years old.[20] It should be noted that recent studies have questioned the single dichotomized definition of hypotension. One multicenter cohort study of more than 5000 patients found an increased mortality at SBP <120 mm Hg, and another analysis of 3844 moderate and severe TBI patients found an inverse linear relationship between mortality and systolic blood pressure.[21,22] Future studies are needed to determine whether MAP goals might be a more appropriate endpoint, because this is more a more direct determinant of ICP.

Neuroimaging

A noncontrast head CT scan should be obtained after initial assessment of airway, breathing, and circulation, and in conjunction with a neurologic examination as already discussed. CT is preferred for its rapidity of image acquisition and ability to detect acute blood products and fractures. The primary purpose of the initial CT scan is to identify lesions requiring surgical intervention. Hematomas are common in moderate to severe TBI, occurring in 5% to 10% and 25% to 35% of patients, respectively.[5] They also occur in up to 15% of patients with a GCS score of 13 to 14.[23] It is therefore recommended that all patients with a history of head injury and GCS of 14 or less undergo head imaging.

Patients who experience head trauma are at significantly greater risk of sustaining spinal injury than patients who experience noncranial trauma, with cervical spine injuries occurring in 6.5% of TBI patients in one recent systematic review.[24] It is therefore recommended that a CT C-spine scan also be obtained.

It is important to recognize that TBI is a dynamic process, and particularly in the first 24 hours of injury, there is risk of hematoma expansion.[25] In patients with diffuse injury on CT, 16% demonstrate deterioration on a later scan.[26] Patients with severe (GCS 3–8) and moderate (GCS 9–12) TBI have an average of 43% and 25% progression on repeat CT imaging, respectively.[27] Patients with mild TBI (GCS 13–15) and an initial CT head scan with an abnormality have an estimated 15.6% progression on repeat imaging.[28] Lesion growth of greater than 5 cm, effacement of basal cisterns on initial CT, and worsened GCS before follow-up scan are strong predictors for late surgical evacuation.[29] For these reasons, a follow-up head CT scan is recommended to evaluate for stability of the lesion.

Magnetic resonance imaging (MRI) is not recommended in the acute setting given the lengthiness of the study and need for metal and device clearance. MRI is more commonly used in the subacute or chronic phases in order to detect DAI and other potential complications of TBI. CT or MR angiography/venography should be considered to evaluate for vascular injury when there is a penetrating head injury, fracture over a venous sinus, select C-spine injuries, or unexplained neurologic deficit.[7]

Reversal of coagulopathy

Coagulopathy is common in TBI with an overall prevalence of 33% and is widely recognized as a risk factor for increased morbidity and mortality.[30] In a retrospective study of more than 3000 patients with isolated TBI, coagulopathy was associated with higher rates of craniotomies, single- and multiple-organ failure, increased length of stay, and an adjusted odds ratio for hospital mortality of 2.97.[31] Identified risk factors include base deficit, lower GCS, severity of head injury, and increased age.[31,32] The pathophysiology is complex and due at least in part to release of tissue factor into the systemic circulation and activated protein C, leading to disseminated intravascular coagulation and platelet dysfunction.[33] Prescribed anticoagulation medications are another major contributing factor, especially in the aging population. It is recommended that measures of coagulation, including prothrombin time, partial thromboplastin time, international normalized ratio, platelet count, fibrinogen, and if available, thromboelastography (TEG) or rotational thromboelastometry (ROTEM), should be routinely obtained in all patients with neurotrauma.[7] Coagulopathy in the acute postinjury period should be rapidly reversed.

What is the evidence for antifibrinolytic therapy?

Tranexamic acid (TXA) is an antifibrinolytic that has been studied in trauma patients and has recently garnered attention as a possible therapy for patients with TBI. To date, there are mixed data regarding its use for isolated TBI. The CRASH-3 trial published in 2019 was an RCT of 12,737 adults with TBI treated within 3 hours of injury with TXA versus placebo. The investigators found no difference in hospital mortality or complications, including vaso-occlusive events or seizures. A pre-planned subgroup analysis however did show a mortality benefit for patients with mild and moderate TBI.[34] The investigators concluded that TXA administration appears to be safe and portend a mortality benefit for patients with mild/moderate TBI. A subsequent RCT of prehospital TXA administration in patients with moderate and severe TBI found no benefit for functional outcomes at 6 months, and a meta-analysis showed no mortality or functional benefit.[35,36] A cohort study of more than 1800 patients in the Netherlands found that prehospital TXA administration was associated with increased mortality in patients with isolated severe TBI.[37] Current guidelines have not yet provided recommendations regarding the use of TXA in TBI.

MANAGEMENT

Management of TBI has become more standardized over time with adherence to national and international guidelines. The BTF has published evidenced-based guidelines on the management of severe TBI, most recently updated in 2016.

The central goal of TBI management is to maintain normal ICP and cerebral perfusion pressure (CPP). CPP is defined as MAP minus ICP. Normal CPP lies between 60 and 80 mm Hg and clinically is obtained as a calculation based on measured MAP and ICP. In the non-brain-injured patient, cerebral blood flow (CBF) is autoregulated, that is, remains constant across a range of perfusion pressures, usually MAP 50 to 150 mm Hg. With changes in perfusion pressure, cerebral blood vessels either dilate or constrict, thus altering blood volume to maintain constant cerebral blood volume. Cerebral autoregulation is impaired or absent in 49% to 87% of patients with severe TBI, such that a fall in systemic blood pressure leads to decreased perfusion pressure, decreased CBF, and ultimately, ischemia.[38] Ischemia can also occur in the setting of raised ICP owing to edema or hemorrhage, and in severe forms leads to cerebral herniation. Current BTF recommendations for CPP are 60 to 70 mm Hg. There has been increased interest in individualizing the target CPP to each patient's autoregulatory range, based on how their ICP changes in response to MAP.[39]

WHAT IS THE ROLE OF INTRACRANIAL PRESSURE MONITORING?

Intracranial hypertension is associated with worse mortality and functional outcomes. BTF guidelines recommend ICP monitoring in all patients with a severe TBI (GCS 3–8) and abnormal CT scan, or GCS 3 to 8 with normal CT and 2 or more of the following: age greater than 40 years, motor posturing, SBP < 90 mm Hg.[20,39] There are different types of invasive ICP monitoring, including monitors in the epidural, subdural, subarachnoid, parenchymal, or intraventricular spaces. Intraventricular drains have the added benefit of providing diagnostic ICP data as well as therapeutic intervention of CSF drainage. Guidelines recommend treatment of ICP sustained greater than 22 mm Hg following a tiered approach (**Fig. 1**). Infection and intracranial hemorrhage are the most common complications.[40]

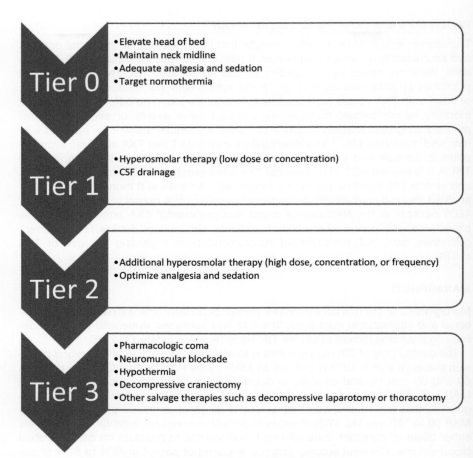

Fig. 1. Tiered approach to management of intracranial hypertension.

MULTIMODALITY MONITORING

One of the major advances in the treatment of TBI is the real-time monitoring of multiple physiologic parameters to provide individualized care. In addition to the standard ICP monitors, these include measures of brain tissue oxygen (PbtO2) and cerebral microdialysis. $Pbto_2$ involves an invasive monitor that measures focal brain oxygen delivery and uptake, with a cutoff of less than 20 mm Hg correlating to CBF 18 mL/100 g/min, the threshold at which ischemia occurs. The ongoing BOOST-3 trial will evaluate the safety and efficacy of treatment based on both ICP and $Pbto_2$ monitoring as compared with ICP monitoring alone. Cerebral microdialysis also requires an invasive monitor to analyze the biochemical makeup of the extracellular fluid, including glucose, lactate and pyruvate, glycerol, and glutamate.[39]

IS THERE AN IDEAL HYPEROSMOLAR THERAPY?

Hypertonic saline (HTS) with concentrations ranging from 3% to 23.4% and 20% mannitol is a hyperosmolar therapy used for the treatment of intracranial hypertension. Studies have shown that hyperosmolar therapy is effective in reducing ICP and radiographic edema but have not demonstrated improvement in mortality or functional outcomes. Both agents create an osmolar gradient that pulls water out of cells into the cerebral vasculature, thereby lowering cerebral blood volume and ICP. These agents also work by reducing blood viscosity, thereby increasing microcirculatory flow and causing arterioles to constrict. These are administered as bolus doses and can be repeated every 4 to 6 hours. It is important to note that 23.4% HTS requires central venous access and acts as a volume expander. Mannitol on the other hand has a profound diuretic effect and may not be the first choice in a patient with hypotension; it can also be associated with hyperkalemia and renal injury. There are data to suggest possible superiority of HTS over mannitol for reducing and sustaining ICP lowering; however, current BTF guidelines do not favor one over the other.[20,41] The recent COBI RCT published in 2021 included 370 adults with moderate to severe TBI and compared treatment with continuous infusion of 20% HTS versus standard care. There was no difference in neurologic outcomes at 6 months, whereas there was a higher proportion of patients with severe hypernatremia (>160 mmol/L) in those who received continuous HTS infusions.[42]

VENTILATION STRATEGIES

In the mechanically ventilated patient, hypoxia should be avoided, and hyperventilation should only be used as a temporizing measure in the patient with elevated ICP or signs of herniation. End-tidal CO_2 ($EtCO_2$) monitoring is recommended as hyperventilation decreases CO_2, which causes cerebral vasoconstriction and decreases CBF. For every 1-mm Hg increase in $PaCO_2$, there is an approximate 4% increase in CBF.[38] Decreasing cerebral metabolism and oxygen use ultimately causes a decrease in ICP. In a patient with signs of herniation, hyperventilation should be targeted to $EtCO_2$ 30 to 35 mm Hg or approximately 20 breaths/min, ideally to clinical effect. Notably, prophylactic hyperventilation should be avoided because there is a risk of secondary ischemia with prolonged vasoconstriction. In one RCT, patients with an initial GCS motor score of 4 to 5 who were prophylactically hyperventilated had worse outcomes.[43]

DECOMPRESSIVE CRANIECTOMY

Surgery should be considered based on the initial injury pattern or as salvage therapy for medically refractory intracranial hypertension. Primary decompressive craniectomy (DC) refers to treatment of acute lesions, including epidural or subdural hematomas. In general, surgery is considered for epidural hematomas greater than 30 mL in volume, subdural hematomas greater than 1 cm in thickness, intraparenchymal hematomas greater than 20 mL in volume, and any lesion associated with greater than 5 mm of midline shift. Parenchymal hematomas without significant mass effect and without signs of neurologic deterioration or elevated ICP can be managed nonoperatively.

Secondary DC remains a controversial topic and refers to delayed surgery for treatment of refractory intracranial hypertension. Two landmark RCTs investigated the use of DC for refractory elevated ICP. The Australian DECRA study published in 2011 compared early bifrontal DC within 72 hours of injury with standard medical therapy for patients with diffuse TBI who had ICP greater than 20 mm Hg for greater than 15 minutes failing tier 1 therapy.[44] The investigators found worse outcomes in the surgical group and no effect on mortality. The surgical group however had more severe injuries, and there was a high cross-over rate, making conclusions difficult to draw. The subsequent RESCUEicp study investigated DC for the treatment of medically refractory intracranial hypertension as tier 3 therapy and found decreased mortality (26.9% vs 48.9% in the medical group), but worse 6-month functional outcomes in those that survived.[45] It thus seems that DC as salvage therapy for refractory elevated ICP is life-saving, but at the expense of increased disability. Based on these studies, current guidelines provide level IIA recommendations for secondary DC for late refractory elevated ICP, but not early refractory intracranial hypertension.

HYPOTHERMIA FOR REFRACTORY INTRACRANIAL HYPERTENSION

There have been 2 RCTs investigating the use of hypothermia in patients with TBI. Eurotherm3235, published in 2015, randomized patients with closed TBI and elevated ICP to either moderate hypothermia (32–35°C) and standard therapy or standard therapy alone. Therapeutic hypothermia actually led to slightly worse mortality and outcomes compared with those with standard therapy alone. The Prophylactic Hypothermia Trial to Lessen Traumatic Brain Injury (POLAR-RCT) included 500 patients randomized to either normothermia or early prophylactic hypothermia (33–35°C) for a minimum of 72 hours and up to 7 days. There was no difference in mortality or outcomes at 6 months.[46] Although hypothermia is effective in reducing ICP, thus still used as a rescue therapy for refractory intracranial hypertension, there is lack of evidence showing benefit in outcomes.

DO ALL PATIENTS NEED SEIZURE PROPHYLAXIS?

The BTF estimates that in severe TBI, clinical seizures occur in up to 12% of patients, and subclinical seizures occur in 20% to 25%.[20] Posttraumatic seizures (PTS) are defined as either early, occurring within 1 week of injury, or late, occurring 7 days of more after injury. Early PTS can contribute to secondary brain injury by causing increased metabolic demand, increased ICP, release of neurotransmitters, and eventual development of hippocampal atrophy.[47–49] Treatment with antiseizure medications however also comes with risk of side effects. A landmark RCT assigning patients to either phenytoin or placebo found significant reduction in early, but not late, PTS.[50] Given the concern for negative long-term neuropsychological impacts from phenytoin, there has been interest in evaluating the safety and efficacy of new antiseizure medications. A 2013 RCT of 813 patients found no difference in clinical early PTS when comparing phenytoin with levetiracetam in brain-injured patients.[51] The American Academy of Neurology (AAN) and BTF currently provide level IIA recommendation for prophylactic phenytoin or levetiracetam for 7 days to decrease the incidence of early PTS.[20] Prophylaxis should be stopped after 7 days if no seizures have occurred. Moreover, given the high rate of subclinical seizures and nonconvulsive status epilepticus, continuous electroencephalographic monitoring should also be considered in comatose patients.

PROGNOSIS

Attempts to accurately predict outcome in TBI remain difficult. The Corticosteroid Randomization After Significant Head injury (CRASH) and International Mission for Prognosis and Analysis of Clinical Trials in Traumatic Brain Injury (IMPACT) models are the most widely used for prognostication and are based on data from patients involved in 2 large clinical trials.[52] Each model predicts 6-month mortality and functional outcomes based on clinical factors (age, pupil response, GCS motor score), CT findings, and laboratory values.

The Transforming Research and Clinical Knowledge in Traumatic Brain Injury (TRACK-TBI) study is a large prospective cohort study that enrolled patients presenting to the ED within 24 hours of injury at 18 level 1 trauma centers in the United States and followed them for 12 months after hospitalization. As part of this study, investigators followed patients' functional outcomes up to 12 months as defined by the Glasgow Outcome Scale-Extended and Disability Rating Scale (DRS). There were 484 patients out of the total 2679 individuals in the study with either moderate or severe TBI. Among those patients, 19.3% of patients with severe TBI, and 32% with moderate TBI reported no disability (DRS score 0) at 12 months. Among participants in a vegetative state at 2 weeks, 62 of 79 (78%) regained consciousness, and 14 of 56 (25%) regained orientation by 12 months.[53] These data suggest that even patients with severe injury may experience a favorable long-term outcome and that clinicians should be wary of prognosticating poor outcomes during the first 2 weeks of injury.

SUMMARY

TBI continues to be a leading cause of morbidity and mortality worldwide with older adults having the highest rate of hospitalizations and deaths. Management in the acute phase is focused on preventing secondary neurologic injury from hypoxia, hypocapnia, hypotension, and elevated ICP. Recent studies on TXA and continuous HTS infusion have not found any difference in neurologic outcomes. Care must be taken in prognosticating TBI outcomes, as recovery of consciousness and orientation has been observed up to 12 months after injury.

CLINICS CARE POINTS

- Care should be taken during intubation to avoid hypoxia and hypotension, both of which worsen outcomes in TBI.
- Decline in GCS of 2 or more points, dilated or nonreactive pupil, and motor posturing should prompt empiric treatment of a herniation syndrome.
- Avoid prolonged or excessive hyperventilation which can lead to cerebral ischemia.
- Hypercapnia results in cerebral vasodilation which can worsen intracranial hypertension.

DISCLOSURE

Drs Salasky and Chang have no disclosures.

REFERENCES

1. Faul M, Coronado V. Epidemiology of traumatic brain injury. Handb Clin Neurol 2015;127:3–13.
2. Faul M, Xu L, Wald MM, et al. Traumatic brain injury in the United States: emergency department visits, hospitalizations, and deaths. Atlanta (GA): Centers for Disease Control and Prevention. National Center for Injury Prevention and Control; 2010. p. 2.
3. Thompson HJ, McCormick WC, Kagan SH. Traumatic brain injury in older adults: Epidemiology, outcomes, and future implications. J Am Geriatr Soc 2006;54(10). https://doi.org/10.1111/j.1532-5415.2006.00894.x.

4. Corps KN, Roth TL, McGavern DB. Inflammation and neuroprotection in traumatic brain injury. JAMA Neurol 2015;72(3). https://doi.org/10.1001/jamaneurol.2014.3558.

5. Maas AI, Stocchetti N, Bullock R. Moderate and severe traumatic brain injury in adults. Lancet Neurol 2008;7(8). https://doi.org/10.1016/S1474-4422(08)70164-9.

6. Badjatia N, Carney N, Crocco TJ, et al. Guidelines for prehospital management of traumatic brain injury 2nd edition. Prehosp Emerg Care 2008;12(SUPPL. 1). https://doi.org/10.1080/10903120701732052.

7. Garvin R, Mangat HS. Emergency Neurological Life Support: Severe Traumatic Brain Injury. Neurocrit Care 2017;27:159–69.

8. Rajajee V, Riggs B, Seder DB. Emergency Neurological Life Support: Airway, Ventilation, and Sedation. Neurocrit Care 2017;27. https://doi.org/10.1007/s12028-017-0451-2.

9. Chang LC, Raty SR, Ortiz J, et al. The Emerging Use of Ketamine for Anesthesia and Sedation in Traumatic Brain Injuries. CNS Neurosci Ther 2013;19(6):390–5.

10. Murray JA, Demetriades D, Berne Tv, et al. Prehospital intubation in patients with severe head injury. J Trauma - Inj Infect Crit Care 2000;49(6). https://doi.org/10.1097/00005373-200012000-00015.

11. Bochicchio Gv, Ilahi O, Joshi M, et al. Endotracheal intubation in the field does not improve outcome in trauma patients who present without an acutely lethal traumatic brain injury. J Trauma 2003;54(2). https://doi.org/10.1097/01.TA.0000046252.97590.

12. Davis DP, Peay J, Sise MJ, et al. The impact of prehospital endotracheal intubation on outcome in moderate to severe traumatic brain injury. J Trauma - Inj Infect Crit Care 2005;58(5). https://doi.org/10.1097/01.TA.0000162731.53812.58.

13. Davis DP, Fakhry SM, Wang HE, et al. Paramedic rapid sequence intubation for severe traumatic brain injury: Perspectives from an expert panel. Prehosp Emerg Care 2007;11(1). https://doi.org/10.1080/10903120601021093.

14. Bernard SA, Nguyen V, Cameron P, et al. Prehospital rapid sequence intubation improves functional outcome for patients with severe traumatic brain injury: A randomized controlled trial. Ann Surg 2010;252(6). https://doi.org/10.1097/SLA.0b013e3181efc15f.

15. Fearnside MR, Cook RJ, Mcdougall P, et al. The Westmead head injury project outcome in severe head injury. A comparative analysis of pre-hospital, clinical and CT variables. Br J Neurosurg 1993;7(3). https://doi.org/10.3109/02688699309023809.

16. Chesnut RM, Chesnut RM, Marshall LF, et al. The role of secondary brain injury in determining outcome from severe head injury. J Trauma - Inj Infect Crit Care 1993;34(2). https://doi.org/10.1097/00005373-199302000-00006.

17. Spaite DW, Hu C, Bobrow BJ, et al. The Effect of Combined Out-of-Hospital Hypotension and Hypoxia on Mortality in Major Traumatic Brain Injury. Ann Emerg Med 2017;69. https://doi.org/10.1016/j.annemergmed.2016.08.007.

18. Cooper DJ, Myles PS, McDermott FT, et al. Prehospital Hypertonic Saline Resuscitation of Patients with Hypotension and Severe Traumatic Brain Injury: A Randomized Controlled Trial. J Am Med Assoc 2004;291(11). https://doi.org/10.1001/jama.291.11.1350.

19. Saline or Albumin for Fluid Resuscitation in Patients with Traumatic Brain Injury. New Engl J Med 2007;357(9). https://doi.org/10.1056/nejmoa067514.

20. Carney N, Totten AM, O'Reilly C, et al. Guidelines for the Management of Severe Traumatic Brain Injury, Fourth edition. Neurosurgery 2017;80(1). https://doi.org/10.1227/NEU.0000000000001432.

21. Fuller G, Hasler RM, Mealing N, et al. The association between admission systolic blood pressure and mortality in significant traumatic brain injury: A multi-centre cohort study. Injury 2014;45(3). https://doi.org/10.1016/j.injury.2013.09.008.

22. Spaite DW, Hu C, Bobrow BJ, et al. Mortality and prehospital blood pressure in patients with major traumatic brain injury: Implications for the hypotension threshold. JAMA Surg 2017;152. https://doi.org/10.1001/jamasurg.2016.4686.

23. Smits M, Dippel DWJ, Steyerberg EW, et al. Predicting intracranial traumatic findings on computed tomography in patients with minor head injury: The CHIP prediction rule. Ann Intern Med 2007;146(6). https://doi.org/10.7326/0003-4819-146-6-200703200-00004.

24. Pandrich MJ, Demetriades AK. Prevalence of concomitant traumatic cranio-spinal injury: a systematic review and meta-analysis. Neurosurg Rev 2020;43(1). https://doi.org/10.1007/s10143-018-0988-3.

25. Narayan RK, Maas AIR, Servadei F, et al. Progression of traumatic intracerebral hemorrhage: A prospective observational study. J Neurotrauma 2008;25(6). https://doi.org/10.1089/neu.2007.0385.

26. Servadei F, Murray GD, Penny K, et al. The value of the "worst" computed tomographic scan in clinical studies of moderate and severe head injury. Neurosurgery 2000;46(1). https://doi.org/10.1093/neurosurgery/46.1.70.

27. Wang MC, Linnau KF, Tirschwell DL, et al. Utility of repeat head computed tomography after blunt head trauma: A systematic review. J Trauma - Inj Infect Crit Care 2006;61(1). https://doi.org/10.1097/01.ta.0000197385.18452.89.

28. Marincowitz C, Lecky FE, Townend W, et al. The risk of deterioration in GCS13-15 patients with traumatic brain injury identified by computed tomography imaging: A systematic review and meta-analysis. J Neurotrauma 2018;35(5). https://doi.org/10.1089/neu.2017.5259.

29. Chang EF, Meeker M, Holland MC. Acute traumatic intraparenchymal hemorrhage: Risk factors for progression in the early post-injury period. Neurosurgery 2006;58(4). https://doi.org/10.1227/01.NEU.0000197101.68538.E6.

30. Harhangi BS, Kompanje EJO, Leebeek FWG, et al. Coagulation disorders after traumatic brain injury. Acta Neurochir (Wien) 2008;150(2). https://doi.org/10.1007/s00701-007-1475-8.

31. Wafaisade A, Lefering R, Tjardes T, et al. Acute coagulopathy in isolated blunt traumatic brain injury. Neurocrit Care 2010;12(2):211-9.

32. Cap AP, Spinella PC. Severity of head injury is associated with increased risk of coagulopathy in combat casualties. J Trauma - Inj Infect Crit Care 2011;71(SUPPL. 1). https://doi.org/10.1097/TA.0b013e3182218cd8.

33. Maegele M. Coagulopathy after traumatic brain injury: Incidence, pathogenesis, and treatment options. Transfusion (Paris) 2013;53(SUPPL. 1). https://doi.org/10.1111/trf.12033.

34. Roberts I, Shakur-Still H, Aeron-Thomas A, et al. Effects of tranexamic acid on death, disability, vascular occlusive events and other morbidities in patients with acute traumatic brain injury (CRASH-3): A randomised, placebo-controlled trial. Lancet 2019;394(10210). https://doi.org/10.1016/S0140-6736(19)32233-0.

35. Rowell SE, Meier EN, McKnight B, et al. Effect of Out-of-Hospital Tranexamic Acid vs Placebo on 6-Month Functional Neurologic Outcomes in Patients with Moderate or Severe Traumatic Brain Injury. JAMA - J Am Med Assoc 2020;324(10). https://doi.org/10.1001/jama.2020.8958.

36. Lawati K, Sharif S, Maqbali S al, et al. Efficacy and safety of tranexamic acid in acute traumatic brain injury: a systematic review and meta-analysis of

randomized-controlled trials. Intensive Care Med 2021;47(1). https://doi.org/10.1007/s00134-020-06279-w.

37. Bossers SM, Loer SA, Bloemers FW, et al. Association between Prehospital Tranexamic Acid Administration and Outcomes of Severe Traumatic Brain Injury. JAMA Neurol 2021;78(3). https://doi.org/10.1001/jamaneurol.2020.4596.

38. Rangel-Castilla L, Gasco J, Nauta HJW, et al. Cerebral pressure autoregulation in traumatic brain injury. Neurosurg Focus 2008;25(4). https://doi.org/10.3171/FOC.2008.25.10.E7.

39. Khellaf A, Khan DZ, Helmy A. Recent advances in traumatic brain injury. J Neurol 2019;266(11). https://doi.org/10.1007/s00415-019-09541-4.

40. Le Roux P. Intracranial pressure monitoring and management. In: Laskowitz G, Grant G, editors. Translational research in traumatic brain injury. Boca Raton, FL: CRC Press/Taylor and Francis Group; 2016. p. 1–36. Chapter 15.

41. Shi J, Tan L, Ye J, et al. Hypertonic saline and mannitol in patients with traumatic brain injury: A systematic and meta-analysis. Medicine 2020;99(35). https://doi.org/10.1097/MD.0000000000021655.

42. Roquilly A, Moyer JD, Huet O, et al. Effect of Continuous Infusion of Hypertonic Saline vs Standard Care on 6-Month Neurological Outcomes in Patients with Traumatic Brain Injury: The COBI Randomized Clinical Trial. JAMA - J Am Med Assoc 2021;325(20). https://doi.org/10.1001/jama.2021.5561.

43. Muizelaar JP, Marmarou A, Ward JD, et al. Adverse effects of prolonged hyperventilation in patients with severe head injury: A randomized clinical trial. J Neurosurg 1991;75(5). https://doi.org/10.3171/jns.1991.75.5.0731.

44. Cooper DJ, Rosenfeld JV, Murray L, et al. Decompressive Craniectomy in Diffuse Traumatic Brain Injury. New Engl J Med 2011;364(16). https://doi.org/10.1056/nejmoa1102077.

45. Hutchinson PJ, Kolias AG, Timofeev IS, et al. Trial of Decompressive Craniectomy for Traumatic Intracranial Hypertension. New Engl J Med 2016;375(12). https://doi.org/10.1056/nejmoa1605215.

46. Cooper DJ, Nichol AD, Bailey M, et al. Effect of Early Sustained Prophylactic Hypothermia on Neurologic Outcomes among Patients with Severe Traumatic Brain Injury. JAMA - J Am Med Assoc 2018;320. https://doi.org/10.1001/jama.2018.17075.

47. Vespa PM, Miller C, McArthur D, et al. Nonconvulsive electrographic seizures after traumatic brain injury result in a delayed, prolonged increase in intracranial pressure and metabolic crisis. Crit Care Med 2007;35(12). https://doi.org/10.1097/01.CCM.0000295667.66853.BC.

48. Vespa PM, McArthur DL, Xu Y, et al. Nonconvulsive seizures after traumatic brain injury are associated with hippocampal atrophy. Neurology 2010;75(9). https://doi.org/10.1212/WNL.0b013e3181f07334.

49. Vespa P, Tubi M, Claassen J, et al. Metabolic crisis occurs with seizures and periodic discharges after brain trauma. Ann Neurol 2016;79(4). https://doi.org/10.1002/ana.24606.

50. Temkin NR, Dikmen SS, Wilensky AJ, et al. A Randomized, Double-Blind Study of Phenytoin for the Prevention of Post-Traumatic Seizures. New Engl J Med 1990;323(8). https://doi.org/10.1056/nejm199008233230801.

51. Inaba K, Menaker J, Branco BC, et al. A prospective multicenter comparison of levetiracetam versus phenytoin for early posttraumatic seizure prophylaxis. J Trauma Acute Care Surg 2013;74(3). https://doi.org/10.1097/TA.0b013e3182826e84.

52. Roozenbeek B, Lingsma HF, Lecky FE, et al. Prediction of outcome after moderate and severe traumatic brain injury: External validation of the International Mission on Prognosis and Analysis of Clinical Trials (IMPACT) and Corticoid Randomisation after Significant Head injury (CRASH) prognostic models. Crit Care Med 2012;40(5). https://doi.org/10.1097/CCM.0b013e31824519ce.
53. McCrea MA, Giacino JT, Barber J, et al. Functional Outcomes over the First Year after Moderate to Severe Traumatic Brain Injury in the Prospective, Longitudinal TRACK-TBI Study. JAMA Neurol 2021;78(8). https://doi.org/10.1001/jamaneurol.2021.2043.

Protect That Neck! Management of Blunt and Penetrating Neck Trauma

Matt Piaseczny, MD, MSc[a],*, Julie La, MD, MESc[b], Tim Chaplin, MD[a], Chris Evans, MD[a]

KEYWORDS

- Neck trauma • Penetrating neck trauma • BCVI • Blunt cerebrovascular injury
- Computed tomography angiography • Vascular injury • Vascular trauma

KEY POINTS

- Blunt cerebrovascular injury can be difficult to appreciate in the acute setting.
- A high index of suspicion for blunt cerebrovascular injury should be maintained depending on the mechanism or pattern of injury.
- Screening guidelines exist for blunt cerebrovascular injury to help risk stratify those at higher risk and need for subsequent imaging.
- Computed tomography angiogram is the diagnostic modality of choice for identifying blunt cerebrovascular injury.
- For penetrating vascular neck injuries, management priorities center around airway management, hemorrhage control, and hemostatic resuscitation.

PART 1. BLUNT CEREBROVASCULAR INJURY

A 60-year-old woman is involved in a high-speed motor vehicle accident. She complains of neck, back, and chest pain. She is hemodynamically stable and after assessment and imaging, her injuries include a few nondisplaced rib fractures and a C2 pedicle fracture. You recall hearing about blunt cerebrovascular injury (BCVI) and consider whether this patient requires further workup for a potential BCVI.

What Is Blunt Cerebrovascular Injury?

Blunt trauma to either the carotid or vertebral arteries is collectively referred to as BCVI.[1,2] BCVI is graded based on the type of injury to vascular structures. The Denver group has created the most widely used grading classification for BCVI (**Box 1**).[2,3] This

---

[a] Department of Emergency Medicine, Victory 3. 76 Stuart St, Kingston, Ontario K7L 2V7, Canada; [b] Division of General Surgery, Victory 3. 76 Stuart St, Kingston, Ontario K7L 2V7, Canada
* Corresponding author.
E-mail address: 13mp25@queensu.ca

Emerg Med Clin N Am 41 (2023) 35–49
https://doi.org/10.1016/j.emc.2022.09.005
0733-8627/23/© 2022 Elsevier Inc. All rights reserved.

grading system has important therapeutic implications and helps to stratify the risk of future stroke, with increasing grade associated with increased stroke risk.

How Common Is Blunt Cerebrovascular Injury?

Although the overall incidence of BCVI is only 1% to 3% among blunt trauma patients, the complications associated with missed or untreated injuries can be significant.[2–6] The challenge in identifying these injuries is that most patients do not present initially with signs or symptoms suggestive of arterial injury. The first symptoms of BCVI are typically of cerebrovascular ischemia, which can often occur in a delayed fashion following the inciting traumatic event. One of the most feared complications of BCVI is stroke, which has been estimated to occur in approximately 20% of cases if left untreated, most often within the first 72 hrs of injury.[3,7] Early diagnosis and management is key to mitigating the risk of stroke.

Pathophysiology and Cerebrovascular Anatomy

The majority of BCVI results from motor vehicle accidents. However, other mechanisms implicated in BCVI include hangings, sporting injuries, falls, direct trauma, or even chiropractic manipulation.[8,9] Blunt injury to vascular structures typically results from shear forces, which commonly occur at junctions between fixed and mobile segments following hyperextension, flexion, or rotational movements of the neck. High-risk injuries involve fractures to C1-3, foramina transversaria involvement, and subluxation.[3,10] Once an injury develops, a dissection flap tends to form, which causes a nidus for platelet aggregation and subsequent vessel occlusion or downstream embolization.[1] Less frequently, a vessel either tears completely or incompletely resulting in pseudoaneurysm formation, which can predispose to rupture.[1,5]

Who Should Be Screened?

Patients presenting with the following signs and symptoms are presumed to have BCVI and should be promptly investigated with computed tomography with angiography (CT-A) from the aortic arch through the neck and cerebral vessels (**Box 2**).[1] The challenge of identifying BCVI in those without classic signs and symptoms is more complex. To address this challenge, many institutions and governing bodies recommend routine screening protocols for BCVI, such as the Expanded Denver Criteria which was updated in 2016.[2,3,11] As of 2020, the Eastern Association for the Surgery of Trauma (EAST) guidelines strongly recommend the use of screening protocols such as the Expanded Denver Criteria to screen for those at high risk for BCVI.[3,12]

Box 1
Blunt carotid and vertebral artery injury grading scale

Grade	Description
I	Luminal irregularity or dissection with 25% luminal narrowing
II	Dissection or intramural hematoma with 25% luminal narrowing, intramural thrombus, or raised intimal flap
III	Pseudoaneurysm
IV	Occlusion
V	Transection with free extravasation

Data from Biffl WL, Moore EE, Offner PJ, *et al.* Blunt carotid arterial injuries: implications of a new grading scale. J Trauma 1999;47(5):845-53.

Box 2
Symptoms suggestive of BCVI warranting emergent CT-A

Suspected arterial hemorrhage from nose, mouth, or neck

Expanding cervical hematoma

Cervical bruit in patient less than 50 years old

Focal neurologic deficit

Neurologic deficit inconsistent with findings on CT or MRI

Stroke identified on CT or MRI

Data from Biffl WL, Cothren CC, Moore EE, et al. Western Trauma Association critical decisions in trauma: screening for and treatment of blunt cerebrovascular injuries. J Trauma Inj Infect Crit Care 2009;67(6):1150–3; and Bromberg WJ, Collier BC, Diebel LN, et al. Blunt cerebrovascular injury practice management guidelines: the Eastern Association for the Surgery of Trauma. J Trauma 2010;68(2):471–7.

(**Box 3**). The authors here agree with the EAST guidelines on screening as this evidence-based approach reflects what is currently done at our institution.

Unfortunately, even with our best current screening guidelines, approximately 5% to 20% of BCVI may be missed according to the literature.[3,13] Although a rare diagnosis, missing BCVI can result in significant morbidity and mortality, especially for missed higher-grade injuries. This has led to the argument for universal screening for BCVI in all trauma patients to prevent significant neurologic sequelae associated with

---

Box 3
Expanded Denver criteria for BCVI

Signs/symptoms of BCVI
    Potential arterial hemorrhage from neck/nose/mouth
    Cervical bruit in patient less than 50 years old
    Expanding cervical hematoma
    Focal neurologic defect: TIA, hemiparesis, vertebrobasilar symptoms, Horner's syndrome
    Neurologic deficit inconsistent with head CT
    Stroke on CT or MRI

Risk factors for BCVI
    High-energy transfer mechanism
    Displaced midface fracture (LeFort II or III)
    Mandible fracture
    Complex skull fracture/basilar skull fracture/occipital condyle fracture
    Severe TBI with GCS less than 6
    Cervical spine fracture, subluxation, or ligamentous injury at any level
    Near hanging with anoxic brain injury
    Clothesline type injury or seat belt abrasion with significant swelling, pain, or altered mental status
    TBI with thoracic injuries
    Scalp degloving
    Thoracic vascular injuries
    Blunt cardiac rupture
    Upper rib fractures

Data from Geddes AE, Burlew CC, Wagenaar AE, *et al.* Expanded screening criteria for blunt cerebrovascular injury: a bigger impact than anticipated. *Am J Surg.* Dec 2016;212(6):1167-1174. https://doi.org/10.1016/j.amjsurg.2016.09.016.

missed injuries.[13] Although universal screening may detect close to 100% of those with BCVI, consequences include increased institutional cost, overtreatment for equivocal findings (particularly grade I injuries, which often resolve spontaneously[14]), as well as radiation and contrast exposure to patients.[3,11,13] That being said, if BCVI screening is done concurrently with the rest of the trauma scan, the concern for additional contrast load and radiation exposure is minimal. Also, generally speaking, equivocal findings can usually be clarified with a repeat CT-A within 48 hrs. Newer studies have looked at hybrid models of screening such as the "Above the Clavicle (ATC)" approach to asymptomatic BCVI screening. In 2021, McCullough and colleagues were able to identify a subset of patients with BCVI that would have been missed by modern screening criteria using the Expanded Denver Criteria. This ATC approach represents a simplified method to screening and offers benefits compared to complicated screening algorithms.[11] However, optimal screening remains contested, and further work is required before deviation from current screening guidelines can be recommended. Until then, there is likely to be variability in how different institutions approach screening for BCVI.

Management Considerations in Blunt Cerebrovascular Injury

The management of BCVI is controversial and based entirely on observational data and expert opinion. Since the last version of *Emergency Medicine Clinics* that discussed BCVI,[1] additional evidence and clinical guidelines addressing the management of these "high-stakes" injuries have emerged, although the general themes remain the same. Specific issues to be considered in BCVI include:

1. Which injuries should be treated?
2. How should these injuries be treated?
3. When should treatment be initiated, particularly in patients with concurrent traumatic brain injury (TBI) or that require urgent surgery?

What types of blunt cerebrovascular injury should be treated?

Available evidence within the literature suggests that all BCVI should be treated, irrespective of injury grade, based on clear reductions in rates of stroke, disability, and death when antithrombotic medications (ATT) are used. A recent meta-analysis reported the stroke risk of untreated BCVI as 25% compared to 8% with ATT, 7% with anticoagulation, and 5% with endovascular therapy.[15] In patients with concurrent TBI, the stroke risk is upwards of 50%, and ATT is similarly effective (reducing stroke risk to approximately 4%), with the caveat that a more nuanced approach to decision making is required to minimize the risk of worsening intracranial bleeding.[15] The EAST guidelines support the treatment of all BCVI with some form of ATT based on demonstrated efficacy in reducing rates of ischemic stroke and mortality.[3]

How should these injuries be treated?

Although it is possible to treat BCVI with endovascular stents and surgical approaches, the mainstay of treatment for nearly all patients is with ATT. **Table 1** summarizes the treatment options for BCVI. For most patients, the decision comes down to treatment with unfractionated heparin (UFH) or a single antiplatelet (AP) agent. The major advantage of UFH over antiplatelets has been its reversibility, which is clearly desirable in the blunt trauma patients who frequently have other extracranial injuries at risk of bleeding and/or requiring surgical intervention or intracranial lesions at risk of hemorrhage. However, newer data from nonrandomized studies have emerged that suggest for most patients, an antiplatelet agent (most often ASA [acetylsalicylic

Table 1
Summary of treatment options for BCVI

Treatment	Advantages	Disadvantages	Dosage
UFH	• Reversible with protamine • Short half-life • At least as effective as AP	• Greater intracranial and extracranial bleeding risks • Risk of heparin-induced thrombocytopenia	• 15 units/kg/h (no bolus) titrated to aPTT 40–50 s
APs	• Newer data suggesting as effective (if not superior) to UFH • Reduced intracranial and extracranial bleeding risks compared to heparin	• Not reversible • Some patients will have allergies, contraindications, or intolerances	• ASA, 325 mg daily, or • Clopidogrel, 75 mg daily
Endovascular	• Thrombectomy can be considered for patients with acute stroke • Embolization could be life-saving for rare patients with grade V injuries	• No role for routine utilization • Very little literature base • Stents also require anticoagulation	
Surgical	• Recommended for the rare patient with grade II • V lesions that are surgically accessible	• Lesions are almost never surgically accessible	

Abbreviations: AP, antiplatelet; ASA, acetylsalicylic acid; UFH, unfractionated heparin.

acid]) is at least as effective for stroke prevention but with fewer hemorrhage-related complications.

Studies comparing AP with UFH have found both treatment strategies to be similarly effective in terms of stroke prevention but found AP medications to be safer with an overall reduced rate of hemorrhagic complications. In fact, AP alone has been shown in some studies to have a lower risk of sustaining a stroke compared to UFH. One explanation for the potential superiority of AP agents in the context of BCVI is that many BCVI-related strokes are caused by artery-to-artery embolic events and that AP agents could be particularly effective for prevention in this context.[16,17] To date, there is no data available to indicate any role for direct oral anticoagulants in the management of BCVI, however, this may evolve over time.

When should treatment for blunt cerebrovascular injury be initiated?
The authors suggest initiation of treatment should be done in consultation with either local experts or a stroke neurologist if available. In general, treatment for BCVI should be initiated as soon as possible, given that the vast majority of BCVI-related strokes occur within the first 72 hours.[16] The challenge, of course, is that these injuries are rarely suffered in isolation. These patients are often at risk of developing progressive intracranial or extracranial hemorrhage, may be hemodynamically unstable, and/or requiring surgery for one or more of their injuries. The timing of when to initiate ATT must therefore be made in the context of the entire patient, including their associated injuries, the management plans for these injuries, as well as the patient's underlying baseline medical comorbidities and premorbid use of AP or anticoagulant

medications. The table below presents possible management strategies for patients with different injury patterns and surgical plans[2,18,19] (**Table 2**).

Regardless of the initial ATT approach undertaken, guidelines suggest all patients with BCVI have interval CT-A imaging at the 7- to 10-day mark.[2] Patients with demonstrated vessel healing can have their ATT discontinued, whereas those with residual injury remain on ATT for a period of 3 to 6 months with further imaging during that period.[2]

Case Resolution

Given the cervical spine fracture identified, you request a CT-A of the neck vasculature. This is positive for a grade II injury to the right internal carotid artery (focal intramural hematoma with 25%–50% narrowing) (**Fig. 1** - left panel). The patient is initiated on ASA and an interval CT-A is performed 1 week later, showing no change in appearance of the lesion. She remains neurologically intact and continues the ASA for 3 months duration before another CT-A is performed, which demonstrates vessel healing, and she is advised to discontinue ASA (see **Fig. 1** - right panel).

PART 2. PENETRATING NECK INJURY

A 35-year-old man presents to the emergency department with multiple penetrating stab wounds to the face and neck after an altercation. He is hemodynamically stable on arrival and rapid primary assessment proceeds. What are your initial management priorities?

Penetrating Neck Injury

Significant penetrating neck injury (PNI) is defined as neck trauma that has violated the platysma muscle. These injuries carry high morbidity and mortality, which is dependent on mechanism, type, extent, and timeliness of diagnosis and management.

Table 2
Management of patients with BCVI based on hemodynamic stability, presence of TBI, and requirement for urgent surgery

Patient Type	Management Strategy
Hemodynamically unstable patient	
All patients	• No ATT until hemodynamics have stabilized and bleeding controlled. • Can then approach as below
Hemodynamically stable patient *with* TBI	
Patient requires urgent surgery	• Confirm with anesthesia and surgeon that bleeding risks are manageable and initiate UFH • Obtain interval CT head postoperatively • Transition patient to ASA if CT findings are stable
Patient does *not* require urgent surgery	• Obtain interval CT head within 6–12 h • Initiate aspirin if CT findings are stable
Hemodynamically stable patient *without* TBI	
Patient requires urgent surgery	• Confirm with anesthesia and surgeon that bleeding risks are manageable and initiate UFH • Obtain interval CT head within 6–12 h • Transition patient to ASA if CT findings are stable
Patient does *not* require urgent surgery	• Initiate aspirin

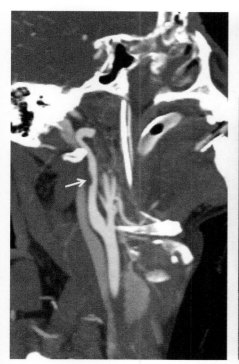 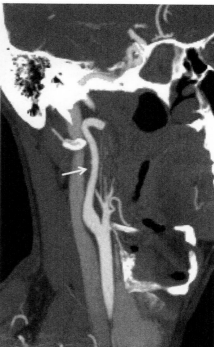

Fig. 1. Grade II BCVI to the right internal carotid artery (focal intramural hematoma with 25-50% narrowing) at presentation (*left panel arrow*) and following 3 months of treatment with ASA (*right panel arrow*). After treatment, the lesion has completely resolved. (Rutman et al. Imaging and management of blunt cerebrovascular injury. Radiographics (2018).)

Globally, the most common mechanism of injury involves stabbing, followed by ballistic trauma (gunshot wounds), motor vehicle collision, and other miscellaneous mechanisms.[20,21] Ballistic trauma is responsible for more complex injury patterns due to high kinetic energy, which can lead to destruction of surrounding structures not in direct contact with the projectile. Conversely, stab wounds have low kinetic energy and cause injury to tissues directly along their path. However, both mechanisms can result in severe injuries with hemorrhagic and neurologic sequelae.[22]

What Are the Anatomic Considerations?

The neck is remarkably vulnerable as it represents a densely packed area of vital anatomy including vascular, neurologic, and aerodigestive structures, with minimal overlying protective tissue. Anatomically, the neck can be described in triangles with the sternocleidomastoid muscles separating the anterior and posterior triangles. The anterior triangle houses major structures including the trachea, larynx, pharynx, esophagus, and major vascular structures. The posterior triangle contains musculature, spinal accessory nerve, and spinal column[23] (**Fig 2**).

PNIs have been traditionally classified into zones according to the entry point of penetrating injury: Zone I (lower) from the clavicles and sternum superiorly to the cricoid cartilage, Zone II (middle) from the cricoid cartilage superiorly to the angle of mandible, and Zone III (upper) from the angle of the mandible superiorly to the base of the skull (**Table 3**).[24,25]

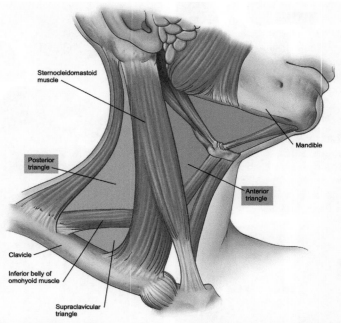

Fig. 2. Anatomy of the anterior and posterior triangles of the neck. (Deslauriers. Anatomy of the Neck and Cervicothoracic Junction. Thoracic surgery clinics (2007).)

Zones Versus No Zones Approach

Anatomic zone-based management algorithms have guided care for over 50 years for PNI. This approach, however, has been called into question, with evidence showing a disconnect between external injury location and injured internal structures identified

Zone	Boundaries	Structures
Table 3 **Summary of the neck zones and potential injuries**		
I (lower)	Clavicles and sternum to the cricoid cartilage	Vascular: subclavian arteries and veins, jugular veins, carotid arteries, vertebral artery Aerodigestive: lungs, trachea, esophagus Neurologic: spinal cord, vagus nerve Other: thoracic duct, thyroid gland
II (middle)	Cricoid cartilage to the angle of the mandible	Vascular: common/internal/external carotid arteries, vertebral arteries, jugular veins Aerodigestive: trachea, larynx, pharynx, esophagus Neurologic: spinal cord, vagus nerve, recurrent laryngeal nerve
III (upper)	Angle of the mandible to the base of the skull	Vascular: internal carotid arteries, vertebral arteries, jugular veins Aerodigestive: pharynx Neurologic: spinal cord, CN IX, X, XI, XI, sympathetic chain Other: salivary glands

intraoperatively.[26] As such, there has been an increasing trend toward CT-A imaging and selective operative management for stable patients without "hard signs" of major vascular or aerodigestive injury.[27,28] Despite this, anatomic zones do continue to be taught in surgical training, are used to guide operative management decisions,[29] and the nomenclature useful as a communication tool. Despite accumulating evidence that a nonzonal approach is superior, there remain real-life challenges with decision making and risks for missing occult injuries.[30,31]

What Are Hard Versus Soft Signs of Penetrating Neck Injury?

One of the priorities during initial assessment of the patient with PNI involves identifying whether "hard signs" of vascular and aerodigestive tract injuries are present (**Box 4**). Their presence should prompt emergent surgical consultation for operative exploration as these injuries have the potential to cause significant morbidity and mortality. Those presenting with hard and soft signs of PNI have a 90% and 30% risk of underlying vascular injury, respectively.

A Practical Approach to Penetrating Neck Injury Management

PNIs present unique challenges to the EM clinician. Here, we will outline an approach to the patient with an isolated PNI and focus on the 2 most common causes of early mortality from PNI: exsanguination and asphyxiation caused by airway obstruction.[32] The concept of prioritizing life-threatening hemorrhage control reflects the significant proportion (50%) of mortality in PNI attributed to exsanguination.[33] While this is performed, IV access, cardiovascular monitoring, and supplemental oxygen should all be applied.

What are my options in the Emergency Department for hemorrhage control in penetrating neck injury?

1. Direct digital pressure. An effective and efficient method of controlling acute hemorrhage that requires minimal resources. Firm focal pressure should be applied directly to the source of hemorrhage, using a single fingertip.
2. Hemostatic dressings. Several products are available that promote hemostasis (Quick Clot combat gauze, Celox, etc). These products are packed tightly into the wound and can be used in conjunction with digital pressure.[34]

Box 4 Hard and soft signs of vascular and aerodigestive injury		
	Hard Signs	**Soft Signs**
Vascular injury	Severe uncontrolled hemorrhage Refractory shock/hypotension Large, expanding, or pulsatile hematoma Unilateral extremity pulse deficit Bruit or thrill Neurologic deficit consistent with stroke	Minor bleeding Small, nonexpanding hematoma Proximity wound
Aerodigestive tract injury	Airway compromise Bubbling through wound Extensive subcutaneous emphysema Stridor Hoarse voice	Mild hemoptysis Mild hematemesis Dysphonia Dysphagia Mild subcutaneous emphysema

Data from Evans C, Chaplin T, Zelt D. Management of Major Vascular Injuries: Neck, Extremities, and Other Things that Bleed. *Emerg Med Clin North Am.* Feb 2018;36(1):181-202. https://doi.org/10.1016/j.emc.2017.08.013.

3. Foley catheter balloon tamponade. Involves inserting a Foley catheter (18 or 20F) into the wound directed toward the source of the bleeding. The balloon is then inflated and the wound is sutured closed until bleeding stops (**Fig 3**).[35] If bleeding continues, placement of a second Foley catheter can be considered.[36]

Once catastrophic hemorrhage is either ruled out or controlled, an assessment of the "hard signs" (see **Box 4**) of vascular and aerodigestive injuries should be performed. Full exposure of the neck is required and the literature supports the safe removal of the cervical spine collar, unless there is a focal neurologic deficit present or a high index of suspicion for spinal cord injury.[37] If hard signs of PNI are present, the priority is safe transport to definitive treatment (eg, the operating room). Although the operating room continues to be the default location for definitive treatment of patients with PNI and hard signs of vascular and/or aerodigestive injury, there is a subgroup of hemodynamically stable patients who may benefit from a CT-A before endovascular treatment of arterial injuries. For example, injuries to the vertebral or subclavian arteries are difficult to access surgically and may be more suitable for endovascular treatment.[38] Before leaving the resuscitation bay, the ED clinician should consider the need for airway management and ongoing hemostatic resuscitation. Any hard signs of vascular injury should prompt a strong consideration for airway management before leaving the resuscitation bay. Although these are considerations for any patient presenting with PNI, the decisions will vary depending on the clinical circumstances, local resources, and experience.

Hemostatic resuscitation
The principles of hemostatic resuscitation include the preservation of tissue perfusion and effective clotting in the patient with severe hemorrhage. This is generally

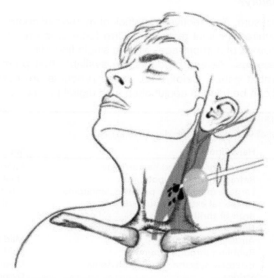

Fig. 3. Foley catheter balloon tamponade of hemorrhage from penetrating neck injury. (Improved mortality from penetrating neck and maxillofacial trauma using Foley catheter balloon tamponade in combat. J Trauma acute Care Surg 2013;75(2):221; with permission; Weppner, Justin DO. Improved mortality from penetrating neck and maxillofacial trauma using Foley catheter balloon tamponade in combat. Journal of Trauma and Acute Care Surgery: August 2013 - Volume 75 - Issue 2 - p 220–224 https://doi.org/10.1097/TA.0b013e3182930fd8.)

accomplished by accepting a lower than physiologic blood pressure (eg, a mean arterial pressure of 50–60 mm Hg),[39,40] early transfusion of red blood cells and clotting factors (plasma, platelets, cryoprecipitate) in a balanced ratio, minimizing use of crystalloids, preventing hypothermia (eg, fluid warmer, Bair Hugger), and administering tranexamic acid.

Airway management

There is no "best" approach to airway management in cases of PNI, and the decision to intubate should be made on a case-by-case basis and consider the clinical context, comfort and skills of the airway provider, and local resources. The threshold to intubate a patient with a PNI may be lower than that for other patients, as injuries of the neck may progress. This is the concept of the "dynamic airway" that may worsen (quickly or slowly) over time. For example, in the case of an expanding hematoma, although an initial airway examination is reassuring, the mass effect may result in the loss of a patent airway over a matter of minutes. We will present 3 approaches to airway management in PNI based on the clinical assessment of the patient's neck:

1. Preserved neck anatomy. Endotracheal intubation using a rapid sequence induction (RSI) is effective and safe in PNI.[41–43] Below, we highlight the unique modifications to RSI in cases of PNI based on the "Ps of RSI" approach:

- Prepare: Anticipate bleeding and distorted anatomy, and plan accordingly. Consider having a double suction set-up, smaller endotracheal tubes, and cricothyroidotomy equipment available.[44]
- Preoxygenate: Oxygenation should be optimized using nasal prongs (at 6LPM) under a nonrebreather (at 15LPM) for a period of at least 3 minutes if allowable. The use of positive pressure via bag-valve-mask or supraglottic device is not recommended as it may cause increased subcutaneous emphysema and further distortion of airway anatomy.
- Pretreatment and paralysis: No specific modifications required.
- Pass the tube: Cricoid pressure and external laryngeal manipulation (eg, the backward, upward, rightward pressure [BURP]) should be avoided as these have the potential to worsen laryngotracheal injuries.
- Postintubation management: No specific modifications required.

2. Distorted neck anatomy. In these challenging cases, an awake fiberoptic intubation is preferred[45] as an RSI may result in loss of airway muscle tone leading to further airway compromise.[46] Consider topical anesthesia of the airway and sedation (eg, IV ketamine) to facilitate the procedure of an awake intubation. This would also be a scenario in which a "double-setup" would be reasonable in case of failed orotracheal intubation. This involves a second physician who is responsible and prepared to perform a cricothyroidotomy. If there is significant anatomy distortion or anticipated difficulty with endotracheal intubation, cricothyroidotomy may be reasonable as a first attempt at securing an airway.

3. Significant laryngotracheal injury. In cases of massive upper airway distortion, significant bleeding that prevents visualization of the glottis or an open, gaping injury to the trachea or larynx, a primary surgical approach is suggested.[47] Ideally, this is achieved using a cricothyroidotomy, but in cases of a large hematoma or crushed larynx, a tracheotomy performed at least one tracheal ring below the injury is indicated. This approach recognizes the risk of creating a false lumen or converting a partial tracheal laceration into a complete transection.[44,48]

If hard signs of PNI are absent, CT-A is the test of choice as it has been shown to be sensitive and specific in identifying vascular and aerodigestive tract injuries.[48] CT-A is also able to define the track of the penetrating trauma and assess for associated injuries. Although CT-A has proved to be a sensitive test in cases of PNI, it may miss small esophageal injuries, or injuries to the thoracic duct or thyroid gland. If CT-A does not reveal any significant injury, but soft signs are present or there is ongoing clinical concern, further diagnostics (eg, laryngoscopy, bronchoscopy, esophagography, esophagoscopy) should be performed in communication with the appropriate service. When both hard and soft signs are absent and CT-A is reassuring, significant injury has effectively been ruled out and these patients can be managed according to local practice.

Case Resolution

Your team efficiently establishes vascular access and initiates cardiorespiratory monitoring. The primary assessment is concerning for an obvious pulsatile bleed just lateral to the larynx. There is an associated hematoma in this area resulting in stridor. You find no other life-threatening injuries and initial vital signs are normal other than sinus tachycardia. You delegate one team member to place firm pressure using a single fingertip over the source of the bleeding, and another to page the trauma or surgical service. You then proceed to secure the patient's airway with an awake intubation strategy and initiate a hemostatic resuscitation plan before definitive care in the OR.

CLINICS CARE POINTS

- Blunt neck trauma patients presenting with stroke symptoms or focal neurologic deficits require computed tomography angiogram imaging to assess for blunt cerebrovascular injury (BCVI).
- High-risk patients for BCVI can be identified using evidence-based screening guidelines such as the Expanded Denver Criteria.
- BCVI is primarily treated with antiplatelet agents or unfractionated heparin.
- Treatment for BCVI should be done in consultation with stroke specialists if available and initiated as soon as injuries are identified.
- Prompt surgical consultation should be made for patients with penetrating neck injuries presenting with hard signs of vascular or aerodigestive injury.
- Direct digital pressure, hemostatic dressings, and Foley catheters can all be used as hemorrhage control options for penetrating neck injuries.
- Airway considerations in penetrating neck trauma will be case and patient specific but should be a top priority in managing these patients.

DISCLOSURE

The authors have nothing to disclose.

REFERENCES

1. Evans C, Chaplin T, Zelt D. Management of Major Vascular Injuries: Neck, Extremities, and Other Things that Bleed. Emerg Med Clin North Am 2018;36(1):181–202.
2. Biffl WL, Cothren CC, Moore EE, et al. Western Trauma Association critical decisions in trauma: screening for and treatment of blunt cerebrovascular injuries. J Trauma 2009;67(6):1150–3.

3. Kim DY, Biffl W, Bokhari F, et al. Evaluation and management of blunt cerebrovascular injury: A practice management guideline from the Eastern Association for the Surgery of Trauma. J Trauma Acute Care Surg 2020;88(6):875–87.

4. Bruns BR, Tesoriero R, Kufera J, et al. Blunt cerebrovascular injury screening guidelines: what are we willing to miss? J Trauma Acute Care Surg 2014;76(3):691–5.

5. Biffl WL, Moore EE, Offner PJ, et al. Blunt carotid arterial injuries: implications of a new grading scale. J Trauma 1999;47(5):845–53.

6. Kerwin AJ, Bynoe RP, Murray J, et al. Liberalized screening for blunt carotid and vertebral artery injuries is justified. J Trauma 2001;51(2):308–14.

7. Burlew CC, Sumislawski JJ, Behnfield CD, et al. Time to stroke: A Western Trauma Association multicenter study of blunt cerebrovascular injuries. J Trauma Acute Care Surg 2018;85(5):858–66.

8. Lee TS, Ducic Y, Gordin E, et al. Management of carotid artery trauma. Craniomaxillofac Trauma Reconstr 2014;7(3):175–89.

9. Biffl WL, Moore EE, Offner PJ, et al. Blunt carotid and vertebral arterial injuries. World J Surg 2001;25(8):1036–43.

10. Geddes AE, Burlew CC, Wagenaar AE, et al. Expanded screening criteria for blunt cerebrovascular injury: a bigger impact than anticipated. Am J Surg 2016;212(6):1167–74.

11. McCullough MA, Cairns AL, Shin J, et al. Above the Clavicle: A Simplified Screening Method for Asymptomatic Blunt Cerebral Vascular Injury. Am Surg 2021. https://doi.org/10.1177/00031348211011141. 31348211011141.

12. Bromberg WJ, Collier BC, Diebel LN, et al. Blunt cerebrovascular injury practice management guidelines: the Eastern Association for the Surgery of Trauma. J Trauma 2010;68(2):471–7.

13. Leichtle SW, Banerjee D, Schrader R, et al. Blunt cerebrovascular injury: The case for universal screening. J Trauma Acute Care Surg 2020;89(5):880–6.

14. Payabvash S, McKinney AM, McKinney ZJ, et al. Screening and detection of blunt vertebral artery injury in patients with upper cervical fractures: the role of cervical CT and CT angiography. Eur J Radiol 2014;83(3):571–7.

15. Murphy PB, Severance S, Holler E, et al. Treatment of asymptomatic blunt cerebrovascular injury (BCVI): a systematic review. Trauma Surg Acute Care Open 2021;6(1):e000668.

16. Ku JC, Priola SM, Mathieu F, et al. Antithrombotic choice in blunt cerebrovascular injuries: Experience at a tertiary trauma center, systematic review, and meta-analysis. J Trauma Acute Care Surg 2021;91(1):e1–12.

17. Foreman PM, Harrigan MR. Blunt Traumatic Extracranial Cerebrovascular Injury and Ischemic Stroke. Cerebrovasc Dis Extra 2017;7(1):72–83.

18. Figueroa JM, Berry K, Boddu J, et al. Treatment strategies for patients with concurrent blunt cerebrovascular and traumatic brain injury. J Clin Neurosci 2021;88:243–50.

19. Catapano JS, Israr S, Whiting AC, et al. Management of Extracranial Blunt Cerebrovascular Injuries: Experience with an Aspirin-Based Approach. World Neurosurg 2020;133:e385–90.

20. Burgess CA, Dale OT, Almeyda R, et al. An evidence based review of the assessment and management of penetrating neck trauma. Clin Otolaryngol 2012;37(1):44–52.

21. Nason RW, Assuras GN, Gray PR, et al. Penetrating neck injuries: analysis of experience from a Canadian trauma centre. Can J Surg 2001;44(2):122–6.

22. Brennan JA, Meyers AD, Jafek BW. Penetrating neck trauma: a 5-year review of the literature, 1983 to 1988. Am J Otolaryngol 1990;11(3):191–7.
23. Alao T WM. Neck Trauma. Treasure Island (FL): StatPealn: StatPearls. Treasure Island (FL): StatPearls Publishing.
24. Roon AJ, Christensen N. Evaluation and treatment of penetrating cervical injuries. J Trauma 1979;19(6):391–7.
25. Monson DO, Saletta JD, Freeark RJ. Carotid vertebral trauma. J Trauma 1969; 9(12):987–99.
26. Fogelman MJ, Stewart RD. Penetrating wounds of the neck. Am J Surg 1956; 91(4):581–93 ; discussion, 593-6.
27. Ko JW, Gong SC, Kim MJ, et al. The efficacy of the "no zone" approach for the assessment of traumatic neck injury: a case-control study. Ann Surg Treat Res 2020;99(6):352–61.
28. Ibraheem K, Khan M, Rhee P, et al. No zone" approach in penetrating neck trauma reduces unnecessary computed tomography angiography and negative explorations. J Surg Res 2018;221:113–20.
29. Feliciano DV, Mattox KL, Moore EE. Trauma. 9th edition. McGraw Hill; 2020.
30. Diaz-Martínez JMJ, Gruezo RB. Review of the penetrating neck Injuries in 279 patients, analysis of a single institution. J Gen Surg 2019;4:2.
31. Bhatt NR, McMonagle M. Penetrating neck injury from a screwdriver: can the No Zone approach be applied to Zone I injuries? BMJ Case Rep 2015;27:2015.
32. O'Brien PJ, Cox MW. A modern approach to cervical vascular trauma. Perspect Vasc Surg Endovasc Ther 2011;23(2):90–7.
33. McConnell DB, Trunkey DD. Management of penetrating trauma to the neck. Adv Surg 1994;27:97–127.
34. Boulton AJ, Lewis CT, Naumann DN, et al. Prehospital haemostatic dressings for trauma: a systematic review. Emerg Med J 2018;35(7):449–57.
35. Gilroy D, Lakhoo M, Charalambides D, et al. Control of life-threatening haemorrhage from the neck: a new indication for balloon tamponade. Injury 1992; 23(8):557–9.
36. Jose A, Arya S, Nagori SA, et al. Management of Life-Threatening Hemorrhage from Maxillofacial Firearm Injuries Using Foley Catheter Balloon Tamponade. Craniomaxillofac Trauma Reconstr 2019;12(4):301–4.
37. Rhee P, Kuncir EJ, Johnson L, et al. Cervical spine injury is highly dependent on the mechanism of injury following blunt and penetrating assault. J Trauma 2006; 61(5):1166–70.
38. Sperry JL, Moore EE, Coimbra R, et al. Western Trauma Association critical decisions in trauma: penetrating neck trauma. J Trauma Acute Care Surg 2013; 75(6):936–40.
39. Tran A, Yates J, Lau A, et al. Permissive hypotension versus conventional resuscitation strategies in adult trauma patients with hemorrhagic shock: A systematic review and meta-analysis of randomized controlled trials. J Trauma Acute Care Surg 2018;84(5):802–8.
40. Dutton RP, Mackenzie CF, Scalea TM. Hypotensive resuscitation during active hemorrhage: impact on in-hospital mortality. J Trauma 2002;52(6):1141–6.
41. Brywczynski JJ, Barrett TW, Lyon JA, et al. Management of penetrating neck injury in the emergency department: a structured literature review. Emerg Med J 2008;25(11):711–5.
42. Mandavia DP, Qualls S, Rokos I. Emergency airway management in penetrating neck injury. Ann Emerg Med 2000;35(3):221–5.

43. Youssef N, Raymer KE. Airway management of an open penetrating neck injury. CJEM 2015;17(1):89–93.
44. Tallon JM, Ahmed JM, Sealy B. Airway management in penetrating neck trauma at a Canadian tertiary trauma centre. CJEM 2007;9(2):101–4.
45. Bhattacharya P, Mandal MC, Das S, et al. Airway management of two patients with penetrating neck trauma. Indian J Anaesth 2009;53(3):348–51.
46. Bent JP 3rd, Silver JR, Porubsky ES. Acute laryngeal trauma: a review of 77 patients. Otolaryngol Head Neck Surg 1993;109(3 Pt 1):441–9.
47. Nowicki JL, Stew B, Ooi E. Penetrating neck injuries: a guide to evaluation and management. Ann R Coll Surg Engl 2018;100(1):6–11.
48. Lee WT, Eliashar R, Eliachar I. Acute external laryngotracheal trauma: diagnosis and management. Ear Nose Throat J 2006;85(3):179–84.

Massive Hemorrhage Protocol

A Practical Approach to the Bleeding Trauma Patient

Andrew Petrosoniak, MD, MSc, FRCPC[a],*,
Katerina Pavenski, MD, FRCPC[b], Luis Teodoro da Luz, MD, MSc[c],
Jeannie Callum, MD, FRCPC[d]

KEYWORDS

- Damage control resuscitation • Trauma • Massive hemorrhage protocol
- Resuscitation

KEY POINTS

- When possible, conduct a team prebriefing to establish a shared mental model for managing a massively hemorrhaging patient.
- Early administration of blood/blood products results in better patient outcomes for bleeding trauma patients.
- No clinical prediction scores are 100% accurate for predicting MHP. A combination of patient factors, clinical course, and response to blood products may be preferrable.
- Regular monitoring of temperature, fibrinogen, and calcium is critical to optimize patient outcomes.
- Massive hemorrhage protocol termination is critical to preserve blood products, and criteria should be established to support this decision.

CASE EXAMPLE

A 57-year-old female involved in a high-speed motor vehicle collision is transported to the emergency department (ED) of a large community hospital in 28 minutes. She is brought into the resuscitation room, and the clinical team begins their assessment and treatment following the principles of Advanced Trauma Life Support. Her vital signs are as follows:

[a] Department of Emergency Medicine, St. Michael's Hospital, 30 Bond Street, Toronto, Ontario M5B 1W8, Canada; [b] Department of Laboratory Medicine, St. Michael's Hospital, 30 Bond Street, Toronto, Ontario M5B 1W8, Canada; [c] Sunnybrook Health Sciences Centre, 2075 Bayview Avenue, Room H1 71, Toronto, Ontario M4N 3M5, Canada; [d] Queen's University, 88 Stuart Street, Kingston, Ontario K7L 3N6, Canada
* Corresponding author.
E-mail address: petro82@gmail.com

Emerg Med Clin N Am 41 (2023) 51–69
https://doi.org/10.1016/j.emc.2022.09.010
0733-8627/23/© 2022 Elsevier Inc. All rights reserved.

Respiratory rate 26 breaths/min,
Blood pressure 88/50,
Heart rate 110 beats/min,
Temperature 34.5°C,
Glasgow Coma Scale is 12.

A focused assessment with sonography in trauma examination is positive for free fluid in the right upper quadrant. There is no evidence of pneumothorax on ultrasound. Her pelvis is stable although suspected to be fractured based on pain during the examination. She has no past medical history, takes no medications, and has no drug allergies. At this point, the clinical team is faced with decisions related to blood product administration, the role of the massive hemorrhage protocol (MHP), and establishing definitive hemostasis.

INTRODUCTION

A damage-control resuscitation strategy represents the standard for the care of the hemorrhaging trauma patient.[1] This 2-pronged approach provides early, ratio-based, blood product administration coupled with definitive and rapid hemostasis. Together, when combined and delivered quickly and effectively, these 2 elements provide improved patient outcomes.[1]

These patients frequently require the initiation of a MHP which is the systematic and coordinated delivery of care to bleeding patients. Previously termed massive transfusion protocols, these early protocols focused predominately on the blood and blood component administration. Emerging evidence supports a more comprehensive approach to caring for these patients, hence the now widely and more aptly termed MHP.

The benefits of MHPs in trauma are numerous, including:[2–6]

1. Decreased variability in treatment
2. Reduced blood product wastage
3. Improved interprofessional communication
4. Standardized process evaluation
5. Faster time to transfusion

Despite the clear benefits of MHPs demonstrated through multiple studies, the details related to the decision-making, the logistics, and the nuances of these protocols remain poorly articulated to the emergency medicine (EM) clinician. As a result, our focus will be to bridge the gap between the evidence and the real-world application of a trauma MHP.

We will address how EM clinicians can practically deliver high-quality, evidence-based care to the bleeding trauma patient through 7 clinically relevant questions. These follow the 7 Ts described by the Ontario MHP group (**Fig. 1**).[7]

Triggers: When Should the Massive Hemorrhage Protocol Be Activated?

The question of when to "trigger" or activate an MHP in trauma is of the utmost importance during the early stages of a trauma resuscitation. There is a clear tension that exists between underactivation (risking preventable exsanguination) and overactivation (resulting in unnecessary transfusion and wasted blood components).[7,8] This tension must be navigated by the emergency or trauma physician during the early stages of the resuscitation and may be complicated by early clinical uncertainty related to the patient's injuries.

Early administration of blood products is linked with improved outcomes among bleeding trauma patients. A delay of 1 minute is associated with a 5% increase in

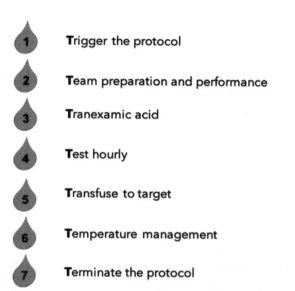

1. **T**rigger the protocol

2. **T**eam preparation and performance

3. **T**ranexamic acid

4. **T**est hourly

5. **T**ransfuse to target

6. **T**emperature management

7. **T**erminate the protocol

Fig. 1. The 7 Ts of massive hemorrhage protocol

odds of death.[9] Some precise and reliable tactics are needed for clinicians to make an informed, evidence-based decision particularly under stress and high cognitive load.

Historically, most MHP activation criteria are evaluated in the context of the traditional definition of massive transfusion such as 10 units of red blood cells (RBCs) in 24 hours.[10] This definition is challenging as it has little clinical relevance during the early stages of resuscitation (**Fig. 2**).

None of these scores are perfectly 100% sensitive and specific, but they do provide guidance in the decision-making process for MHP activation (**Table 1**).[17] The recently developed RABT score likely offers the greatest utility by combining the shock index (SI), components of the ABC score, and the addition of pelvic fracture.[15]

Many patients with hypotension or hypoperfusion, however, will stabilize following 1 to 2 units of RBCs, and only a subset will require additional blood products.[18] In most cases, our preferred approach to MHP activation is a 2-tiered process whereby the clinician calls for and administers up to 3 units of uncross-matched RBCs (**Fig. 3**). Should this critical administration threshold be surpassed (or predicted to be), then MHP is activated.[16,18]

In our opinion, there are some circumstances under which MHP activation can be considered even before any blood products are administered:

1. The clinician predicts ≥3 units of blood products will be required based on the injury mechanism and initial available clinical information[16] (eg, profound prehospital hypotension [systolic blood pressure <60 mm Hg], prehospital traumatic cardiac arrest, hemodynamic instability, and transmediastinal gunshot wound).
2. Institutions whereby the only way to acquire immediate blood products is through MHP activation.
3. The patient is receiving blood products via EMS or at the transferring facility and has ongoing hemodynamic instability.

Finally, based on our collective experience, we consider several high-risk conditions or circumstances that lower our threshold for MHP activation. While evidence is

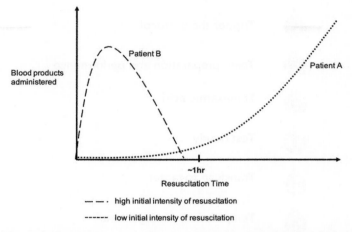

Fig. 2. Patient A who receives 2 units in the emergency department (ED) and 10 units 4 hours later during a trauma laparotomy while considered a "massive transfusion" (MT) by the traditional definition has a more delayed resuscitation trajectory. In contrast, patient B who requires 4 red blood cells (RBCs) and 3 fresh frozen plasma within 60 minutes of ED arrival before stabilizing, while not meeting the typical MT threshold, benefits more from immediate blood products, and hence early massive hemorrhage protocol (MHP) activation. Patients with similar trajectories to patient B are those who the ED clinician wishes to quickly identify for MHP activation.

lacking to provide specific recommendations in such circumstances, we have repeatedly observed rapid clinical deterioration and suggest that the presence of 1 or more of these components lower the threshold to activate the MHP:[19–21]

1. Anticoagulation
2. Prehospital hypotension or shock index ≥ 1.0
3. Geriatric population (typically >65 years).

Team: How Can Team Performance During a Massive Hemorrhage Protocol Be Leveraged to Optimize Patient Outcomes?

An MHP is a specialized, complex yet highly effective strategy to rapidly deliver blood components and coordinate patient care in the setting of traumatic hemorrhage. This protocolized delivery of interventions requires a multidisciplinary (and often ad hoc) team to function seamlessly in a time-sensitive manner. Mini-teams form at the bedside, in the transfusion department, hematology laboratory, and in the transportation of blood products. MHP performance is critical to patient outcomes.

A high-performing team during an MHP is akin to the pit crew in Formula 1.[22] Each individual or mini-team functions semi-autonomously in their defined roles, yet together they strive toward a common goal. For a Formula 1 pit crew, the goal is to prepare the car to head back on the track as fast as possible. During an MHP, the goal is to deliver the necessary blood components and other care interventions as efficiently as possible. To achieve these goals, there are several aspects that lead to a successful MHP team performance:[23–26]

1. Prebriefing and debriefing for each MHP to establish a shared mental model and promote future improvement by tracking quality metrics over time.

Table 1
Massive hemorrhage protocol prediction tools, components, and sensitivity/specificity for massive transfusion (>10U/24 h)

Score/Tool	Components	Sensitivity	Specificity
ABC score[11-14] (≥2 predicts MT)	1. Heart rate (HR) > 120 2. Systolic blood pressure (sBP) < 90 mm Hg 3. Focused abdominal sonography in trauma (FAST) positive 4. Penetrating trauma	47%-90%	67%-90%
Shock Index[14,15] (≥1.0 predicts MT)	HR/sBP	68%	81%
RABT score[15] (≥2 predicts MT)	1. Shock Index ≥ 1.0 2. Pelvic fracture 3. FAST positive 4. Penetrating trauma	78%	91%
Resuscitation intensity (RI)[16]	Total number of products in first 30 min of arrival (eg, 1U RBC, 1U FFP, 1L crystalloid, 500 cc colloid). Typical threshold is ≥4 (RI4)	80%[a]	37%[a]
Critical administration threshold[16]	3U RBC during 1-h period within 24 h after arrival	90%[a]	26%[a]
Narrow pulse pressure[17]	Systolic arterial pressure - diastolic arterial pressure < 30 mm Hg	52.8%	82.7%

Abbreviation: ABC, assessment of blood consumption; FFP, fresh frozen plasma; MT, massive transfusion; RABT, revised assessment of bleeding and transfusion.
[a] Predicting 24-h mortality.

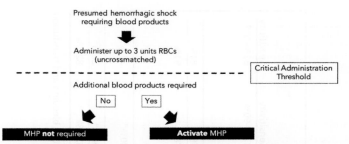

Fig. 3. Two-tiered approach to massive hemorrhage protocol (MHP) activation using the critical administration threshold.

2. Regular practice through case-based education or preferably simulation-based training.
3. Focus on evidence-based communication techniques including closed-loop communication, standardized lexicon of MHP terms, role clarity, and regular situation-assessment updates.

Testing: What Lab Tests Are Needed Initially and Throughout the Process?

Throughout an MHP, laboratory tests are necessary to monitor the adequacy of treatment and evolving complications. High-quality clinical studies are scarce, and there is considerable real-life heterogeneity about which tests are ordered, at what intervals, and how the results impact further management. It remains uncertain whether point-of-care viscoelastic testing such as thromboelastography (TEG) and rotational thromboelastometry (ROTEM) can effectively guide resuscitation of bleeding patients in trauma.[27] Recognizing these limitations, our group recently developed best-practice recommendations on laboratory testing during MHP.[7] These are summarized below:

- Prioritize the collection of samples for ABO/typing and compatibility testing.
- Laboratory testing should include complete blood count, coagulation testing (INR, activated partial thromboplastin time [aPTT], and fibrinogen), electrolytes, calcium (preferably, ionized), arterial or venous blood gas, and lactate.
- TEG or ROTEM represent an alternative for managing coagulopathy; however, these tests lack a clear benefit while increasing the frequency of transfusion.[27]
- A prespecified sequence of sample acquisition eliminates the risk of tube anticoagulant/additive cross-contamination (**Fig. 4**).
- Hourly laboratory testing until the termination of the protocol.
- Required tubes should be assembled into bundles, along with prechecked requisitions, labeled, and attached to the MHP cooler.
- Prioritized results that may have a direct impact on clinical care (eg, hemoglobin, electrolytes).
- Aim for a lab turn-around-time of 20 minutes for all tests.
- Direct communication of laboratory results to clinicians is essential (ie, passive communication such as uploading to a hospital information system, faxing, or emailing is not acceptable during MHP).
- Consider MHP phone attached to the first MHP cooler with a direct line for clinicians to the laboratory.

BLOOD DRAW TOOL

Lab tests[1]		Adult	Pediatric	Baseline	#1	#2	#3	#4	#5
				MHP Blood Draw and Testing Protocol					
INR, aPTT (baseline only), Fibrinogen	Sodium Citrate (Blue)	2.7mL	1.8 mL	x	x	x	x	x	x
ROTEM/TEG	Sodium Citrate (Blue)	2.7 mL	1.8 mL	x	x	x	x	x	x
Na, K, Cl, Mg, Urea	Serum (Red/Gold)	4.5 mL	2.0 mL	x	x	x	x	x	x
Glucose (baseline only)	Serum (Red/Gold)	NA		x	NA	NA	NA	NA	NA
Ionized Calcium[2]	Serum (Gold)	4.5 mL	2.0 mL	x	x	x	x	x	x
Venous Lactate[3]	Lithium Heparin (Green)	4.5 mL	2.0 mL	x	x	x	x	x	x
G&S (baseline only)[3]	EDTA (Pink)	6.0 mL	1.0 mL[4]	x	x	x	x	x	x
CBC	EDTA (Lavender)	4.0 mL	1.0 mL	x	NA	NA	NA	NA	NA
Venous Lactate	Lithium Heparin (Syringe)	-	-	x	x	x	x	x	x
Arterial Lactate	Lithium Heparin (Syringe)	-	-	x	x	x	x	x	x
Blood gas (pH and base excess)	Lithium Heparin (Syringe)	-	-	x	x	x	x	x	x
Ionized Calcium	Lithium Heparin (Syringe)	-	-	x	x	x	x	x	x
Na, K, Cl	Lithium Heparin (Syringe)	-	-	x	x	x	x	x	x

[1]Lab draws appear in appropriate draw order - Sodium Citrate should always be draw n first.
[2]Can be bundled up (i.e., done together with a blood gas sample, if device/analyzer is available).
[3]Follow facility specific policies regarding ABO confirmation and requirement for second specimen.
[4]500uL for neonates
Prioritize samples as per MHP lead and as available at your facility - vacutainer/microtainers may differ depending on facility and patient population.

Fig. 4. Massive hemorrhage protocol blood draw tool including sequence of sample acquisition (credit ORBCoN).

Tranexamic Acid: What Is the Role of Tranexamic Acid in a Massive Hemorrhage Protocol?

Tranexamic acid (TXA) has been shown in definitive trials to prevent bleeding-related mortality in cases of traumatic injury,[28,29] traumatic brain injury,[30,31] and postpartum hemorrhage.[32] It is most effective in reducing mortality rates if given within 60 minutes of injury or onset of hemorrhage.[28,29,33] An adult total dose of 2 to 3 g appears sufficient[29] and can be given as a single infusion to minimize complexity of care[30] or as 2 intravenous pushes.[34,35] In traumatic injury, prehospital administration of TXA is superior to delaying treatment till hospital arrival,[29,30] has been proven to be logistically possible, is safe, and should be a goal for prehospital transport teams.

In the future, once high-quality bioavailability studies have been performed, intramuscular administration is likely to be an alternative route of administration for patients where intravenous access cannot be secured.[36] In contrast to all other patient groups, TXA is of no benefit in patients with gastrointestinal hemorrhage and increases the risk of thromboembolic complications (in the high doses used in the trial [4 g]).[37] TXA cannot be withheld or its dose cannot be personalized based on currently available laboratory testing, including viscoelastic testing, due to its poor sensitivity.[38] Investigators have put forward analyses from nonrandomized studies suggesting the need to withhold TXA for patients with "fibrinolytic shutdown" (abnormal hypofibrinolysis) due to concerns regarding an increased risk of thromboembolic complications[39]; however, this concern has not been confirmed in other retrospective studies and remains a theoretic concern.[40,41] TXA improves the coagulopathy seen in severely injured trauma patients,[35] for example, when employed before arriving at the hospital, it abrogates trauma-induced coagulopathy.[42] The cost of treatment is minimal (approximately $20 USD per patient), and hence, it is highly cost-effective.[43] The risk of adverse events from a single dose is low, with only an elevated risk of seizures being identified from the randomized trials.[30] Systematic reviews find no increased risk of arterial or venous thromboembolism,[44] with the exception of patients with gastrointestinal hemorrhage receiving high doses (4 g).[37]

Temperature: How Should the Patient's Temperature Be Managed During the Massive Hemorrhage Protocol?

Monitoring and managing temperature is essential for every MHP. In a hypothermic patient, an increase in core temperature of 1°C is associated with a 10% reduction in RBC transfusion.[45] In addition, hypothermia is an independent predictor of mortality in trauma and causes increased blood loss and higher transfusion requirements.[45,46] Furthermore, the administration of blood components stored at temperatures between 2° C and 6° C can worsen hypothermia if the patient is massively transfused.[47] In this section, we will provide practical recommendations on how to manage temperature in actively bleeding trauma patients focusing on:

1. How to accurately monitor temperature,
2. What techniques to use to maintain or increase temperature, and
3. Practical tips to apply these techniques.

How to monitor the patient's temperature?

The thermal resistor of an intravascular pulmonary catheter is the gold standard for temperature monitoring. However, given the need for specific technical skills for placement and potential complications associated with its use, these catheters are not recommended as a standard tool.[48,49] The use of esophageal, rectal, or bladder thermometer is the technique recommended.[49–52] The selected modality should be informed by the clinical situation and local resources. Thermometers that are accurate at temperatures less than 34° C are recommended to measure the core temperature given the concern for hypothermia during massive hemorrhage resuscitation.[53] Peripheral thermometers (axillary, oral, tympanic membrane, or temporal artery) are less accurate with a margin of error of 2° C, especially at extremes of temperature.[50,51] Based on the best available evidence, we recommend the following:

- The use of a tympanic membrane thermometer until a central monitor is in place.[54,55]
- Initial temperature measurement within 15 minutes of patient arrival or protocol activation.
- Continuous temperature measurement during active rewarming[56] (if not possible, then at least every 30 minutes).

Techniques to maintain or increase a patient's temperature

Prevention of heat loss is important as rewarming hypothermic patients is challenging. Multiple methods should be applied to prevent hypothermia and rewarm the patient, including passive external warming, active external rewarming, and active internal rewarming.[49]

Passive rewarming methods such as removing wet clothing, increasing room temperature, and applying warm blankets should be used to avoid heat loss. However, in isolation, none of these methods are effective to manage significant hypothermia.

Forced-air warmer devices should be used as one of the active external rewarming methods covering a larger area, to be more effective.[57] They are easy and safe to use, decrease heat loss, provide heat to the body, and should be continued in the operating room.[57] Resistive heating devices can increase thermal comfort and maintain the core temperature when physical and logistical challenges limit other methods, such as in prehospital setting and intrahospital transport.[58,59]

Routine use of intravenous fluid warmers should be adopted to avoid worsening of hypothermia due to resuscitation with cold fluids. They should deliver components at normothermia at both low and high flow rates. The temperature should be set ideally at 41.5° C to effectively avoid hypothermia[58]; however, not higher than 43° C to avoid the risk of hemolysis and air embolism.[60]

Intubated patients have a higher risk of heat loss from the airway.[61] Heat and moisture exchange filters should be used to reduce evaporative heat loss from the airway of these patients.

Finally, for patients with temperatures below 32° C who have impaired thermogenesis, the previous cited interventions will possibly be insufficient to raise the core temperature. In these scenarios, clinicians should refer to local guidelines to treat severe hypothermia and investigate other causes aside from massive hemorrhage or transfusion.

Practical tips to apply passive and active rewarming techniques

1. Using shears, as soon as it is safe, remove wet clothing, linens, dressings, and dry the patient thoroughly.[62]
2. Cover the patient with warm blankets
3. The patient's head should also be covered with a warm towel to avoid additional heat loss.[62,63]
4. Forced-air warmer blankets should be in direct contact with the patient, with the perforated side facing the patient, and be secured to avoid it from blowing off the patient as it inflates.

Targets: Once the Massive Hemorrhage Protocol Is Activated, What Resuscitation Targets Should Be Used?

Since bleeding trauma patients may be coagulopathic on arrival and laboratory tests take time, the recommended approach to the transfusion therapy during MHP is ratio-based and is associated with decreased mortality, and faster time to transfusion was associated with better outcomes.[64] The PROPPR trial demonstrated no difference between approaches using 1:1:1 and 1:1:2 ratios.[65] The commonly used and guideline-recommended ratio is 1:1:2 (1 adult dose of platelets (pool of 4 or 1 apheresis unit), 4 units of plasma for every 2 units of RBCs.[66] **Fig. 5** illustrates a prototypical option for configuring MHP packs or coolers. Ratio-based resuscitation may, however, result in inadequate management of coagulopathy, and periodic coagulation tests or viscoelastic assays during MHP is imperative.[67] These tests may allow for a more precise assessment of coagulopathy and enable provision of targeted and personalized hemostatic treatment. The evidence on laboratory targets of transfusion is sparse, with no high-quality clinical trials. Once hemorrhage control is achieved, we recommend to switch to laboratory-based resuscitation.

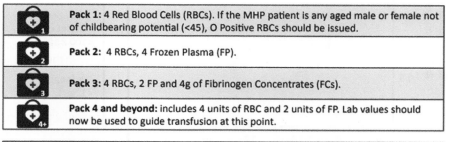

Fig. 5. Example of massive hemorrhage protocol cooler packs composition. (credit ORBCoN).

Thresholds to transfuse red blood cells

RBC transfusion optimizes the oxygen-carrying capacity and provides volume to bleeding patients. In general, numeric thresholds for RBC transfusion are not relevant in the early phases of trauma resuscitation. Rather, we follow the more commonly utilized approach of RBCs when volume is required following the ratios described above.

Thresholds to transfuse platelets

During massive bleeding, platelets usually fall to critical levels only after substantial blood loss and hours of resuscitation (**Fig. 6**). In contrast to the ratio-based approach described above, it may be reasonable to delay platelet transfusion until levels are available. If so, then platelets are transfused when the level is <100 × 10⁹/L in patients with intracranial/spinal hemorrhage and less than 50 × 10⁹/L for all other bleeding patients. These thresholds are based on a study from 1972, which demonstrated nearly normal bleeding time at a platelet count of greater than 100 × 10⁹/L and a steep prolongation in bleeding time as platelets fell below 50 × 10⁹/L.[68] These thresholds were widely adopted, and there are no recent high-quality clinical studies to update these recommendations. We recommend platelet transfusion when the level falls below 50 × 10⁹/L rather than following a ratio-based approach for platelets.[7]

Platelet count is only able to assess for quantitative deficiency of platelets. In injured patients, platelet dysfunction may result from injury itself, the use of antiplatelet agents, or congenital defects. If platelet dysfunction is suspected, platelet transfusion may be indicated even in the presence of an adequate platelet count.[69] We strongly recommend consultation with hematology/transfusion medicine regarding an optimal platelet transfusion strategy for complex patients. Viscoelastic assays have an

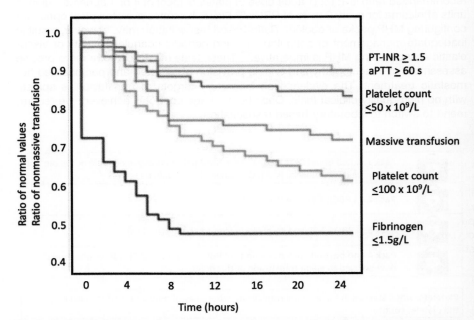

Fig. 6. Kaplan-Meier curves for severely injured trauma patients from emergency department arrival to reaching critical levels of routine coagulation parameters and criteria for massive transfusion (MT) (≥ 10U RBCs). Fibrinogen decreases before platelets, INR, activated partial thromboplastin time (aPTT), and need for MT. (With permission from author).[81]

advantage to assess for the presence of platelet dysfunction.[70] Evidence on how to use their results to guide transfusion therapy is being analyzed. If using ROTEM, reduced EXTEM A10 or MCF (35 mm or below) may signal the need for a platelet transfusion. To correct MCF, in addition to platelets, fibrinogen supplementation may be necessary.[71]

Thresholds to transfuse plasma (or prothrombin complex concentrate)

About 25% of severely injured patients are coagulopathic on admission to ED.[72] Moreover, conventional coagulation tests such as INR are inaccurate to diagnose acute coagulopathy of trauma. More sensitive tests include viscoelastic testing and thrombin generation assays; however, these are not widely available.

It is reasonable to consider plasma transfusion for an INR $\geq$1.8 as it may not be possible to decrease the INR to <1.8 despite large volumes of plasma transfusion.[73,74] Moreover, at INR <1.8, there remain sufficient quantities of clotting factors to effect hemostasis. In the absence of ready availability of plasma, a prothrombin complex concentrate (PCC) may be used.[75,76] The PCC, as compared to plasma, is associated with reduced mortality in bleeding trauma patients and reduced blood loss in bleeding cardiac surgery patients.[76,77]

In some patients, abnormal coagulation tests may also signal the presence of anticoagulant medications or a congenital bleeding disorder. Discussion of these topics is outside the scope of this article. A summary of common drugs that may impair hemostasis and their antidotes is provided in **Table 2**.

Thresholds to transfuse fibrinogen concentrate

Fibrinogen is the first factor to reach critically low levels during massive bleeding.[81] Fibrinogen levels less than 1.5 g/L are associated with increased mortality in massively bleeding trauma patients.[82] Guidelines typically recommend to replace fibrinogen at levels $\leq$1.5 g/L.[66,83] If using rTEG, then a functional fibrinogen (FF)-TEG maximum amplitude less than 20 mm may inform the need for fibrinogen replacement. If using ROTEM, the FIBTEM clot amplitude at 5 min (CA5) may assist with this decision.[71] Evidence-based thresholds have not been established.

Termination: What Factors Should Guide the Clinical Team to Stop the Massive Hemorrhage Protocol?

Similar to the decision to activate the MHP, it is important to have standardized criteria for "stepping down" the protocol. In contrast to the prolific literature on when to activate the MHP, there is very little science to guide the termination of the MHP. Premature termination of the MHP could lead to delays in transfusion, laboratory testing, and transportation. In addition, premature termination can lead to a need to "reactivate" the MHP and to reassemble all team member and leads to confusion within the laboratory as to whether to recommence with pack 1 of blood or continue on from the last pack issued. Similarly, delayed termination can lead to unnecessary transfusions, loss of valuable blood products, continued preparation of blood products by the laboratory staff, and delayed transfusions for other patients within the hospital.

Based on our experience and the best available evidence,[84] it is suggested to consider protocol termination when any of the following occurs:

1. There is definitive hemorrhage control (or a substantial deceleration in blood loss).
2. The patient's hemodynamics and coagulation profile are improving.
3. Inotropes can be reduced or stopped.

At a system level, a protocolized, proactive call from the transfusion laboratory to the clinical team should be integrated into the process if there has been no request

Table 2
Anticoagulant and antiplatelet medications and antidotes

Drug	Antidote	Dosage
Warfarin	PCC IV Vitamin K	INR 1.5 to 2.9–1000 IU INR 3.0 to 5.0–2000 IU INR > 5.0–3000 IU INR unknown – 2000 IU PLUS vitamin K 10 mg IV
Dabigatran (Pradaxa)	Idarucizumab (Praxbind)	5 g IV Repeat at 24 h if PTT up and ongoing bleeding risk
All Xa inhibitors (eg, apixaban [Eliquis], edoxaban [Savaysa], rivaroxaban [Xarelto])[a]	PCC (Note: andexanet not widely available)	2000 IU Repeat at 1 h if ongoing hemorrhage
Low molecular weight heparin (eg, dalteparin, enoxaparin, danaparoid, tinzaparin)	Contact hematology/ transfusion medicine for advice	N/A
ASA	Nothing[b]	N/A
Clopidogrel	Nothing[b] Consider platelet transfusion if ongoing bleeding and other coagulopathies have been corrected	N/A
Ticagrelor	Nothing[b] (Note: bentracimab not yet available)	N/A

Abbreviation: ASA, Acetylsalicylic acid; DOAC, direct acting oral anticoagulants; ICH, intracranial hemorrhage; N/A, not applicable.
[a] Reversal of DOACs is to be considered for a period of 24 h following the last dose.
[b] Clinical studies failed to confirm a benefit of platelet transfusions for ASA/Clopidogrel-treated patients with gastrointestinal bleeding and spontaneous ICH and raised concern regarding harm (use platelet transfusions with caution).[78–80]

for blood within 60 minutes to reaffirm the need to continue the MHP. Failure to terminate the protocol is a common failure point.[85] The MHP almost always commences with formula-based transfusion support and then transitions to laboratory-guided transfusion resuscitation. It remains unknown whether institutions utilizing bedside viscoelastic testing have better clinical outcomes.[27] Some MHPs are designed to be terminated at this transition to lab-based resuscitation; however, we believe that the 2 transitions may not align temporally. Hence, it is acceptable to start lab-guided resuscitation before terminating the MHP. The hospital MHP needs to have a termination protocol to ensure prompt return of blood products, return of the MHP phone or other equipment, safe handover to the intensive care team, and end of protocol blood work. Unnecessary transfusions can occur if this handoff is not structured (ie, failing to communicate that 4 units of RBC were transfused after the last hemoglobin of 6.4 g/dL, leading to additional unnecessary units before a hemoglobin repeat).

An easy, practical, and high-yield tactic to continually improve MHP performance is the integration of a team debrief or huddle to the MHP protocol termination, including a process of reporting processes that did not go as planned to ensure continuous quality improvement. Finally, to objectively and systematically optimize the MHP, we recommend tracking key process quality indicators including, but not limited to, the following:[7]

1. Proportion of patients receiving TXA within 1 hour of protocol activation.
2. Proportion of patients in whom RBC transfusion is initiated within 15 minutes of protocol activation.
3. Proportion of patients without any blood component wastage.

Case Resolution: Integration of Massive Hemorrhage Protocol Principles

This article provides a detailed review of key MHP principles using the 7T framework. Using the case presented in the introduction of a 57-year-old female involved in a high-speed MVC, we provide a summary for the application of the 7 Ts.

Team: Prior to arrival, the trauma team leader (TTL) conducted a prebriefing "time out" to create a shared mental model, stablish care priorities, and assign tasks. This includes discussion on MHP preactivation, which was not deemed necessary at this point. Instead, the TTL requested 4 units of RBCs to be brought to the trauma bay/ ED by a dedicated team member (in case they are not readily and locally available).

Trigger: On arrival, 3 prediction tools were positive (shock index > 1.0, ABC score = 2, and RABT score = 2). However, the team opted to use the critical administration threshold. They transfused 2 units of RBCs while progressing with patient assessment. Two sources of bleeding were identified: (1) intra-abdominal (positive focused assessment with sonography in trauma) and (2) anteroposterior compression fracture of the pelvis on pelvic x-ray. Blood pressure did not improve (90 mm Hg) with the 2 units transfused. The third unit was initiated, and the MHP was activated.

Tranexamic acid: During the prebriefing, the TTL requested TXA (2 g IV bolus), which was prepared and promptly administered following patient's admission. Importantly, the team learned that the patient was using Rivaroxaban for chronic atrial fibrillation. This prompted the administration of PCC (requested urgently and administered while the patient had been taken to the CT scanner suite).

Testing: Following handover from paramedics, the circulating nurse collected blood samples as a new intravenous access was being catheterized prioritizing ABO typing and compatibility testing. Bed-side bundled supplies for minimal laboratory testing were used. Laboratory tests were requested using an established order set, and a team member transported the samples immediately to the laboratory and blood bank. Results with critical values were communicated as they were released by the laboratory staff via phone calls to the trauma bay and operating room (OR) where the patient was transported to following the care provided in the trauma bay/ED. Using a Trauma Resuscitation Checklist to guide postactivation best practices, further blood samples were collected hourly until MHP was called off.

Targets: Following intermittent improvement of the hemodynamic status, the patient was transferred to a hybrid OR for trauma laparotomy, angiography, and possible pelvic angioembolization. At this point, the patient had received the third MHP pack (12 RBCs, 6 plasmas, and 4 g of fibrinogen concentrate [for a fibrinogen level of 1.0 mg/ dL]). Platelet level was 157.000/mm^3, and INR was 1.49, not requiring correction. The anesthesiologist switched to a lab-guided strategy by the end of the procedures as the resuscitation moved forward and the patient's hemodynamic status and coagulopathy improved (see Targets section for details).

Temperature: The admission temperature was 34.8°C measured by a tympanic membrane thermometer and at each 30 minutes, subsequently. Two rapid infusers had been primed prior to patient arrival as part of the prebriefing checklist to infuse blood products at 41.5°C. The patient was promptly exposed with removal of clothes followed by placement of warmed blankets. Following primary and secondary assessments, prior to OR transfer, a forced warm air device was applied. The patient was intubated, warm blankets were placed around the head, and heat and moisture exchange filters were used to reduce further heat loss.

Termination: In the operating room, evacuation of 2 L of blood from the abdominal cavity, splenectomy, liver packing, angiography with embolization, and an external pelvic fixation were performed in a damage-control fashion. By the end of these procedures, the patient's hemodynamic status and coagulopathy had improved considerably, prompting the anesthesiologist to call off the MHP before transfer to the intensive care unit.

SUMMARY

A well-designed MHP is essential in the care of injured and bleeding patients. This article proposes the application of a structured approach using the 7 Ts of MHP to guide this complex process. A successful resuscitation requires a high-performing team following evidence-based metrics. At an institutional level, each MHP requires review to promote areas of success and opportunities for improvement. We believe the 7 Ts of MHP approach is practical, feasible, and customizable across all ED sizes and circumstances. Optimized MHP strategies will inevitably improve outcomes for bleeding trauma patients and reduce the cognitive load for the clinical team.

CLINICS CARE POINTS

- To assist with the decision for MHP activation, the RABT score or critical administration threshold (>3 units/h) is useful.
- When hemorrhage is suspected in a trauma patient, 2 g of TXA should be administered within 3 hours and ideally <1 hour from the injury.
- Upon patient arrival, temperature measurement is essential.
- After the administration of 3 units of RBCs, begin FFP administration to achieve a 2:1 ratio (RBC:FFP).

DISCLOSURE

A. Petrosoniak is cofounder of Advanced Performance Healthcare Design. J. Callum has received research funding from Canadian Blood Services and Octapharma. L.T. da Luz has received funds from Octapharma. K. Pavenski has no relevant disclosures.

ACKNOWLEDGMENTS

The authors thank the Ontario Regional Blood Coordinating Network (ORBCoN) for their support in creating the Ontario massive hemorrhage protocol toolkit.

REFERENCES

1. Cannon JW, Khan MA, Raja AS, et al. Damage control resuscitation in patients with severe traumatic hemorrhage: A practice management guideline from the

Eastern Association for the Surgery of Trauma. J Trauma Acute Care Surg 2017; 82:605–17.

2. Cotton BA, Dossett LA, Au BK, et al. Room for (performance) improvement: provider-related factors associated with poor outcomes in massive transfusion. J Trauma 2009;67:1004–12.

3. Khan S, Allard S, Weaver A, et al. A major haemorrhage protocol improves the delivery of blood component therapy and reduces waste in trauma massive transfusion. Injury 2013;44:587–92.

4. Milligan C, Higginson I, Smith JE. Emergency department staff knowledge of massive transfusion for trauma: the need for an evidence based protocol. Emerg Med J 2011;28:870–2.

5. Nunez TC, Young PP, Holcomb JB, et al. Creation, implementation, and maturation of a massive transfusion protocol for the exsanguinating trauma patient. J Trauma 2010;68:1498–505.

6. Lim G, Harper-Kirksey K, Parekh R, et al. Efficacy of a massive transfusion protocol for hemorrhagic trauma resuscitation. Am J Emerg Med 2018;36:1178–81.

7. Callum JL, Yeh CH, Petrosoniak A, et al. A regional massive hemorrhage protocol developed through a modified Delphi technique. CMAJ Open 2019;7:E546–61.

8. Narayan SE, Poles D, eaobotSHoTSS Group. The 2020 Annual SHOT Report. Serious Hazards of Transfusion (SHOT) 2021. Available at: https://www.shotuk. org/wp-content/uploads/myimages/SHOT-REPORT-2020.pdf. Accessed April 1, 2022.

9. Meyer DE, Vincent LE, Fox EE, et al. Every minute counts: Time to delivery of initial massive transfusion cooler and its impact on mortality. J Trauma Acute Care Surg 2017;83:19–24.

10. Pham HP, Shaz BH. Update on massive transfusion. Br J Anaesth 2013; 111(Suppl 1):i71–82.

11. Brockamp T, Nienaber U, Mutschler M, et al. Predicting on-going hemorrhage and transfusion requirement after severe trauma: a validation of six scoring systems and algorithms on the TraumaRegister DGU. Crit Care 2012;16:R129.

12. Cotton BA, Dossett LA, Haut ER, et al. Multicenter validation of a simplified score to predict massive transfusion in trauma. J Trauma 2010;69(Suppl 1):S33–9.

13. Nunez TC, Voskresensky IV, Dossett LA, et al. Early prediction of massive transfusion in trauma: simple as ABC (assessment of blood consumption)? J Trauma 2009;66:346–52.

14. Schroll R, Swift D, Tatum D, et al. Accuracy of shock index versus ABC score to predict need for massive transfusion in trauma patients. Injury 2018;49:15–9.

15. Hanna K, Harris C, Trust MD, et al. Multicenter Validation of the Revised Assessment of Bleeding and Transfusion (RABT) Score for Predicting Massive Transfusion. World J Surg 2020;44:1807–16.

16. Meyer DE, Cotton BA, Fox EE, et al. A comparison of resuscitation intensity and critical administration threshold in predicting early mortality among bleeding patients: A multicenter validation in 680 major transfusion patients. J Trauma Acute Care Surg 2018;85:691–6.

17. Warren J, Moazzez A, Chong V, et al. Narrowed pulse pressure predicts massive transfusion and emergent operative intervention following penetrating trauma. Am J Surg 2019;218:1185–8.

18. Savage SA, Sumislawski JJ, Zarzaur BL, et al. The new metric to define large-volume hemorrhage: results of a prospective study of the critical administration threshold. J Trauma Acute Care Surg 2015;78:224–9 [discussion: 229–30].

19. Damme CD, Luo J, Buesing KL. Isolated prehospital hypotension correlates with injury severity and outcomes in patients with trauma. Trauma Surg Acute Care Open 2016;1:e000013.

20. Kheirbek T, Martin TJ, Cao J, et al. Prehospital shock index outperforms hypotension alone in predicting significant injury in trauma patients. Trauma Surg Acute Care Open 2021;6:e000712.

21. Ohmori T, Kitamura T, Tanaka K, et al. Bleeding sites in elderly trauma patients who required massive transfusion: a comparison with younger patients. Am J Emerg Med 2016;34:123–7.

22. Martinetti A, Awadhpersad P, Singh S, et al. Gone in 2s: a deep dive into perfection analysing the collaborative maintenance pitstop of Formula 1. J Qual Maintenance Eng 2021;27:550–64.

23. Bogdanovic J, Perry J, Guggenheim M, et al. Adaptive coordination in surgical teams: an interview study. BMC Health Serv Res 2015;15:128.

24. Hicks C, Petrosoniak A. The Human Factor: Optimizing Trauma Team Performance in Dynamic Clinical Environments. Emerg Med Clin North Am 2018; 36:1–17.

25. Mathieu J, Goodwin G, Heffner T, et al. The Influence of Shared Mental Models on Team Process and Performance. Joural Appl Psychol 2000;85:273–83.

26. Westli HK, Johnsen BH, Eid J, et al. Teamwork skills, shared mental models, and performance in simulated trauma teams: an independent group design. Scand J Trauma Resuscitation Emerg Med 2010;18:47.

27. Baksaas-Aasen K, Gall LS, Stensballe J, et al. Viscoelastic haemostatic assay augmented protocols for major trauma haemorrhage (ITACTIC): a randomized, controlled trial. Intensive Care Med 2021;47:49–59.

28. collaborators C-t, Shakur H, Roberts I, et al. Effects of tranexamic acid on death, vascular occlusive events, and blood transfusion in trauma patients with significant haemorrhage (CRASH-2): a randomised, placebo-controlled trial. Lancet 2010;376:23–32.

29. Guyette FX, Brown JB, Zenati MS, et al. Tranexamic Acid During Prehospital Transport in Patients at Risk for Hemorrhage After Injury: A Double-blind, Placebo-Controlled, Randomized Clinical Trial. JAMA Surg 2020;156(1):11–20.

30. Rowell SE, Meier EN, McKnight B, et al. Effect of Out-of-Hospital Tranexamic Acid vs Placebo on 6-Month Functional Neurologic Outcomes in Patients With Moderate or Severe Traumatic Brain Injury. JAMA 2020;324:961–74.

31. collaborators C-t. Effects of tranexamic acid on death, disability, vascular occlusive events and other morbidities in patients with acute traumatic brain injury (CRASH-3): a randomised, placebo-controlled trial. Lancet 2019;394:1713–23.

32. Collaborators WT. Effect of early tranexamic acid administration on mortality, hysterectomy, and other morbidities in women with post-partum haemorrhage (WOMAN): an international, randomised, double-blind, placebo-controlled trial. Lancet 2017;389:2105–16.

33. Gayet-Ageron A, Prieto-Merino D, Ker K, et al. Effect of treatment delay on the effectiveness and safety of antifibrinolytics in acute severe haemorrhage: a meta-analysis of individual patient-level data from 40 138 bleeding patients. Lancet 2018;391:125–32.

34. Ageron FX, Coats TJ, Darioli V, et al. Validation of the BATT score for prehospital risk stratification of traumatic haemorrhagic death: usefulness for tranexamic acid treatment criteria. Scand J Trauma Resusc Emerg Med 2021;29:6.

35. Morrison JJ, Dubose JJ, Rasmussen TE, et al. Military Application of Tranexamic Acid in Trauma Emergency Resuscitation (MATTERs) Study. Arch Surg 2012;147: 113–9.
36. Kane Z, Picetti R, Wilby A, et al. Physiologically based modelling of tranexamic acid pharmacokinetics following intravenous, intramuscular, sub-cutaneous and oral administration in healthy volunteers. Eur J Pharm Sci 2021;164:105893.
37. Collaborators H-IT. Effects of a high-dose 24-h infusion of tranexamic acid on death and thromboembolic events in patients with acute gastrointestinal bleeding (HALT-IT): an international randomised, double-blind, placebo-controlled trial. Lancet 2020;395:1927–36.
38. Dixon AL, McCully BH, Rick EA, et al. Tranexamic acid administration in the field does not affect admission thromboelastography after traumatic brain injury. J Trauma Acute Care Surg 2020;89:900–7.
39. Moore EE, Moore HB, Gonzalez E, et al. Rationale for the selective administration of tranexamic acid to inhibit fibrinolysis in the severely injured patient. Transfusion 2016;56(Suppl 2):S110–4.
40. David JS, Lambert A, Bouzat P, et al. Fibrinolytic shutdown diagnosed with rotational thromboelastometry represents a moderate form of coagulopathy associated with transfusion requirement and mortality: A retrospective analysis. Eur J Anaesthesiol 2020;37:170–9.
41. Gomez-Builes JC, Acuna SA, Nascimento B, et al. Harmful or Physiologic: Diagnosing Fibrinolysis Shutdown in a Trauma Cohort With Rotational Thromboelastometry. Anesth Analg 2018;127:840–9.
42. Stein P, Studt JD, Albrecht R, et al. The Impact of Prehospital Tranexamic Acid on Blood Coagulation in Trauma Patients. Anesth Analg 2018;126:522–9.
43. Guerriero C, Cairns J, Perel P, et al. Cost-effectiveness analysis of administering tranexamic acid to bleeding trauma patients using evidence from the CRASH-2 trial. PLoS One 2011;6:e18987.
44. Al-Jeabory M, Szarpak L, Attila K, et al. Efficacy and Safety of Tranexamic Acid in Emergency Trauma: A Systematic Review and Meta-Analysis. J Clin Med 2021; 3:10.
45. Lester ELW, Fox EE, Holcomb JB, et al. The impact of hypothermia on outcomes in massively transfused patients. J Trauma Acute Care Surg 2019;86:458–63.
46. Rajagopalan S, Mascha E, Na J, et al. The effects of mild perioperative hypothermia on blood loss and transfusion requirement. Anesthesiology 2008;108:71–7.
47. Poder TG, Pruneau D, Dorval J, et al. Effect of warming and flow rate conditions of blood warmers on red blood cell integrity. Vox Sang 2016;111:341–9.
48. Marik PE. Obituary: pulmonary artery catheter 1970 to 2013. Ann Intensive Care 2013;3:38.
49. Perlman R, Callum J, Laflamme C, et al. A recommended early goal-directed management guideline for the prevention of hypothermia-related transfusion, morbidity, and mortality in severely injured trauma patients. Crit Care 2016; 20:107.
50. Barnett BJ, Nunberg S, Tai J, et al. Oral and tympanic membrane temperatures are inaccurate to identify Fever in emergency department adults. West J Emerg Med 2011;12:505–11.
51. Niven DJ, Gaudet JE, Laupland KB, et al. Accuracy of peripheral thermometers for estimating temperature: a systematic review and meta-analysis. Ann Intern Med 2015;163:768–77.
52. O'Grady NP, Barie PS, Bartlett JG, et al. Guidelines for evaluation of new fever in critically ill adult patients: 2008 update from the American College of Critical Care

Medicine and the Infectious Diseases Society of America. Crit Care Med 2008;36: 1330–49.

53. Soar J, Perkins GD, Abbas G, et al. European Resuscitation Council Guidelines for Resuscitation 2010 Section 8. Cardiac arrest in special circumstances: Electrolyte abnormalities, poisoning, drowning, accidental hypothermia, hyperthermia, asthma, anaphylaxis, cardiac surgery, trauma, pregnancy, electrocution. Resuscitation 2010;81:1400–33.

54. Asadian S, Khatony A, Moradi G, et al. Accuracy and precision of four common peripheral temperature measurement methods in intensive care patients. Med Devices (Auckl) 2016;9:301–8.

55. Uleberg O, Eidstuen SC, Vangberg G, et al. Temperature measurements in trauma patients: is the ear the key to the core? Scand J Trauma Resusc Emerg Med 2015;23:101.

56. Tsuei BJ, Kearney PA. Hypothermia in the trauma patient. Injury 2004;35:7–15.

57. Brauer A, Quintel M. Forced-air warming: technology, physical background and practical aspects. Curr Opin Anaesthesiol 2009;22:769–74.

58. Kober A, Scheck T, Fulesdi B, et al. Effectiveness of resistive heating compared with passive warming in treating hypothermia associated with minor trauma: a randomized trial. Mayo Clin Proc 2001;76:369–75.

59. Lundgren P, Henriksson O, Naredi P, et al. The effect of active warming in prehospital trauma care during road and air ambulance transportation - a clinical randomized trial. Scand J Trauma Resusc Emerg Med 2011;19:59.

60. Poder TG, Nonkani WG, Tsakeu Leponkouo E. Blood Warming and Hemolysis: A Systematic Review With Meta-Analysis. Transfus Med Rev 2015;29:172–80.

61. Alam A, Olarte R, Callum J, et al. Hypothermia indices among severely injured trauma patients undergoing urgent surgery: A single-centred retrospective quality review and analysis. Injury 2018;49:117–23.

62. Sedlak SK. Hypothermia in trauma: the nurse's role in recognition, prevention, and management. Int J Trauma Nurs 1995;1:19–26.

63. Lawson LL. Hypothermia and trauma injury: temperature monitoring and rewarming strategies. Crit Care Nurs Q 1992;15:21–32.

64. Meneses E, Boneva D, McKenney M, et al. Massive transfusion protocol in adult trauma population. Am J Emerg Med 2020;38:2661–6.

65. Holcomb JB, Tilley BC, Baraniuk S, et al. Transfusion of plasma, platelets, and red blood cells in a 1:1:1 vs a 1:1:2 ratio and mortality in patients with severe trauma: the PROPPR randomized clinical trial. JAMA 2015;313:471–82.

66. Vlaar APJ, Dionne JC, de Bruin S, et al. Transfusion strategies in bleeding critically ill adults: a clinical practice guideline from the European Society of Intensive Care Medicine. Intensive Care Med 2021;47:1368–92.

67. Caspers M, Maegele M, Frohlich M. Current strategies for hemostatic control in acute trauma hemorrhage and trauma-induced coagulopathy. Expert Rev Hematol 2018;11:987–95.

68. Harker LA, Slichter SJ. The bleeding time as a screening test for evaluation of platelet function. N Engl J Med 1972;287:155–9.

69. Anderson TN, Schreiber MA, Rowell SE. Viscoelastic Testing in Traumatic Brain Injury: Key Research Insights. Transfus Med Rev 2021;35:108–12.

70. Da Luz LT, Nascimento B, Shankarakutty AK, et al. Effect of thromboelastography (TEG(R)) and rotational thromboelastometry (ROTEM(R)) on diagnosis of coagulopathy, transfusion guidance and mortality in trauma: descriptive systematic review. Crit Care 2014;18:518.

71. Brill JB, Brenner M, Duchesne J, et al. The Role of TEG and ROTEM in Damage Control Resuscitation. Shock 2021;56:52–61.

72. Frith D, Davenport R, Brohi K. Acute traumatic coagulopathy. Curr Opin Anaesthesiol 2012;25:229–34.

73. Abdel-Wahab OI, Healy B, Dzik WH. Effect of fresh-frozen plasma transfusion on prothrombin time and bleeding in patients with mild coagulation abnormalities. Transfusion (Paris) 2006;46:1279–85.

74. Holland LL, Brooks JP. Toward rational fresh frozen plasma transfusion: The effect of plasma transfusion on coagulation test results. Am J Clin Pathol 2006;126: 133–9.

75. Kao TW, Lee YC, Chang HT. Prothrombin Complex Concentrate for Trauma Induced Coagulopathy: A Systematic Review and Meta-Analysis. J Acute Med 2021;11:81–9.

76. van den Brink DP, Wirtz MR, Neto AS, et al. Effectiveness of prothrombin complex concentrate for the treatment of bleeding: A systematic review and meta-analysis. J Thromb Haemost 2020;18:2457–67.

77. Karkouti K, Bartoszko J, Grewal D, et al. Comparison of 4-Factor Prothrombin Complex Concentrate With Frozen Plasma for Management of Hemorrhage During and After Cardiac Surgery: A Randomized Pilot Trial. JAMA Netw Open 2021; 4:e213936.

78. Baharoglu MI, Cordonnier C, Al-Shahi Salman R, et al. Platelet transfusion versus standard care after acute stroke due to spontaneous cerebral haemorrhage associated with antiplatelet therapy (PATCH): a randomised, open-label, phase 3 trial. Lancet 2016;387:2605–13.

79. Godier A, Garrigue D, Lasne D, et al. Management of antiplatelet therapy for non-elective invasive procedures or bleeding complications: Proposals from the French Working Group on Perioperative Haemostasis (GIHP) and the French Study Group on Thrombosis and Haemostasis (GFHT), in collaboration with the French Society for Anaesthesia and Intensive Care (SFAR). Arch Cardiovasc Dis 2019;112:199–216.

80. Yorkgitis BK, Tatum DM, Taghavi S, et al. Eastern Association for the Surgery of Trauma Multicenter Trial: Comparison of pre-injury antithrombotic use and reversal strategies among severe traumatic brain injury patients. J Trauma Acute Care Surg 2022;92:88–92.

81. Hayakawa M, Gando S, Ono Y, et al. Fibrinogen level deteriorates before other routine coagulation parameters and massive transfusion in the early phase of severe trauma: a retrospective observational study. Semin Thromb Hemost 2015; 41:35–42.

82. Bouzat P, Ageron FX, Charbit J, et al. Modelling the association between fibrinogen concentration on admission and mortality in patients with massive transfusion after severe trauma: an analysis of a large regional database. Scand J Trauma Resusc Emerg Med 2018;26:55.

83. Levy JH, Welsby I, Goodnough LT. Fibrinogen as a therapeutic target for bleeding: a review of critical levels and replacement therapy. Transfusion (Paris) 2014;54:1389–405 [quiz: 1388].

84. Foster JC, Sappenfield JW, Smith RS, et al. Initiation and Termination of Massive Transfusion Protocols: Current Strategies and Future Prospects. Anesth Analg 2017;125:2045–55.

85. Margarido C, Ferns J, Chin V, et al. Massive hemorrhage protocol activation in obstetrics: a 5-year quality performance review. Int J Obstet Anesth 2019;38:37–45.

Resuscitative Endovascular Balloon Occlusion of the Aorta: A Practical Review

Zaffer Qasim, MD, FRCEM, EDIC

KEYWORDS

- REBOA • Hemorrhage • Resuscitation

KEY POINTS

- Noncompressible torso hemorrhage remains a significant contributor to potentially preventable trauma mortality.
- REBOA presents a minimally invasive technique to temporarily control noncompressible torso hemorrhage in exsanguinating patients until they can get to definitive care.
- REBOA carries the risks of end-organ ischemia and vascular injury.
- Within an appropriate system of care, REBOA can be a useful adjunct in the resuscitation team's toolbox.

CASE

Emergency medical services (EMS) bring in a 42-year-old male bicyclist who has been struck by a bus. EMS report that the bus had run over the victim's lower torso, pinning him, and he required extrication. They noted him to be progressively confused en route to the emergency department (ED).

In the ED, that patient appears confused but with an intact airway. There are no signs of injury to the chest, but his respiratory rate is 44 breaths per minutes, and his oxygen saturation is 94% on room air. The abdomen is tense in the lower quadrants, and there is a tire track visible over the lower abdomen. Careful evaluation of the pelvis reveals gross instability, and there is blood noted at the urethral meatus. The patient's skin is cool and clammy. The nurse notifies the team that the patient's remaining vital signs including heart rate (HR) 134 beats/min and blood pressure (BP) 74/50 mm Hg.

The team leader requests bilateral large bore intravenous access, initiation of blood product resuscitation, and activation of the massive transfusion protocol. The peripheral veins are noted to be collapsed; therefore, a subclavian central venous line is

Department of Emergency Medicine, Perelman School of Medicine at the University of Pennsylvania, 51N 39th Street, Ground Floor Myrin Building, Philadelphia, PA 19104, USA
E-mail address: Zaffer.qasim@pennmedicine.upenn.edu

Emerg Med Clin N Am 41 (2023) 71–88
https://doi.org/10.1016/j.emc.2022.09.011
0733-8627/23/© 2022 Elsevier Inc. All rights reserved.

placed. A pelvic binder is applied for a suspected pelvic fracture. A chest x-ray is obtained, which reveals no obvious intrathoracic injuries. Following the administration of the second unit of packed red blood cells, the patient's repeat vital signs are HR 140 beats/min and BP 65/49 mm Hg. The patient is much more somnolent, and his airway is being supported with jaw thrust and face-mask oxygen. A focused assessment with sonography in trauma (FAST) examination reveals free fluid in the right upper quadrant and pelvis.

The trauma team leader, suspecting both an open-book pelvic fracture and possible intraabdominal injury, with no response to initial appropriate resuscitative measures, decides to proceed with resuscitative endovascular balloon occlusion of the aorta (REBOA). They hand off team leadership to the airway attending. Ultrasound is used to identify the right common femoral artery (CFA), and a 7-French introducer sheath is placed on first pass. The REBOA catheter is prepared and inserted to a depth consistent with zone 1. The balloon is slowly inflated while monitoring BP on the monitor. Appropriate occlusion is achieved, and the BP improves to 101/71. The catheter is secured, and the time of inflation is documented.

The trauma team leader resumes command of the resuscitation and directs for the patient to be intubated and transferred urgently to the operating room (OR). Operative findings include a large pelvic hematoma, a grade 3 liver injury, and bleeding from mesenteric vessels. The pelvis is packed, and other points of bleeding are addressed while the anesthesiology team continues resuscitation. Once hemostasis appears to have been achieved, and the trauma surgeon, in close coordination with the anesthesiology team, slowly deflates the REBOA balloon. There does not appear to be any ongoing active bleeding, and the patient's hemodynamics remain relatively stable. The total balloon occlusion time is 38 minutes. The patient is transferred to the interventional radiology (IR) suite where a branch of left internal iliac artery is embolized.

INTRODUCTION

Hemorrhage remains the leading cause of trauma-related mortality in the United States and globally.[1] Hemorrhage can occur from compressible sites, such as a distal extremity wound. These sites allow direct control through compression, packing, or tourniquet application. Controlling bleeding from noncompressible sites is much more challenging. These sites can include the thorax, abdomen, and pelvis, areas where it is very difficult if not impossible to apply direct pressure. In addition, junctional sites of hemorrhage, such as at the axillae, neck, and groin, often cannot be controlled through tourniquet application. Noncompressible torso hemorrhage (NCTH), therefore, represents a significant challenge in the management of the trauma patient.

NCTH in fact has been the most significant contributor to potentially preventable hemorrhage-related mortality in both military and civilian populations.[2,3] In the military setting, NCTH accounts for up to 60% of potentially preventable deaths.[2,4] Figures in the civilian population lie in the 60% to 70% range for all potentially preventable prehospital deaths (when traumatic brain injuries [TBIs] are excluded).[5]

Patients with NCTH require rapid intervention or risk progressing to traumatic cardiac arrest. High-grade NCTH deaths typically occur within a short time period (30 minutes to 1 hour). The primary means to achieve control is rapid surgical control in the OR. Should they arrest, inflow control can be achieved by cross-clamping the aorta through a resuscitative thoracotomy (RT).[6] This is associated with significant disadvantages, including poor neurologically-intact survival rates, physiologic stress of opening an additional body cavity, and risks to the clinician.[7,8]

In an attempt to address this challenge, numerous techniques have been developed including the use of junctional and abdominal tourniquets, as well as REBOA.

REBOA is a mechanism of NCTH control based on endovascular principles.[9] It requires a balloon catheter be inserted through the femoral artery and then threaded up the abdominal aorta above the suspected source of hemorrhage. The balloon is then inflated to occlude the aorta, providing inflow control. The concept was first described in Korea and subsequently in case series in the United States in the 1980s.[10–12] The recent conflicts in Afghanistan and Iraq highlighted the need to further study this as a feasible option for hemorrhage control.

Numerous animal studies demonstrated the potential benefit of REBOA. White and colleagues showed that, when compared to RT, REBOA achieved hemostasis with a lower need for fluid and vasoactive medication support.[13] Early civilian human case series proved the feasibility of using REBOA for NCTH, with no hemorrhage-related mortality.[14–16] The American Association for the Surgery of Trauma prospective observational trial, Aortic Occlusion for Resuscitation in Trauma and Acute Care Surgery (AORTA), reported in 2016 that the mortality rates were similar between RT and REBOA.[17]

With the demonstration of feasibility, focus changed to the equipment required for REBOA. Modern catheters have moved beyond the wire-based systems requiring large vascular introducer sheaths to wire-free devices that can be inserted through 7-French or even 4-French sheaths.[18]

In Which Patient Should We Consider Resuscitative Endovascular Balloon Occlusion of the Aorta?

REBOA remains an adjunctive tool in major hemorrhage resuscitation. The focus should be on ensuring the basics of hemorrhagic shock resuscitation are addressed alongside the consideration for REBOA.

REBOA is indicated in:

- Subdiaphragmatic source of NCTH (abdomen, pelvis, retroperitoneum, or groin junctional)
- Transient responder or nonresponder to blood product resuscitation.

REBOA is contraindicated in:

- Major supradiaphragmatic injuries
  - Pericardial tamponade
  - Massive hemothorax
  - Neck or axillary junctional vascular injuries
- High suspicion of aortic injury
- Inability to move to a definitive hemorrhage-control intervention within 30 minutes of placement.

Many programs have developed algorithms for the use of REBOA.[14,19] **Fig. 1** shows the one developed at the R Adams Cowley Shock Trauma Center in Baltimore, Maryland.[14] Such algorithms often delineate the appropriate patient as having a systolic BP (SBP) less than or equal to 90 mm Hg. While this may represent an objective indication of malperfusion, in clinical practice, this isolated number is problematic to identify the truly exsanguinating patient and may manifest late in the clinical course.[20,21] In addition, in a patient with baseline hypertension as a comorbid condition, a pressure under 110 mm Hg may represent true hypotension for that patient.[22]

In the absence of a TBI, many trauma clinicians may find a SBP of 90 mm Hg to be reasonable in the setting of concern for active hemorrhage.[23,24] The balance is of

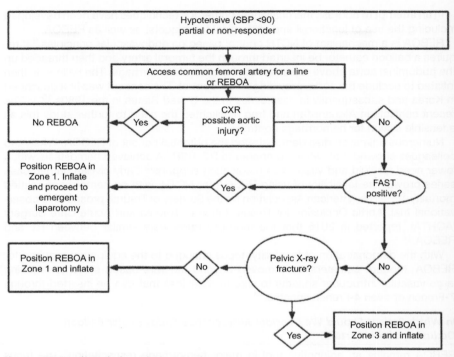

Fig. 1. REBOA clinical algorithm. CXR, chest x-ray.

reasonable perfusion of vital organs versus allowing hemostasis to begin without disruption of a fragile clot through a high arterial pressure. Signs of appropriate perfusion include the presence of a central and peripheral pulse and normal mental status.

Some characteristics may define the truly exsanguinating patient and include diaphoresis, pallor, collapsed veins, altered mental status, hypotension, tachycardia or bradycardia, falling or low end-tidal CO_2, and air hunger.[25] These changes may develop very rapidly and be challenging to identify. The early placement of an arterial line (ideally in the CFA) would assist in the clinical diagnosis of progressive hemorrhagic shock and should be considered in all critically injured patients. Early placement may actually infer a survival advantage.[26]

What Does the Clinician Using Resuscitative Endovascular Balloon Occlusion of the Aorta Need to Understand About the Anatomy?

Placement of REBOA requires an understanding of groin vascular as well as aortic anatomy.

Groin Vascular Anatomy

In order to gain access to the aorta, an introducer sheath needs to be inserted into the CFA. The CFA is a continuation of the external iliac artery as it crosses the inguinal ligament. It lies lateral to the common femoral vein and is about 4 cm in length. It ends by dividing into the superficial femoral artery (SFA) and the profunda femoris.

The CFA is a relatively-large-diameter groin artery. Placement of an introducer sheath in this vessel minimizes the risk of iatrogenic vascular injury, especially when larger introducer sheaths are placed. A potentially significant error can occur if the SFA is accessed in error. This requires an understanding of both the surface and ultrasound anatomy of the CFA.

The inguinal ligament spans from the anterior superior iliac spine laterally to the pubic tubercle medially. Note that this is higher than the inguinal crease, which is often erroneously used as a surface landmark. The CFA forms just medial of the midpoint of the inguinal ligament and can be reliably accessed 1-2 cm below this point. Given the short length of the CFA, using the inguinal crease as a landmark will inevitably cause the operator to access the SFA.

Aorta Anatomy

The aorta originates at the aortic orifice of the left ventricle. It has a short ascending segment which continues as the arch (beginning at the level of the second sterno-costal joint and ending at the level of the T4 vertebra). The arch has 3 major branches: the brachiocephalic trunk, the left common carotid artery, and the left subclavian artery. The descending aorta comprises a thoracic and abdominal segment. The abdominal aorta terminates around the level of T12 as the right and left common iliac arteries.

The REBOA catheter's balloon is typically inflated in either the descending thoracic or abdominal aorta. For the purposes of occlusion, the aorta is divided into 3 zones (**Table 1**). These correlate reliably to external landmarks based on imaging and cadaveric studies.[27,28]

How Do You Actually Do the Procedure?

Regardless of which make of REBOA catheter is used, the general principles remain the same. While efforts should be made to ensure this procedure is done in as sterile manner as possible, ultimately this is a life-saving procedure where time remains of the essence.

- Obtain CFA access
  - This is the rate-limiting step for REBOA (and any endovascular procedure). The clinician should consider obtaining access early, even before a definitive decision has been made to proceed with REBOA. As the patient progresses in hemorrhagic shock, the target vessel will continue to vasoconstrict and, hence, become more difficult to access. There remains a survival advantage to obtaining this access early.[26]
  - The introducer sheath and catheter are placed using the Seldinger technique. The available introducer sheaths and catheters are placed over a wire with a

Table 1
Aortic zones and surface external landmarks for use during placement of REBOA

Aortic Zone	Demarcation	External Landmark	Average Distance from the Common Femoral Artery
Zone 1	Left subclavian artery to celiac trunk	Midsternal line	45–50 cm
Zone 2	Celiac trunk to lowest renal artery	NA	NA
Zone 3	Lowest renal artery to aortic bifurcation	Umbilicus	25 cm

0.035-inch diameter. In order to prevent the need for a second arterial puncture, the initial arterial catheter should have a large-enough internal diameter
to accommodate a wire of this size. This typically translates to at least an
18-gauge or 4-French catheter.
  ○ Once the introducer sheath is placed, close the side-arm valve to ensure blood
    is not lost through this route.
- Prepare the catheter according to the manufacturer's requirements.
- Measure the length of insertion required based on clinical information and using
  external landmarks.
  ○ Regardless of the type of device used, place the bottom of the balloon against
    the external landmark to ensure an appropriate distance of insertion.
  ○ If a wire is required for the type of device used, this must also be measured for
    appropriate insertion length.
- Place the catheter through the introducer sheath.
  ○ If any resistance is met, stop the procedure and ensure the sheath is appropri-
    ately placed in the vessel.
- Once the appropriate depth of insertion is achieved, slowly inflate the balloon
  (with volumes according to the manufacturer's recommendations).
  ○ Only inflate using sterile water or saline. Using air risks an air embolism if the
    balloon were to rupture.
  ○ A 50:50 mix of saline and iodinated contrast can be used but is not strictly
    necessary.
  ○ The aortic diameter decreases from zone 1 to zone 3; hence, less volume is
    required to occlude at zone 3.
  ○ Monitor patient response; once appropriate occlusion is achieved, there is
    often a dramatic change in hemodynamics.
  ○ Stop inflating if you meet resistance.
- If time permits, confirm the position with plain x-ray imaging.
- Secure the catheter, noting the depth of insertion.
- Document the time of inflation, volume in the balloon, and depth of insertion.
- Expedite transfer to definitive care.
  ○ Once the balloon is inflated, the risk of ischemia is present. Therefore, despite
    the relative comfort of improved hemodynamics, it is important for the clinician
    not to be lulled into a false sense of security. All efforts should be made to
    expedite to definitive hemorrhage control.

What Happens After the Balloon Is Up?

Successful hemodynamic response to balloon inflation represents a breath of fresh air
to the clinician managing an exsanguinating patient who would very likely have deteriorated to traumatic arrest. While the collective tone in the room may relax somewhat,
it is important not be lulled into a false sense of security. The BP response is somewhat
artificial and remains at the cost of the impending ischemic burden being produced by
occluding blood flow to critical organs.

Assessment of Response

The hemodynamic response can be dramatic once the aorta is occluded, especially at
zone 1.[29,30] There is a marked increase in systemic vascular resistance, reflected in an
improvement in systolic and mean arterial pressure. The HR may also improve.
  Clinically, the patient may manifest improved responsiveness as the brain receives
improved perfusion. The trauma team should be aware of this, as the patient may

suddenly become aware of their surroundings. Skin perfusion may improve, and diaphoresis resolve.

Complete occlusion, especially at zone 1, may produce a supranormal BP. While most otherwise healthy individuals may be able to tolerate this, the rapid increase in BP may lead to inadvertent adverse effects, including the possibility of worsening of a previously relatively minor TBI, or precipitating cardiac failure in those with a preexisting cardiac disease.[31]

Therefore, the principle of permissive hypotension can be followed when using REBOA. Achieving a SBP of 80 to 90 mm Hg may be sufficient until definitive hemostasis is achieved. Adjustments can be made for the patient with suspected concomitant TBI or for those with comorbid conditions such as hypertension.

Physiology of Balloon Occlusion

Balloon occlusion in the setting of continuing fluid resuscitation leads to a marked and almost immediate improvement in hemodynamics and a profound rise in left ventricular (LV) afterload.[32] Zone 1 occlusion produces a more dramatic response. Although it seems likely that more distal occlusion will be better tolerated, early studies in a swine model did not demonstrate a difference in mortality or neurologic injury (paraplegia), based on zone 1 versus zone 3 occlusion.[33] However, evolving clinical observation seems to support better tolerance at zone 3.

Zone 1 balloon occlusion produces acute changes in cardiovascular physiology and organ perfusion, as predicted by the existing body of literature related to aortic cross-clamping for vascular surgeries. The physiologic response to zone 1 balloon occlusion, in a patient with a previously normal ventricle, is an increase in LV afterload, wall tension, and mean central aortic pressure, with an associated increase in the subendocardial oxygen demand. In a swine model of hemorrhagic shock, these changes were variable over time, based on the duration of balloon occlusion.[34] In elective vascular surgery patients, Roizen and colleagues described greater changes in physiology with more proximal aortic occlusion: occluding the descending thoracic aorta increased the mean arterial pressure (MAP) by 35% to 84%, pulmonary capillary wedge pressure by 90% to 190%, and central venous pressure by 35%.[35] Conversely, supraceliac occlusion increased end-diastolic and end-systolic area pressures by 28% and 69%, respectively, with decreases in ejection fraction and cardiac index of 38% and 29%, respectively.[35] Wall motion abnormalities were present in 92% of patients after occlusion.

Zone 3 occlusion does not typically produce the same profound cardiovascular changes as seen in zone 1 occlusion. In vascular surgery patients, infrarenal aortic cross-clamping leads to a mild increase in MAP (2%–8%), no change in pulmonary capillary wedge pressure or central venous pressure, and increases in end-diastolic and end-systolic area of 9% and 11%, respectively.[35] There is limited evidence of wall motion abnormalities in patients undergoing infrarenal occlusion, in contrast to those with more proximal occlusion.[35,36]

Aortic cross-clamping induces damage to the vascular endothelium.[36,37] Compared to aortic cross-clamping, REBOA may be a favorable alternative.[38] In particular, the concept of partially occluding the aorta is being explored. Russo and colleagues demonstrated that complete REBOA (C-REBOA) compared to partial REBOA aorta (P-REBOA) was accompanied by supraphysiologic proximal pressures in the C-REBOA group.[39] Supraphysiologic pressure was defined as a MAP greater than 110 mm Hg for the duration of balloon occlusion. Pressure gradients were maintained consistently between proximal and distal systolic pressures in each group. Pressure gradients averaged 90% in the C-REBOA group, 50% in the P-REBOA group, and

10% in the control group (no intervention). Lactate concentrations rose more rapidly in the C-REBOA group, and histologic changes in the duodenum (ischemic necrosis) and renal parenchyma (acute tubular necrosis) were observed.[39]

In a different animal model of hemorrhagic shock, the maximum tolerated duration for zone 1 balloon occlusion was about 60 minutes.[40] Both organ ischemia and mortality increased as the occlusion time approached 90 minutes. Maintaining proximal MAP near the normal physiologic target with P-REBOA may decrease the incidence of cerebral edema, respiratory failure, and cardiac dysfunction when compared to sustained aortic occlusion, but this hypothesis has not yet been prospectively studied in humans.

Hemodynamic instability after balloon deflation is reduced in patients undergoing P-REBOA versus C-REBOA, with less duodenal ischemia in the P-REBOA group despite equivalent visceral MAP.[16,41] This effect may be attributed to a phenomenon similar to ischemic preconditioning.[42]

Consideration should be given to having 2 arterial lines set up to measure BP above and below the balloon. This can take the form of having a radial arterial line, as well as a transducer attached to the side arm of the femoral access sheath. One manufacturer of REBOA does allow proximal aortic pressure to be measured directly through the balloon catheter.

As with traditional aortic cross-clamping for vascular surgeries, an increase in MAP with aortic occlusion does not imply correction of hypovolemia or resolution of distal bleeding. The circulating volume is essentially contracted above the point of occlusion. Full resuscitative measures should continue until the surgeon has identified and controlled the source of hemorrhage. While case-controlled data are limited, it seems clinically prudent to deliberately increase preload during aortic occlusion, in anticipation of balloon release.

Safe Occlusion Times

The safe duration of balloon occlusion in humans remains a challenge to define. There is to date no high-quality evidence in humans to support setting specific limits. The animal studies are however clearer in that prolonged balloon occlusion, especially at more proximal aortic sites, has a time-dependent effect on ischemia.[40] Prolonged occlusion inevitably leads to irreversible end-organ injury and multi-system organ failure.

For complete occlusion, consensus expert opinion advises occlusion at zone 1 for no longer than 60 minutes.[43] Many consider 30 minutes to be a safer goal. Zone 3 occlusion is likely to be better tolerated in clinical practice, and there are case reports of zone 3 occlusion times beyond 60 minutes without adverse outcomes. However, maintaining a rule-of-thumb of "shorter is better" allows the clinician to maintain a momentum toward rapid definitive hemorrhage control.

Likely, as our ability to perform P-REBOA improves, there will be better tolerance of more prolonged partial occlusion.

How Should You Let the Balloon Down?

REBOA balloon deflation is a tenuous time. The balloon may be deflated when hemostasis is achieved or to check for ongoing hemorrhage. Deflation is akin to releasing an aortic cross-clamp. A lactic acid load will accumulate in direct relation to the duration of occlusion. There is growing evidence to support the presence of hypocalcemia and hyperkalemia in both hemorrhagic shock and particularly following periods of balloon occlusion.[44] Along with the accompanying myocardial depression, release may result in decreases of LV afterload of 70% to 80% with resultant drops in MAP.[35,40] Coronary blood flow and LV end-diastolic volume also decrease by as much as 50%. This combination of lactic acid load, change in cardiac function, and ongoing hemorrhagic shock can lead to profound hypotension at the time of balloon deflation.

The resuscitation clinician (often the anesthesiologist at this point) should be prepared to administer further blood products, calcium, and potentially sodium bicarbonate as indicated.[44] Clear team communications are required. Balloon deflation should be gradual, allowing the surgeon to check for potential continued hemorrhage while the anesthesiologist monitors perfusion. If rapid deterioration occurs, the balloon can be reinflated to allow additional time for reassessment and planning. Once all hemorrhage is controlled and the patient is hemodynamically stable with the balloon deflated, resuscitation should be completed in accordance with usual practice. Monitoring of serum lactate is recommended as a guide to successful reversal of shock.

Are There Ways to Limit the Ischemic Burden from Resuscitative Endovascular Balloon Occlusion of the Aorta (and Prolong Occlusion Times)?

Limiting the ischemic burden of REBOA is a key question that is vexing clinicians. As reviewed above, there is ongoing animal work to develop an ideal balance of hemorrhage control and organ perfusion. Two techniques are under consideration. Intermittent REBOA (or I-REBOA) requires a period of complete occlusion, followed by variable periods of complete deflation which is either defined by reaching a certain BP or time duration. P-REBOA requires a period of complete occlusion (to allow clot formation to be initiated) followed by a graduated deflation of the balloon to allow a small amount of flow beyond the balloon to vital organs. Of note, of the currently available commercial devices, only one allows precise-enough control of the balloon volume for true P-REBOA. Most other devices provide an "all or nothing" approach to occlusion, essentially I-REBOA. The additional challenge is that the terms P-REBOA and I-REBOA are used somewhat variably in the literature, limiting generalizability of some of the results.[45]

A recent swine model by Kuckelman and colleagues compared I-REBOA using either pressure- or time-based strategies.[46] The pressure-based approach allowed a drop of MAP to 40 mm Hg, and the time-based approach used a cycle of 10 minutes of complete occlusion followed by 3 minutes of deflation. They concluded that I-REBOA presented a viable alternative to C-REBOA; the time-based regimen allowed higher survival and more prolonged occlusion times, but the pressure-based model was associated with the lowest degree of ischemic end-organ injury.

Hoareau and colleagues reached slightly different conclusions.[47] They compared (in swine) either I-REBOA or P-REBOA, each modality being used after 15 minutes of complete occlusion. They concluded that both techniques had a similar mortality rate, but the P-REBOA group required a lower period of time at full occlusion and had lower blood product needs. Follow on work from Johnson and colleagues showed that P-REBOA showed reduced time spent at full occlusion as well as fewer precipitous drops in MAP than I-REBOA.[48] P-REBOA also delivered more distal aortic blood flow without increasing the total blood loss. Again, mortality in this swine model was similar for both techniques.

It is important to understand the limitations of animal studies. Although swine anatomy can be a surrogate for humans, the presence of collateral circulation may limit their use. Bleeding is typically controlled and from a single injury site in many animal studies, and the follow-up period is relatively short before the animals are sacrificed. Most animal studies also have small numbers, again limiting generalizability.

Nevertheless, it is clear that to mitigate the effects of distal ischemia, a protocol should be established for implementation of a form of incomplete occlusion.[45] In clinical experience, due to the limitations of existing devices, this is best done by having accurate monitoring of arterial pressure both proximal and distal to the balloon. Proximal measurements can be obtained by placing a radial arterial line or by obtaining direct pressures through a suitable balloon catheter. Distal measurements, obtained by transducing the side arm of the introducer sheath, can target specific low pressures to ensure some flow is achieved across the balloon. It is recommended that all cases undergoing these techniques be enrolled into existing registries to determine clinical effectiveness.

What Other Complications Does the Clinical Team Need to Be Aware About?

Complications with the REBOA procedure can be divided into access-related, equipment-related, and procedural complications.[49]

Access-Related Complications

The primary challenge with the procedure is obtaining arterial access. This is often done with the patient in extremis, with limited time to optimize your surroundings and the technique before proceeding. In a retrospective review of patients who survived at least 48 hours after undergoing REBOA, there was an incidence of access-related complications of 8.6%.[50]

Access-related injuries can include direct arterial injury, often damaging the intima and creating pseudoaneurysms; distal thromboembolism; limb ischemia as a result of vessel occlusion; and retroperitoneal hemorrhage, especially if the artery is accessed above the inguinal ligament.[51]

Specific factors related to increased risk of injury include the use of large-caliber introducer sheaths and catheters, accessing smaller caliber vessels (eg, SFA) and requiring a cutdown to access the CFA (18.51). Complex groin-area injury may also predispose to an increased risk of vascular injury.

Mitigation techniques should be adopted to minimize the risk of access-related injury. The clinician placing REBOA should be intimately aware of the anatomy. The CFA should be the preferred vessel to access. Ultrasound-guided vascular access may limit the possibility of injury. Early vascular access should be strongly considered—this has the benefit of having a higher caliber vessel available before progression to worsening hemorrhagic shock. Lower-profile devices, if available, should be used. The catheter and sheath should be removed as soon as feasible. Limb perfusion must be regularly checked after the procedure for at least 24 hours—any concern should be appropriately interrogated and managed.

Equipment-Related Complications

The available equipment ranges from catheters used primarily by IR or vascular surgery colleagues to purpose-built catheters designed for use in trauma. Wire-based catheters carry the risk of wire-misplacement (in particular, entering branch vessels) or direct vascular injuries.

The balloon on each catheter is designed to accommodate a particular volume of fluid. Overinflation risks rupture of the balloon (and vascular injury). The balloon also may suffer damage while it traverses the introducer sheath.

The balloon, once inflated, may migrate downward as the pressure head above it pushes down on the balloon. This is a particular concern with zone 1 occlusion and with the use of smaller-profile catheters. Care must be taken to ensure migration has not occurred once the balloon is inflated, and the catheter should be secured rapidly once the appropriate occlusion and position has been achieved.

Procedural/Technique-Related Complications

Numerous potential complications can be ascribed to the technique. The primary complication is as a result of end-organ ischemia secondary to prolonged occlusion.[40,43,49,52] This has been detailed above, and the consequences include bowel ischemia, renal embarrassment, and spinal cord ischemia leading to paralysis. In patients with a preexisting cardiac disease, sudden increases in afterload may precipitate cardiac ischemia and failure.

Care must always be taken to exclude a supradiaphragmatic major vascular injury before balloon inflation. It is possible such an injury, such as a massive hemothorax or neck junctional injury, is inadvertently missed but made worse by balloon occlusion of the aorta. Clinical history, thorough examination, and simple adjuncts such as plain chest radiography and sonography can assist in identifying these injuries.

Are there opportunities to use resuscitative endovascular balloon occlusion of the aorta closer to the point of injury?

There remains a significant burden of potentially preventable prehospital death from torso hemorrhage worldwide. For example, the updated AORTA trial data included about 60% of patients who had prehospital cardiac arrest from torso hemorrhage.[53] Additional studies continue to highlight this burden.[54,55] Therefore, there has been much discussion about being able to use REBOA at the point of injury.

This however requires significant system-level support. The challenges include not only ensuring a prehospital team is able to do the procedure but also that transport to definitive care is expedited to minimize the burden of ischemic injury. Systems in London and Paris have overcome these obstacles and incorporated REBOA into a well-governed prehospital care system.[56,57] They provide key lessons for introducing similar innovations into existing agencies.

The military has also thought it is prudent to bring REBOA far-forward to combat the potentially preventable deaths from torso hemorrhage.[58] To date, the US Air Force and Belgian Special Operations Surgical Teams have used REBOA successfully close to the front line, including in mass casualty incidents.[59–61]

Elements of the procedure along with other advanced trauma-critical care concepts can be successfully brought closer to the point of injury if clinical teams are not able to fully incorporate REBOA.[62] This includes early ultrasound-guided CFA access. Placing the arterial line in the field will allow this key rate-limiting step to be accomplished earlier in the course of the patient's clinical journey and likely at a time when shock has not progressed to a point where the vessel is markedly vasoconstricted and difficult to access. This reinforces the importance of obtaining early vascular access.

In North America, many areas of the country may not have immediate access to a level-1 or level-2 trauma center. REBOA may allow a means to temporize bleeding when critically injured patients with NCTH present to level-3 centers. This could allow either the on-call but off-site surgeon to arrive to the hospital and take the patient to the OR or facilitate transport of the patient to a higher level of care.[63] The latter has been described within a US critical care transport system where REBOA was placed (but the balloon not inflated) by the physician team at a level-3 facility and the flight team was instructed on how to manage the catheter en route.[64] This included inflating the balloon should the patient's hemodynamics worsen. Given the current landscape (geographically and logistically) of trauma systems in North America, this could prove the most beneficial role for REBOA.

Can We Use Resuscitative Endovascular Balloon Occlusion of the Aorta for Other Indications?

NCTH is not isolated to traumatic injuries. Similar catastrophic situations can arise when the bleeding is from a gastrointestinal (GI) source (such as a bleeding gastric ulcer), nonaortic aneurysmal rupture, or obstetric source (such as from abnormal placentation, a ruptured ectopic pregnancy, or other causes of postpartum hemorrhage). All these could be temporarily controlled by REBOA.[65] Note that as the catheter is placed blindly, use in ruptured aortic aneurysms is not recommended because the catheter may easily traverse the thin wall of the aneurysm rather than stay in the lumen.

The use of REBOA for GI-source hemorrhage has been described in case series, primarily from Japan.[66] Of note, the bleeding source should not be from the portal venous system—it is unclear whether using REBOA in this instance may actually inadvertently worsen venous source bleeding. Typical catheter placement for GI-source hemorrhage is zone 1.

Obstetric-source hemorrhage presents an important opportunity to intervene with REBOA. Postpartum hemorrhage is still a very significant contributor to maternal mortality worldwide. In order to reduce the burden of death among this group of young, otherwise healthy women, REBOA was introduced in some centers (often in a coordinated fashion between obstetric and surgical teams) for both elective cases (when a known case of abnormally adherent placenta is known) and emergency cases.[67,68] Evolving international evidence supports the use of REBOA for this indication, with lower rates of hysterectomy and lower blood transfusion requirements than the standard therapy.

Another area of current investigation is the role of REBOA in nontraumatic cardiac arrest.[69] Out-of-hospital cardiac arrest remains a significant contributor to mortality around the world. The premise is that a form of mechanical support to the heart may improve cardiocerebral perfusion and improve the chance of achieving a return of spontaneous circulation (ROSC). Numerous animal studies have shown the potential benefit of using aortic balloon occlusion for this purpose. Recent prospective observational human data from Europe have shown the feasibility of applying this in humans, showing both increased end-tidal carbon dioxide levels and ROSC in their small cohort.[70] It is currently the subject of trials in both Europe and North America.[71] If the results are positive, this may allow an adjunct to advanced cardiac life support and may be an interim step before proceeding to the extracorporeal membrane oxygenation support.

Are there human factors to consider with the use of resuscitative endovascular balloon occlusion of the aorta?

REBOA is a potentially life-saving procedure in the appropriate patient. Equally, if used inappropriately, it can worsen morbidity and mortality. While the procedural steps are easy to learn, it is much more complex to implement this within the trauma system to allow maximal patient safety. Doing so requires an interprofessional, multidisciplinary approach involving all stakeholders. Leading the effort should be a physician champion who can "own" the process and ensure appropriate quality assurance and review all cases undergoing REBOA.[72]

All proceduralists (regardless of specialty) should ideally undertake an approved training course for REBOA. In the author's opinion, a cadaver-based course is most appropriate. Secondary training should then be done at the local institution. This allows local factors to be taken into account, including the logistics of equipment storage, practice with arterial line monitoring, ensuring an appropriate documentation template is used, and identifying the acute time taken to transfer to the OR. By reviewing all these processes, simple solutions can be identified to shorten the time to definitive care. Such marginal gains, driven by input from the entire care team, can assist in reducing the time of aortic occlusion. Simulation can play a key role in assisting with identifying challenges and opportunities, as well as in maintaining skills in this procedure.

All members of our interprofessional team, including physicians and nurses from the ED, trauma surgery, vascular surgery, and anesthesiology, play key roles in the safe delivery of REBOA. Important support is also provided by radiology and OR staff. Therefore, each of these members must receive directed training to understand their own role and that of the wider health care team when a patient undergoes REBOA.

The resuscitation room in particular can allow an interplay of roles. The emergency physician, proficient in ultrasound, may be tasked to perform the FAST examination or even obtain ultrasound-guided arterial access. If the trauma surgeon is the only one trained to place REBOA, they can hand off the resuscitation team leadership to the emergency physician. This prevents the trauma surgeon from losing situational awareness of the resuscitation as they become task-focused in the procedure.

Similarly in the OR, as the surgeon becomes task-focused with achieving hemorrhage control, they may lose situational awareness of the duration of balloon occlusion. Ensuring the anesthesiology team understands the principles of REBOA can allow them to keep track of the balloon inflation time and continually relay this information to the surgeon. This offloads a crucial task from the surgeon so that their main focus can remain on achieving hemorrhage control.

REBOA is a rarely performed procedure, and there is a possibility of cognitive overload remembering the setup of the equipment and the procedural steps when this procedure is called for. Developing a checklist and algorithm for the procedure is helpful to recall the order of tasks in the moment. In order to offload the cognitive task of remembering how the various pieces of equipment should be laid out, they can be labeled numerically or alphabetically. This allows very rapid access to all the items needed in the order that they are to be used for the procedure.

It is strongly recommended that a robust quality-assurance program is in place to monitor competency and patient safety within a REBOA program. Centers implementing a REBOA program should develop a local database as well as contribute to any national/international studies concerning REBOA. As with other high-acuity low-occurrence procedures, skills for REBOA should be maintained and refreshed at regular intervals, as this can deteriorate rapidly if the procedure is not done for long periods.[73]

SUMMARY

There remains a continuing challenge of addressing potentially preventable death from NCTH. REBOA presents one option to add to the resuscitation toolbox for subdiaphragmatic exsanguinating hemorrhage. It carries the benefit of being a minimally invasive, proactive resuscitation tool that builds on principles of the Seldinger-technique vascular access. It carries the benefit of arresting hemorrhage to allow for transition to definitive care although at the potential cost of limb and organ ischemia if the aorta is inadvertently left occluded for prolonged periods of time. Evolution in both equipment and technique likely will allow safer duration of balloon occlusion through the use of P-REBOA and lower risk of vascular injury through the development of lower profile devices. There is also a potential for use in nontraumatic hemorrhage and even medical cardiac arrest. Nevertheless, underpinning successful utilization of REBOA is a system-based multidisciplinary approach to ensure safe utilization and optimal patient outcomes.

CLINICS CARE POINTS

- When evaluating major trauma patients, it is important to identify patients with noncompressible torso hemorrhage who will be at high risk of early death. These patients will have major injury in the chest, abdomen, and/or pelvis.
- The global management of these patients involves attention to oxygenation/ventilation and blood-product resuscitation, but the clinician should consider placing an early common femoral arterial line to allow close monitoring, as well as ease of progressing to endovascular procedures like REBOA.
- REBOA may be used to temporarily stop noncompressible torso hemorrhage in the abdomen of the pelvis.
- REBOA is contraindicated with major supradiaphragmatic vascular injuries, including neck and axillary arterial bleeding, tamponade, and massive hemothorax.
- Once the REBOA balloon is inflated, the trauma team must be expeditious about moving the patient to definitive care so as to minimize the adverse effects of ischemia related to aortic occlusion.
- Teamwork and attention to task saturation and its prevention must be incorporated in order for the trauma team to safely and effectively use REBOA.

DISCLOSURE

The authors have nothing to disclose.

REFERENCES

1. Kauvar DS, Lefering R, Wade CE. Impact of hemorrhage on trauma outcome: an overview of epidemiology, clinical presentations, and therapeutic considerations. J Trauma 2006;60(6 Suppl):S3–11.
2. Eastridge BJ, Mabry RL, Seguin P, et al. Death on the battlefield (2001-2011): implications for the future of combat casualty care. J Trauma Acute Care Surg 2012; 73(6 Suppl 5):S431–7.
3. Morrison JJ, Rasmussen TE. Noncompressible torso hemorrhage: a review with contemporary definitions and management strategies. Surg Clin North Am 2012;92(4):843–58.
4. Morrison J, Stannard A, Rasmussen TE, et al. Injury pattern and mortality of noncompressible torso hemorrhage in UK combat casualties. J Trauma Acute Care Surg 2013;75(2):S263–8.
5. Kisat M, Morrison JJ, Hashmi ZG, et al. Epidemiology and outcomes of noncompressible torso hemorrhage. J Surg Res 2013;184(1):414–21.
6. Ledgerwood AM, Kazmers M, Lucas CE. The role of thoracic aortic occlusion for massive hemoperitoneum. J Trauma 1976;16(8):610–5.
7. Hughes M, Perkins Z. Outcomes following resuscitative thoracotomy for abdominal exsanguination, a systematic review. Scand J Trauma Resusc Emerg Med 2020;28(1):9.
8. Seamon MJ, Shiroff AM, Franco M, et al. Emergency department thoracotomy for penetrating injuries of the heart and great vessels: an appraisal of 283 consecutive cases from two urban trauma centers. J Trauma 2009;67(6):1250–7.

9. Starnes BW, Quiroga E, Hutter C, et al. Management of ruptured abdominal aortic aneurysm in the endovascular era. J Vasc Surg 2010;51:9–18.
10. Hughes CW. Use of an intra-aortic balloon catheter tamponade for controlling intra-abdominal hemorrhage in man. Surgery 1954;36(1):65.
11. Low RB, Longmore W, Rubinstein R, et al. Preliminary report on the use of the Percluder occluding aortic balloon in human beings. Ann Emerg Med 1986;15:1466–9.
12. Gupta BK, Khaneja SC, Flores L, et al. The role of intra-aortic balloon occlusion in penetrating abdominal trauma. J Trauma 1989;29(6):861–5.
13. White JM, Cannon JW, Stannard A, et al. Endovascular balloon occlusion of the aorta is superior to resuscitative thoracotomy with aortic clamping in a porcine model of hemorrhagic shock. Surgery 2011;150(3):400–9.
14. Brenner ML, Moore LJ, DuBose JJ, et al. A clinical series of resuscitative endovascular balloon occlusion of the aorta for hemorrhage control and resuscitation. J Trauma Acute Care Surg 2013;75(3):506–11.
15. Moore LJ, Brenner M, Kozar RA, et al. Implementation of resuscitative endovascular balloon occlusion of the aorta as an alternate to resuscitative thoracotomy for noncompressible truncal hemorrhage. J Trauma Acute Care Surg 2015;79(4):523–30.
16. Norii T, Crandall C, Terasaka Y. Survival of severe blunt trauma patients treated with resuscitative endovascular balloon occlusion of the aorta compared with propensity score-adjusted untreated patients. J Trauma Acute Care Surg 2015;78(4):721–8.
17. DuBose JJ, Scalea TM, Brenner M, et al, AAST AORTA Study Group. The AAST prospective Aortic Occlusion for Resuscitation in Trauma and Acute Care Surgery (AORTA) registry: data on contemporary utilization and outcomes of aortic occlusion and resuscitative balloon occlusion of the aorta (REBOA). J Trauma Acute Care Surg 2016;81(3):409–19.
18. Teeter WA, Matsumoto J, Idoguchi K, et al. Smaller introducer sheaths for REBOAmay be associated with fewer complications. J Trauma Acute Care Surg 2016;81(6):1039–45.
19. Napolitano LM. Resuscitative endovascular balloon occlusion of the aorta: indications, outcomes, and training. Crit Care Clin 2017;33(1):55–70.
20. Parks JK, Elliott AC, Gentilello LM, et al. Systemic hypotension is a late marker of shock after trauma: a validation study of Advanced Trauma Life Support principles in a large national sample. Am J Surg 2006;192(6):727–31.
21. Edelman DA, White MT, Tyburski JG, et al. Post-traumatic hypotension: should systolic blood pressure of 90-109 mmHg be included? Shock 2007;27(2):134–8.
22. Eastridge BJ, Salinas J, McManus JG, et al. Hypotension begins at 110 mm Hg: redefining "hypotension" with data. J Trauma 2007;63(2):291–7.
23. Woodward L, Alsabri M. Permissive hypotension vs. conventional resuscitation in patients with trauma or hemorrhagic shock: a review. Cureus 2021;13(7):e16487.
24. Tran A, Yates J, Lau A, et al. Permissive hypotension versus conventional resuscitation strategies in adult trauma patients with hemorrhagic shock: a systematic review and meta-analysis of randomized controlled trials. J Trauma Acute Care Surg 2018;84(5):802–8.
25. Lendrum R, Perkins Z, Chana M, et al. Reply to: Prehospital REBOA: time to clearly define the relevant indications. Resuscitation 2019;142:191–2.
26. Matsumura Y, Matsumoto J, Kondo H, et al. Early arterial access for resuscitative endovascular balloon occlusion of the aorta is related to survival outcome in trauma. J Trauma Acute Care Surg 2018;85(3):507–11.

27. Morrison JJ, Stannad A, Midwinter MJ, et al. Prospective evaluation of the correlation between torso height and aortic anatomy in respect of a fluoroscopy free aortic balloon occlusion system. Surgery 2014;155(6):1044–51.

28. Eliason JL, Derstine BA, Horbal SR, et al. Computed tomography correlation of skeletal landmarks and vascular anatomy in civilian adult trauma patients: implications for resuscitative endovascular balloon occlusion of the aorta. J Trauma Acute Care Surg 2019;87(1S Suppl 1):S138–45.

29. Qasim ZA, Sikorski RA. Physiologic considerations in trauma patients undergoing resuscitative endovascular balloon occlusion of the aorta. Anesth Analg 2017; 125(3):891–4.

30. Engdahl AS, Parrino CR, Wasicek PJ, et al. Anesthetic management of patients after traumatic injury with resuscitative endovascular balloon occlusion of the aorta. Anesth Analg 2019;129(5):e146–9.

31. Uchino H, Tamura N, Echigoya R, et al. REBOA"-is it really safe? A case with massive intracranial hemorrhage possibly due to endovascular balloon occlusion of the aorta (REBOA). Am J Case Rep 2016;17:810–3.

32. Russo RM, Neff LP, Johnson MA, et al. Emerging endovascular therapies for noncompressible torso hemorrhage. Shock 2016;46:12–9.

33. Long KN, Houston RIV, Watson JD, et al. Functional outcome after resuscitative endovascular balloon occlusion of the aorta of the proximal and distal thoracic aorta in a swine model of controlled hemorrhage. Ann Vasc Surg 2015;29: 114–21.

34. Markov NP, Percival TJ, Morrison JJ, et al. Physiologic tolerance of descending thoracic aortic balloon occlusion in a swine model of hemorrhagic shock. Surgery 2013;153:848–56.

35. Roizen MF, Beaupre PN, Alpert RA, et al. Monitoring with twodimensional transesophageal echocardiography. Comparison of myocardial function in patients undergoing supraceliac, suprarenal-infraceliac, or infrarenal aortic occlusion. J Vasc Surg 1984;1:300–5.

36. Gelman S. The pathophysiology of aortic cross-clamping and unclamping. Anesthesiology 1995;82:1026–60.

37. Geenens R, Famaey N, Gijbels A, et al. Arterial vasoreactivity is equally affected by in vivo cross-clamping with increasing loads in young and middle-aged mice aortas. Ann Thorac Cardiovasc Surg 2016;22:38–43.

38. Abe T, Uchida M, Nagata I, et al. Resuscitative endovascular balloon occlusion of the aorta versus aortic cross clamping among patients with critical trauma: a nationwide cohort study in Japan. Crit Care 2016;20:400.

39. Russo RM, Neff LP, Lamb CM, et al. Partial resuscitative endovascular balloon occlusion of the aorta in swine model of hemorrhagic shock. J Am Coll Surg 2016; 223:359–68.

40. Morrison JJ, Ross JD, Markov NP, et al. The inflammatory sequelae of aortic balloon occlusion in hemorrhagic shock. J Surg Res 2014;191:423–31.

41. Saito N, Matsumoto H, Yagi T, et al. Evaluation of the safety and feasibility of resuscitative endovascular balloon occlusion of the aorta. J Trauma Acute Care Surg 2015;78:897–903.

42. Ulus AT, Yavas S, Sapmaz A, et al. Effect of conditioning on visceral organs during indirect ischemia/reperfusion injury. Ann Vasc Surg 2014;28:437–44.

43. Bulger EM, Perina DG, Qasim Z, et al. Clinical use of resuscitative endovascular balloon occlusion of the aorta (REBOA) in civilian trauma systems in the USA, 2019: a joint statement of the American College of Surgeons Committee on Trauma, the American College of Emergency Physicians, the National

Association of Emergency Medical Services Physicians, and the National Association of Emergency Medical Technicians. Trauma Surg Acute Care Open 2019; 4(1):e000376.

44. Abid M, Neff LP, Russo RM, et al. Reperfusion repercussions: A review of metabolic derangements following resuscitative endovascular balloon occlusion of the aorta. J Trauma Acute Care Surg 2020;89(2S Suppl 2):S39–44.

45. Russo RM, White JM, Baer DG. Partial resuscitative endovascular balloon occlusion of the aorta: a systematic review of the preclinical and clinical literature. J Surg Res 2021;262:101–14.

46. Kuckelman J, Derickson M, Barron M, et al. Efficacy of intermittent versus standard resuscitative endovascular balloon occlusion of the aorta in a lethal solid organ injury model. J Trauma Acute Care Surg 2019;87(1):9–17.

47. Hoareau G, Caples C, Spruce M, et al. Extending the golden hour: intermittent versus partial REBOA for prolonged hemorrhage control. Ann Emerg Med 2019;74(4 Suppl):S135.

48. Johnson MA, Hoareau GL, Beyer CA, et al. Not ready for prime time: Intermittent versus partial resuscitative endovascular balloon occlusion of the aorta for prolonged hemorrhage control in a highly lethal porcine injury model. J Trauma Acute Care Surg 2020;88(2):298–304.

49. Davidson AJ, Russo RM, Reva VA, et al. The pitfalls of resuscitative endovascular balloon occlusion of the aorta: risk factors and mitigation strategies. J Trauma Acute Care Surg 2018;84(1):192–202.

50. Laverty RB, Treffalls RN, McEntire SE, et al. Life over limb: arterial access-related limb ischemic complications in 48-hour REBOA survivors. J Trauma Acute Care Surg 2022;92(4):723–8.

51. Wasicek PJ, Teeter WA, Yang S, et al. Life over limb: lower extremity ischemia in the setting of resuscitative endovascular balloon occlusion of the aorta (REBOA). Am Surg 2018;84(6):971–7.

52. Joseph B, Zeeshan M, Sakran JV, et al. Nationwide analysis of resuscitative endovascular balloon occlusion of the aorta in civilian trauma. JAMA Surg 2019; 154(6):500–8.

53. Brenner M, Inaba K, Aiolfi A, et al. Resuscitative endovascular balloon occlusion of the aorta and resuscitative thoracotomy in select patients with hemorrhagic shock: early results from the American Association for the Surgery of Trauma's Aortic Occlusion for Resuscitation in Trauma and Acute Care Surgery registry. J Am Coll Surg 2018;226(5):730–40.

54. Kalkwarf KJ, Drake SA, Yang Y, et al. Bleeding to death in a big city. An analysis of all trauma deaths from hemorrhage in a metropolitan area during 1 year. J Trauma Acute Care Surg 2020;89(4):716–22.

55. Davis JS, Satahoo SS, Butler FK, et al. An analysis of prehospital deaths: who can we save? J Trauma Acute Care Surg 2014;77(2):213–8.

56. Lendrum R, Perkins Z, Chana M, et al. Pre-hospital resuscitative endovascular balloon occlusion of the aorta (REBOA) for exsanguinating pelvic hemorrhage. Resuscitation 2019;135:6–13.

57. Lamhaut L, Qasim Z, Hutin A, et al. First description of successful use of zone 1 resuscitative endovascular balloon occlusion of the aorta in the prehospital setting. Resuscitation 2018;133:e1–2.

58. Butler FK Jr, Holcomb JB, Shackelford S, et al. Advanced resuscitative care in tactical combat casualty care: TCCC guidelines change 18-01:14 October 2018. J Spec Oper Med 2018;18(4):37–55.

59. Lyon RF, Northern DM. REBOA by a non-surgeon as an adjunct during MASCAL. Am J Emerg Med 2018;36(6):1121.e5–6.
60. Northern DM, Manley JD, Lyon R, et al. Recent advances in austere combat surgery: use of aortic balloon occlusion as well as blood challenges by special operations medical forces in recent combat operations. J Trauma Acute Care Surg 2018;85(1S Suppl 2):S98–103.
61. De Schoutheete JC, Fourneau I, Waroquier F, et al. Three cases of resuscitative endovascular balloon occlusion of the aorta (REBOA) in austere pre-hospital environment-technical and methodological aspects. World J Emerg Surg 2018; 13:54.
62. Qasim Z, Butler FK, Holcomb JB, et al. Selective prehospital advanced resuscitative care-developing a strategy to prevent prehospital deaths from noncompressible torso hemorrhage. Shock 2022;57(1):7–14.
63. Yamamoto R, Alarhayem A, Muir MT, et al. Gaining or wasting time? Influence of time to operating room on mortality after temporary hemostasis using resuscitative endovascular balloon occlusion of the aorta. Am J Surg 2022;224(1 Pt A): 125–30, epub ahead of print.
64. Weir R, Lee J, Almroth S, et al. Flying with a safety net: use of REBOA to enable safe transfer to a level 1 trauma center. J Endovasc Trauma Management 2021; 5(3):122–8.
65. Hoehn MR, Hansraj NZ, Pasley AM, et al. Resuscitative endovascular balloon occlusion of the aorta for non-traumatic intra-abdominal hemorrhage. Eur J Trauma Emerg Surg 2019;45(4):713–8.
66. Sano H, Tsurukiri J, Hoshiai A, et al. Resuscitative endovascular balloon occlusion of the aorta for uncontrollable nonvariceal upper gastrointestinal bleeding. World J Emerg Surg 2016;11:20.
67. Riazanova OV, Reva Va, Fox KA, et al. Open versus endovascular REBOA control of blood loss during cesarean delivery in the placenta accreta spectrum: a single-center retrospective case control study. Eur J Obstet Gynecol Reprod Biol 2021;258:23–8.
68. Kamijo K, Nakajima M, Shigemi D, et al. Resuscitative endovascular balloon occlusion of the aorta for life-threatening postpartum hemorrhage: a nationwide observational study in Japan. J Trauma Acute Care Surg 2022;93(3):418–23. Epub ahead of print.
69. Daley J, Morrison JJ, Sather J, et al. The role of resuscitative endovascular balloon occlusion of the aorta (REBOA) as an adjunct to ACLS in non-traumatic cardiac arrest. Am J Emerg Med 2017;35(5):731–6.
70. Gamberini L, Coniglio C, Lupi C, et al. Resuscitative endovascular balloon occlusion of the aorta (REBOA) for refractory out of hospital cardiac arrest. An Utstein-based Case Series Resuscitation 2021;165:161–9.
71. Brede JR, Skulberg AK, Rehn M, et al. REBOARREST, Resuscitative endovascular balloon occlusion of the aorta in non-traumatic out-of-hospital cardiac arrest: a study protocol for a randomized parallel group, clinical multicenter trial. Trials 2021;22(1):511.
72. Qasim Z, Bradley K, Panichelli H, et al. Successful interprofessional approach to development of a resuscitative endovascular balloon occlusion of the aorta program at a community trauma center. J Emerg Med 2018;54(5):419–26.
73. Hatchimonji JS, Sikoutris J, Smith BP, et al. The REBOA dissipation curve: training starts to wane at 6 months in absence of clinical REBOA cases. J Surg Educ 2020;77(6):1598–604.

Extracorporeal Life Support for Trauma

Joseph Hamera, MD*, Ashley Menne, MD

KEYWORDS

• ECMO • ARDS • Respiratory failure • ECPR

KEY POINTS

- Extracorporeal membrane oxygenation (ECMO) is a lifesaving intervention for support of trauma patients suffering from post-injury severe respiratory failure.
- With training, the technical skills of ECMO cannulation are accessible to most surgeons and intensivists involved in the care of trauma patients.
- Using a systematic approach and with readily available bedside equipment, most ECMO circuit troubleshooting can be accomplished bedside by a trained intensivist.
- In general, the risk of hemorrhage is not a contraindication to ECMO for trauma patients as current technologies and data permit conservative or anticoagulation-free strategies.

INTRODUCTION

Extracorporeal membrane oxygenation (ECMO) has achieved widespread adoption for a variety of medically refractory cardiac and pulmonary conditions. Although most of the ECMO performed worldwide is for non-traumatic conditions, the first applications of ECMO in the adult population were for traumatic acute respiratory distress syndrome (ARDS).[1] Currently, despite expanding indications and increased utilization, the application of ECMO for trauma represents less than 1% of all ECMO runs.[2] Despite the relatively infrequent presentation of trauma patients suitable for ECMO, this therapy results in reasonable outcomes and has been suggested to improve survival.[3–7]

Evidence and Epidemiology

In the most robust description of ECMO utilization to date, traumatic indications account for approximately 1% of all ECMO runs greater than [2(p3),3]. However, the overall trauma ECMO volumes increased substantially in the latter portion of the analysis, mirroring global trends in increasing the use of ECMO for non-traumatic disease after the

Department of Emergency Medicine, R Adams Cowley Shock Trauma Center, University of Maryland School of Medicine, 22 South Greene Street, Baltimore MD 21201, USA
* Corresponding author. 155 N Fresno St, Fresno CA 93701.
E-mail address: jhamera@gmail.com

Emerg Med Clin N Am 41 (2023) 89–100
https://doi.org/10.1016/j.emc.2022.09.012
0733-8627/23/© 2022 Elsevier Inc. All rights reserved.

2009 H1N1 pandemic. Veno-venous (VV) ECMO was the most commonly used configuration of ECMO and the most common indication was therefore respiratory failure.[2] A minority of ECMO runs in trauma were configured as veno-arterial (VA) ECMO for either traumatic cardiac failure or extracorporeal CPR (ECPR). The most common traumatic indication for ECMO is respiratory failure resulting from blunt thoracic trauma.[3]

Most published descriptions of ECMO in trauma report generally favorable prognosis and comparable survival to non-traumatic ECMO.[3] Propensity-matched studies suggest superior survival when VV ECMO is used in appropriately selected trauma patients with severe ARDS, but due to the rarity of the disease, heterogeneous patient population and ethical considerations randomized clinical trial data do not exist.[8,9]

Extracorporeal Membrane Oxygenation Circuit Components

The ECMO circuit is a simplified and miniaturized version of the cardiopulmonary bypass machine used in cardiac surgery. Recent developments in materials and component engineering have greatly simplified the implantation of the ECMO circuit. A conceptual diagram of the VA and VV ECMO circuits is shown in **Fig. 1**. Individual programs will use equipment from various manufacturers and configure circuits slightly differently; an example of one center's equipment is shown in **Fig. 2**.

Blood is drained from the body through a large-diameter multistage cannula (known commonly as either the drainage, outflow, or venous cannula). For most patients, this is inserted into one of the femoral veins either percutaneously or by surgical cutdown and advanced as close as possible to the right atrium (RA) and inferior vena cava (IVC) junction.

Blood then travels through the tubing to the pump head. Most contemporary adult pumps are magnetically suspended centrifugal flow rotary pumps. The operator sets the RPM of the pump head and the flow depends on the adequate supply of blood to the pump head as well as the pressure downstream. Even with modern magnetically

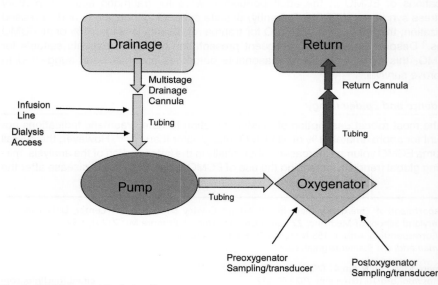

Fig. 1. ECMO conceptual circuit.

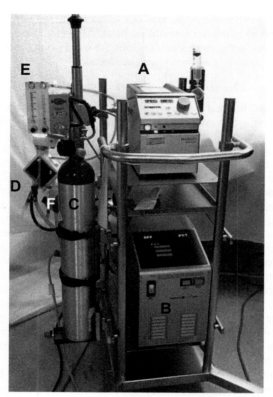

Fig. 2. Example of ECMO Machinery[33](*A*) Control Console (*B*) Heat Exchanger (*C*) Backup/ transport gas source (*D*) Oxygenator (*E*) Gas Blender (*F*) Emergency hand crank.

suspended pumps, a higher pump RPM will increase shear stress and thermal injury resulting in increasingly unacceptable levels of hemolysis.

From the pump head blood then passes through the oxygenator. Modern oxygenators consist of thousands of gas-porous microfiber tubules arranged in parallel to provide a compact and efficient surface for gas exchange. Connected to the oxygenator is the gas supply, which flows fresh gas through the air side of the membrane lung. The rate of this gas flow is referred to as the "sweep." Built into most oxygenators is a heat exchanger.

After passing through the membrane lung, the blood path then goes into the return cannula (also referred to as "arterial") and back into the patient. In VV ECMO, this is placed into the venous circulation, typically into the right internal jugular vein. In peripheral VA ECMO, the return cannula is typically placed into the femoral artery and ends in the abdominal aorta, pumping blood into the central circulation in a retrograde fashion.

Various customization options exist for circuit configuration. Of particular interest to trauma, infusion limbs can be placed pre-pump allowing extremely rapid volume administration. Renal replacement therapy can be performed directly through the circuit as well. Stopcocks placed at various points along the blood path allow infusion of medications and sampling. Increased connectors within a circuit increase failure points, increase complexity, increase infection risk, and increase the risk of blood stasis and clotting. In general, while the connection points should be minimized as much as practical, splicing in necessary access points later requires temporary discontinuation of support and all of the accompanying risks.[10] Balancing the merits of ensuring the circuit is properly configured for any anticipated needs with the risk of excessively complicated circuit design is an individualized decision.

Veno-Venous vs Veno-Arterial

The initiation of ECMO is a complex process requiring staff with various skills. First, the surgical skills of cannulation are described below. Although the general principles will be very familiar to emergency physicians and intensivists, there are several nuances and cautions described for the placement of such large cannulae. Second, as described above, the ECMO circuit is a formidably complex apparatus. Because of this, specially qualified staff in the form of perfusionists and/or ECMO specialists assist in the procedure to facilitate rapid and seamless initiation. Finally, ECMO initiation is a time of rapid hemodynamic changes as tissue oxygen delivery is restored. Careful monitoring and anticipation of hemodynamic changes by critical care nurses and physicians are important to avoid complications. A general approach to the organization and responsibilities of a cannulation team is shown in **Fig. 3**.

The dominant form of ECMO used in the setting of trauma is VV, representing at least 70% of the total ECMO runs. The indication for VV ECMO is pulmonary failure resulting in an inability to provide adequate oxygenation with a mechanical ventilator, most commonly in trauma caused by ARDS or tracheobronchial tree injury.[2,3,7,9,11] No specific criteria for trauma exist and the initiation criteria can be largely extrapolated from the general ARDS population in combination with clinical judgment. As posttraumatic ARDS is not commonly a hyperacute phenomenon. The mean time to initiation of ECMO is measured in days.

A variety of configuration options exist for VV ECMO, of which the simplest is a peripherally inserted two-cannula configuration. Access can be accomplished percutaneously with ultrasound guidance or via surgical cutdown. Percutaneous ultrasound-guided technique is more commonly used and is a relatively straightforward elaboration on skills possessed by critical care and emergency physicians. There

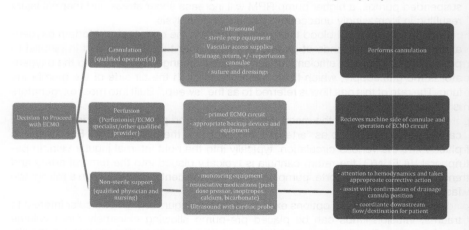

Fig. 3. Diagram of the ECMO cannulation process. Starting at the decision to initiate ECMO, the second level describes the three major task groups consisting of cannulating operators, skilled circuit management, and resuscitation staff. The third level gives an abbreviated list of equipment each role requires. The third level gives a general description of the tasks each personnel group should be ready to perform to ensure a safe cannulation.

are a few technical considerations relative to conventional central vascular access. First, in the femoral vessels, specific cannulation of the common femoral vein (for VV ECMO) or common femoral artery (for VA ECMO) is essential to ensure the safe accommodation of the very large cannulae. Second, puncture at the 12-o'clock position is likewise essential for the same reason. Finally, a relatively shallow angle of approach is desired to avoid kinking and sharp turns with the less flexible dilators and cannulae during insertion.[12,13]

The drainage cannula is typically inserted into the common femoral vein. Under ultrasound guidance, an initial vascular catheter or sheath is placed. After confirmation of puncture of the appropriate vessel and satisfactory access technique, a long wire is then passed through the sheath and ideally visualized passing through the intrahepatic IVC with ultrasound or fluoroscopy. A generous skin incision is made and serial dilation is performed to accommodate the multistage drainage cannula. Under real-time fluoroscopic or ultrasound guidance, the cannula is advanced to the cavoatrial junction and secured.

The return cannula can be placed in either the right internal jugular or the contralateral femoral vein. Subclavian positioning is uncommon due to the placement of a large cannula in a non-compressible site, and the turns required to position in the left internal jugular are undesirable. The access technique is largely similar, with the caveat that positioning is less particular as blood returned to the superior vena cava (SVC) will be entrained by the right atrium. In general, some separation between the drainage and return cannulae is desired, but close positioning does not guarantee that recirculation will occur. ECMO support is then initiated.

Another option for VV ECMO is the dual lumen cannula, incorporating the drainage and return into one device. These are typically placed in the right internal jugular vein. The return lumen is directed out of one side of the cannula. To avoid recirculation or vascular injury, the jet of the return blood must be carefully directed toward the tricuspid valve. For this reason, transesophageal echo is often used during cannulation to guide positioning. Care must be taken when securing and managing the cannula to prevent migration of cannula depth or rotational migration of the cannula.

Veno-Arterial Extracorporeal Membrane Oxygenation and Procedural Technique

For primary cardiac failure as a result of trauma, VA ECMO is the modality of choice. VA ECMO in trauma carries higher mortality than VV ECMO in most series, likely as a reflection of more acute and difficult-to-manage underlying injury such as cardiac contusion or post-arrest myocardial dysfunction.[13] VA ECMO is also a possible therapy for cardiac arrest ECPR in the management of traumatic injuries. Because of the high blood flow rates and efficient heat exchangers on ECMO circuits, VA ECMO is a potent tool for managing cardiac arrest secondary to hypothermia.[14]

The initial cannulation for VA ECMO is broadly similar to the above-described steps for VV ECMO cannulation. In place of a venous return cannula, a smaller diameter return cannula is usually placed in the femoral artery. Owing to the relatively large size of the cannula, distal perfusion of the leg is at risk with an incidence of up to 10% to 70% with the need for fasciotomy in up to 8%.[15–17] The risk of ischemia is reduced by the placement of a distal perfusion cannula (DPC). The decision to place DPC prophylactically at the time of cannulation versus placement upon evidence of limb hypoperfusion is program specific but is recommended by extracorporeal life support organization (ELSO).[13,18] Distal perfusion is accomplished with a smaller bore arterial sheath (typically 6 French diameter) inserted antegrade into the superficial femoral artery (SFA). The arterial puncture site should be as close as possible to the cannula entry site to minimize the low-flow zone and avoid missing perfusion of branch arteries.

The DPC is attached to the arterial return cannula via a side port and the flow down the DPC should be monitored to ensure that flow is adequate and that it is not excessive to detract from delivery to the rest of the body.

Monitoring and Support on Extracorporeal Membrane Oxygenation

Patients on ECMO require continuous monitoring of their physiology, machine function, and constant attendance by trained staff. At a minimum, all patients should have continuous telemetry monitoring, pulse oximetry, and invasive arterial blood pressure monitoring.[11,19] Serial radiographs should be followed to monitor the cannula position and the development of other complications. Staff trained in the management of system failure should be present at all times; depending on local program protocols, this can include perfusionists, specifically trained ECMO specialists, or nursing staff with demonstrated competency.

From a machinery perspective, at minimum continuous monitoring of rpm and flow are necessary. Various newer generation systems can continuously monitor access pressures and pre-oxygenator oxygen saturation, although with some marginal added expense. Oxygenator function should be assessed in a protocolized manner with regular assessment of post-oxygenator blood gasses. If the oxygenator is failing to deliver gas or is suspected to be responsible for a flow issue, a transmembrane pressure can be displayed or transduced to evaluate for obstruction. The cannula position should be assessed regularly to detect migration or failure of securing sutures.

For patients on VV ECMO, the adequacy of support is assessed by patient blood gas and pulse oximetry. Blood gas analysis should be performed per protocol and with clinical changes and adjustments should be made to sweep accordingly.[11] On VA ECMO, consideration should be given to advanced continuous hemodynamic monitoring. A pulmonary artery catheter is especially useful in the weaning phase to assess hemodynamic response as support is weaned. The right upper extremity arterial monitoring is necessary to monitor for the north–south syndrome, a condition in which poorly oxygenated blood moving through the native circulation is ejected by the heart into the most proximal aortic branches supplying the myocardium and right cerebral circulation.[13,20]

Specific physiologic targets on VV ECMO are not clearly defined by the medical literature. In principle, the objective of VV ECMO is to deliver sufficient gas exchange to sustain life, ideally while maintaining non-injurious ventilator settings.[21,22] The ELSO guidelines advise maintaining a $SaO_2 > 80\%$ and suggest that a circuit blood flow of 50 to 80 mL/kg/min should be targeted to achieve this.[20] At least initially, sweep gas flow should be titrated to maintain normal pH and Pco_2 (ELSO guidelines). Many centers aim for a so-called ultra-lung protective strategy if possible, with plateau pressures of 20 to 25 cmH$_2$O, a driving pressure of 10, and tidal volumes well under 6 mL/kg/IBW.[11,22]

Significant hemodynamic changes can be observed with the initiation of ECMO. Exposure to the foreign substance of the ECMO circuit can cause an acute vasodilatory process similar to the systemic inflammatory response syndrome but it usually abates rapidly. Alternatively or subsequently, with the initiation of extracorporeal support with improved oxygen delivery in the case of VV ECMO or restoration of flow with VA support rapid improvement of hemodynamics is often seen and vigilant down-titration of vasoactive support is indicated to avoid hypertensive complications. There exists no consensus on hemoglobin targets for ECMO patients, but many centers adopt the general critical care target of 7 mg/dL[11].

Anticoagulation is preferred in all ECMO settings to avoid the risk of thromboembolism. A loading dose is typically given around the time of cannulation as there is a high risk of stasis around the time of cannulation before the initiation of ECMO flow. Maintenance of anticoagulation during the ECMO run decreases the risk of thromboembolism, prolongs circuit component life, and decreases the risk of catastrophic circuit component clotting.[23,24] However, VV ECMO embolization to the pulmonary circulation poses less risk of catastrophic complication than systemic embolization risk in VA ECMO. Additionally, the use of heparin-bonded circuits in contemporary equipment decreases the risk of circuit failure. Collectively this means that VV ECMO can be run safely without systemic anticoagulation for prolonged periods after a risk–benefit analysis of particular use in the trauma population.[25,26] However, most of the trauma ECMO patients can be anticoagulated without clinically significant or surgical bleeding.[9,27]

Extracorporeal Membrane Oxygenation Troubleshooting

The magnitude of support possible for circulation or oxygenation in an ECMO circuit is proportional to the maximal achievable flow. Like a ventricular assist device, the pump in an extracorporeal life support (ECLS) circuit can be thought of as preload dependent and afterload sensitive. Recalling this principle can assist the bedside physician in addressing low-flow situations that can be lethal in a patient dependent on extracorporeal support. **Table 1** summarizes the causes of low-flow states and possible corrective actions are described below.

The availability of blood in the venous side is often the rate-limiting component of the overall ECMO circuit flow. The movement of blood through the circuit creates a significant suction force that can result in the collapse of the IVC around the drainage cannula. Therefore, positioning as much of the drainage cannula as possible within the non-compressible intrahepatic IVC and cavoatrial junction is desirable. Ensuring adequate intravascular volume is also essential to prevent the collapse of the IVC around the drainage cannula and is of particular concern in the early phase of trauma. On the other extreme and pertinent to the trauma population is the possibility of increased intraabdominal pressure leading to extrinsic compression of the IVC and flow starvation of the circuit. This can be because of over-resuscitation and third spacing or mass effect from intraperitoneal or retroperitoneal hemorrhage. Kinking or other restrictions of the drainage cannula at any point along its internal or

Table 1		
Extracorporeal membrane oxygenation low-flow alarms		
Low-Flow Alarms	**Causes**	**Corrective Action**
Pre-pump	Hypovolemia	Resuscitation
	Cannula kinking/obstruction	Limb positioning, loosening of constricting sutures or connectors
	Misplaced cannula	Cannula advancement/retraction
	Increased pressure around cannula	Rule out abdominal compartment syndrome or mass occupying lesions
	Low cardiac output	Resuscitation
	Inadequate drainage cannula size	Cannula replacement
Pump	Controller power failure	Manual crank, replace unit/power supply
	Pump embolism/thrombosis	Pump exchange
Post-pump	Arterial hypertension (VA)	Blood pressure management
	Oxygenator clotting	Oxygenator exchange
	Inadequate return cannula size	Cannula replacement

extracorporeal course can also result in circuit preload issues. Externally, this is often observed as "chugging" (intermittent shaking motion of the cannula) and manifested as transient or sustained flow drops. In the acute phase of a trauma ECLS run, simultaneous assessment of several possibilities should be undertaken. Particularly with the trauma population, the intravascular volume should be assessed for hypovolemia and corrected. Increased intrabdominal pressure may require either surgical decompression or evacuation. External circuit components should be evaluated for kinking, restrictive connectors, or excessively tight securing sutures. Ensure appropriate positioning of the limb where the drainage cannula is located (often an individualized trial and error process). Appropriate positioning of the drainage cannula should be verified. Reference to daily measurements of external cannula length or chest radiograph can be of use. A bedside ultrasound, particularly the subxiphoid/IVC window, can visualize the hyperechoic cannula tip in the appropriate position. Drainage cannulae that are too small or too large for the patient can either restrict flow or increase predilection for chugging and can be replaced if technically feasible. If unsuitable, a second drainage cannula can be placed.[20]

Flow decreases can also be seen due to issues intrinsic to the pump. Pump failure can be caused by an interruption of the power supply or failure of the control console. All ECLS circuits should have a mechanism for docking the pump to a manual hand crank in the event of catastrophic failure. Mechanical failure of the pump or embolized thrombus entrainment can also cause abrupt pump failure requiring emergency pump replacement. In situ thrombus development will cause a more gradual degradation in pump efficiency and also necessitates replacement.

The final class of flow failure on ECMO relates to increased pump afterload. In both VV and VA circuits, this can be caused by clot formation in the oxygenator or mechanical kinking of any other downstream component. In these cases, the oxygenator can be changed and any restricting elements removed. In VA ECMO, elevated arterial blood pressure will result in increased pump afterload and decreased extracorporeal flow. The use of vasodilators targeting a normal mean arterial pressure may be necessary to restore extracorporeal flow in hypertensive patients.

Hypoxemia on VV ECMO despite adequate flow raises many possibilities. As described above, extracorporeal oxygenation potential depends on blood flow through the ECMO circuit. The first possibility, when confronted with a hypoxemic ECMO patient, is that the circuit flow is insufficient for the patient's needs. If the flow achieved has dropped below what the patient had previously maintained, the above evaluation should be performed to diagnose the cause of decreased flows. There are two significant additional issues while on VV ECMO: recirculation and insufficient capture. Recirculation occurs when blood from the return limb is entrained by the drainage cannula instead of going through the right ventricle (RV) and on through the lungs to the systemic circulation. This can be diagnosed by either observation of failure of color change between the drainage and return tubing or by an inappropriately high oxygen saturation on a pre-oxygenator blood gas. The first step in management is often counterintuitively lowering the pump rpm, which should decrease the suction pressure on the drainage limb, and therefore, decrease entrainment of the arterialized blood. As long as the patient oxygenates appropriately with the reduced flow, no further action is required. If this fails, retraction of the cannula to increase separation is usually indicated. Another possibility, especially in recovering or infected trauma patients with healthy hearts, is decreased capture fraction. Even well-functioning ECMO circuits seldom flow greater than approximately 6 L per minute; cardiac output in excess of the ECMO circuit flow is functionally shunted if there is negligible native lung function. Generally, a ratio of ECMO flow to total cardiac output above 0.6 will provide sufficient oxygen.[21,28]The first objective is to ascertain appropriate oxygen targets; patients on ECMO will often tolerate lower oxygen saturation. Next, in cases where perfusion is adequate, suppression of cardiac output with either anxiolysis or beta-blockade is an option. These interventions have a dual effect of decreasing oxygen demand.

The lifespan of individual ECMO circuit components is not clearly defined or consistent. The most vulnerable component of the circuit to failure is the oxygenator, which by virtue of the turbulent flow sectors created as blood partitions between the microfibers and the numerous internal small channels with resultant high surface area to volume ratio is prone to macroscopic and microscopic clot formation and degradation over time. Visual inspection may reveal clots, but these usually do not mandate intervention unless significant and on the arterialized side of the oxygenator. The function of an oxygenator can be interrogated by measurement of post-oxygenator blood gas and measurement of transmembrane pressure. A decrease of the post-oxygenator Po_2 below a certain threshold or elevation of the transmembrane pressure suggests oxygenator failure and an indication for replacement. Depending on the circuit/manufacturer, the oxygenator can be replaced individually or may be replaced as a unit with the pump head.

Catastrophic failure of ECMO circuit components is uncommon but potentially lethal. Despite the track record of safe and prolonged support, ECMO circuit components are not rated for indefinite support.[29] Catastrophic failure would be most easily addressed by the replacement of the entire circuit to simplify the process. Failures at the cannula level mandate emergent re-cannulation.

Future Directions

Selective aortic arch perfusion (SAAP) is an underdeveloped extracorporeal support technique with applications in medical and traumatic cardiac arrest. SAAP is a balloon catheter inserted via the femoral artery retrograde into the aorta. The tip of the catheter contains a large bore infusion port. When inflated, the device functions much like a resuscitative balloon occlusion of the aorta with added functionality for infusion of vasoactives and blood products targeting the central circulation.[30] SAAP has been assessed in several animal models of traumatic cardiac arrest with good outcomes but has yet to be deployed in humans.

Emergency preservation and resuscitation is another experimental concept in the early pilot phase. This procedure borrows from the data and experience with deep hypothermic circulatory arrest in cardiac surgery and involves either open or endovascular descending thoracic aortic cross-clamp followed by clamshell thoracotomy to allow the introduction of a cannula directly into the proximal aorta. Ice cold fluid is administered to achieve a profoundly low upper body temperature of 10° Celsius and the patient is placed on full cardiopulmonary bypass.[31] Expectations based on animal data suggest that up to 2 hours of cold ischemic time can then be well tolerated while definitive hemorrhage control is obtained with good neurologic outcome.[32]

Each of these described experimental technologies should not be attempted outside of research protocols.

CLINICS CARE POINTS

- Trauma surgeons and non-surgical experienced physicians can, within an appropriately supported program, use ECMO to rescue refractory respiratory and circulatory failure in trauma patients.

- ECMO cannulation can be accomplished bedside either as the preferred technique or in patients too unstable to move.
- Cannulation requires knowledgeable and skilled vascular access skills to ensure an appropriate approach and entry point to the target vessels.
- VV ECMO can be safely managed at least temporarily with minimal or no anticoagulation, and as such, trauma is not a contraindication to ECMO.
- Maintaining adequate flow through the ECMO circuit is the most essential task of maintaining adequate extracorporeal support while on ECMO.

DISCLOSURE

The authors have nothing to disclose.

REFERENCES

1. Hill JD, O'Brien TG, Murray JJ, et al. Prolonged extracorporeal oxygenation for acute post-traumatic respiratory failure (shock-lung syndrome). Use of the Bramson membrane lung. N Engl J Med 1972;286(12):629–34.
2. Hu PJ, Griswold L, Raff L, et al. National estimates of the use and outcomes of extracorporeal membrane oxygenation after acute trauma. Trauma Surg Acute Care Open 2019;4(1):e000209.
3. Swol J, Brodie D, Napolitano L, et al. Indications and outcomes of extracorporeal life support in trauma patients. J Trauma Acute Care Surg 2018;84(6). Available at: https://journals.lww.com/jtrauma/Fulltext/2018/06000/Indications_and_outcomes_of_extracorporeal_life.1.aspx.
4. Menaker J, Tesoriero RB, Tabatabai A, et al. Veno-Venous Extracorporeal Membrane Oxygenation (VV ECMO) for Acute Respiratory Failure Following Injury: Outcomes in a High-Volume Adult Trauma Center with a Dedicated Unit for VV ECMO. World J Surg 2018;42(8):2398–403.
5. Banfi C, Pozzi M, Siegenthaler N, et al. Veno-venous extracorporeal membrane oxygenation: cannulation techniques. J Thorac Dis 2016;8(12):3762–73.
6. Cordell-Smith JA, Roberts N, Peek GJ, et al. Traumatic lung injury treated by extracorporeal membrane oxygenation (ECMO). Injury 2006;37(1):29–32.
7. Michaels AJ, Schriener RJ, Kolla S, et al. Extracorporeal life support in pulmonary failure after trauma. J Trauma 1999;46(4):638–45.
8. Kruit N, Prusak M, Miller M, et al. Assessment of safety and bleeding risk in the use of extracorporeal membrane oxygenation for multitrauma patients: A multicenter review. J Trauma Acute Care Surg 2019;86(6):967–73.
9. Wang C, Zhang L, Qin T, et al. Extracorporeal membrane oxygenation in trauma patients: a systematic review. World J Emerg Surg 2020;15(1):51.
10. Lequier L, Horton SB, McMullan DM, et al. Extracorporeal Membrane Oxygenation Circuitry. Pediatr Crit Care 2013;14(5 0 1):S7–12.
11. Tonna JE, Abrams D, Brodie D, et al. Management of Adult Patients Supported with Venovenous Extracorporeal Membrane Oxygenation (VV ECMO): Guideline from the Extracorporeal Life Support Organization (ELSO). ASAIO J 2021;67(6):601–10.
12. Burrell AJC, Ihle JF, Pellegrino VA, et al. Cannulation technique: femoro-femoral. J Thorac Dis 2018;10(Suppl 5):S616–23.
13. Lorusso R, Shekar K, MacLaren G, et al. ELSO Interim Guidelines for Venoarterial Extracorporeal Membrane Oxygenation in Adult Cardiac Patients. ASAIO J Am Soc Artif Intern Organs 2021;67(8):827–44.

14. Attou R, Redant S, Preseau T, et al. Use of Extracorporeal Membrane Oxygenation in Patients with Refractory Cardiac Arrest due to Severe Persistent Hypothermia: About 2 Case Reports and a Review of the Literature. Case Rep Emerg Med 2021;2021:5538904.

15. Yen CC, Kao CH, Tsai CS, et al. Identifying the Risk Factor and Prevention of Limb Ischemia in Extracorporeal Membrane Oxygenation with Femoral Artery Cannulation. Heart Surg Forum 2018;21(1):E018–22.

16. Bonicolini E, Martucci G, Simons J, et al. Limb ischemia in peripheral venoarterial extracorporeal membrane oxygenation: a narrative review of incidence, prevention, monitoring, and treatment. Crit Care 2019;23(1):266.

17. Foley PJ, Morris RJ, Woo EY, et al. Limb ischemia during femoral cannulation for cardiopulmonary support. J Vasc Surg 2010;52(4):850–3.

18. Lamb KM, DiMuzio PJ, Johnson A, et al. Arterial protocol including prophylactic distal perfusion catheter decreases limb ischemia complications in patients undergoing extracorporeal membrane oxygenation. J Vasc Surg 2017;65(4): 1074–9.

19. Merkle J, Azizov F, Fatullayev J, et al. Monitoring of adult patient on venoarterial extracorporeal membrane oxygenation in intensive care medicine. J Thorac Dis 2019;11(Suppl 6):S946–56.

20. Extracorporeal Life Support: The ELSO Red Book. 5th edition. Extracorporeal Life Support Organization.

21. Delnoij TSR, Driessen R, Sharma AS, et al. Venovenous Extracorporeal Membrane Oxygenation in Intractable Pulmonary Insufficiency: Practical Issues and Future Directions. Biomed Res Int 2016;2016:9367464.

22. Marhong JD, Munshi L, Detsky M, et al. Mechanical ventilation during extracorporeal life support (ECLS): a systematic review. Intensive Care Med 2015;41(6): 994–1003.

23. Sklar M, Sy E, Lequier L, et al. Anticoagulation Practices during Venovenous Extracorporeal Membrane Oxygenation for Respiratory Failure. A Systematic Review. Ann Am Thorac Soc 2016;13:2242–50.

24. McMichael ABV, Ryerson LM, Ratano D, et al. 2021 ELSO Adult and Pediatric Anticoagulation Guidelines. ASAIO J 2022;68(3):303–10.

25. Olson SR, Murphree CR, Zonies D, et al. Thrombosis and Bleeding in Extracorporeal Membrane Oxygenation (ECMO) Without Anticoagulation: A Systematic Review. ASAIO J 2021;67(3):290–6.

26. Wood KL, Ayers B, Gosev I, et al. Venoarterial-Extracorporeal Membrane Oxygenation Without Routine Systemic Anticoagulation Decreases Adverse Events. Ann Thorac Surg 2020;109(5):1458–66.

27. Bedeir K, Seethala R, Kelly E. Extracorporeal life support in trauma: Worth the risks? A systematic review of published series. J Trauma Acute Care Surg 2017;82(2):400–6.

28. Schmidt M, Tachon G, Devilliers C, et al. Blood oxygenation and decarboxylation determinants during venovenous ECMO for respiratory failure in adults. Intensive Care Med 2013;39(5):838–46.

29. Philipp A, De Somer F, Foltan M, et al. Life span of different extracorporeal membrane systems for severe respiratory failure in the clinical practice. PLoS ONE 2018;13(6):e0198392.

30. Barnard EBG, Manning JE, Smith JE, et al. A comparison of Selective Aortic Arch Perfusion and Resuscitative Endovascular Balloon Occlusion of the Aorta for the management of hemorrhage-induced traumatic cardiac arrest: A translational model in large swine. Plos Med 2017;14(7):e1002349.

31. Tisherman SA, Alam HB, Rhee PM, et al. Development of the emergency preservation and resuscitation for cardiac arrest from trauma clinical trial. J Trauma Acute Care Surg 2017;83(5):803–9.
32. Tisherman SA. Emergency preservation and resuscitation for cardiac arrest from trauma. Ann N Y Acad Sci 2022;1509(1):5–11.
33. Rector R. University of Maryland ECMO Circuit.

Intimate Partner Violence and Human Trafficking
Trauma We May Not Identify

Kari Sampsel, MD, MSc, FRCP[a],*,
Julianna Deutscher, MD, PGY-5, FRCP-EM[b],
Emma Duchesne, MD, PGY-4, FRCP-EM[c]

KEYWORDS

- Intimate partner violence • Human trafficking • Trauma • Trauma-informed care

KEY POINTS

- Defining intimate partner violence and human trafficking as a subset of trauma patients.
- Recognizing these presentations in and out of the trauma bay.
- Implementing trauma-informed care.
- Creating a pathway to screen and provide resources.

INTRODUCTION

Case 1: While awaiting imaging after a high-speed motor vehicle collision, the patient is asking how much longer she needs to be in hospital because she is concerned her partner will be upset that he has not heard from her. You explain that there is ongoing concern for possible serious injuries based on her abdominal pain. She becomes increasingly anxious and is requesting her telephone, repeating that her partner is going to be upset if she cannot reach him. You reassure the patient that you will provide her a telephone to call her partner after she is taken to computed tomography (CT).

Several barriers have been previously identified regarding emergency department (ED) screening and management of patients experiencing intimate partner violence (IPV) and human trafficking (HT). This article

[a] Sexual Assault and Partner Abuse Care Program, The Ottawa Hospital, University of Ottawa, 1053 Carling Avenue, Ottawa, Ontario K1Y 4E9, Canada; [b] Department of Medicine, Faculty of Medicine, University of Toronto, C. David Naylor Building, 6 Queen's Park Crescent West, Third Floor, Toronto, Ontario M5S 3H2, Canada; [c] Department of Emergency Medicine, Kingston Health Sciences Centre, 76 Stuart Street, Victory 3, Kingston, Ontario K7L 2V7, Canada
* Corresponding author:
E-mail address: ksampsel@toh.ca
Twitter: @KariSampsel (K.S.); @jul_deutscher (J.D.)

Emerg Med Clin N Am 41 (2023) 101–116
https://doi.org/10.1016/j.emc.2022.09.013
0733-8627/23/© 2022 Elsevier Inc. All rights reserved.
emed.theclinics.com

1. Describes the diverse spectrum of ED presentations related to IPV and HT
2. Improves clinicians' knowledge regarding trauma-informed care, screening tools, and management steps
3. Facilitates development of evidence-based approaches to care for individuals who screen positive for IPV or HT, especially in the setting of traumatic injuries

INTIMATE PARTNER VIOLENCE: WHO IS IT AND WHAT IS IT

IPV is defined as any behavior within an intimate relationship that causes harm to those in the relationship.[1] These acts may be committed by a current or previous partner, regardless of whether these partners have lived together.[2] Examples are listed next:

- Physical violence: Any forms of abuse involving intentional use of force against a partner, such as physical assault (eg, having objects thrown at them) or threat of physical assault (eg, being threatened with a weapon).[2]
- Psychological violence: Any forms of abuse targeting psychological or financial well-being or threatening sense of safety.[2,3] Examples include jealous or manipulative behavior, public humiliation, confinement, or harassment.
  Spiritual abuse refers to using a partner's religion, faith, or beliefs to exert power and control.[3]
  Financial abuse refers to using money or property to control or exploit someone else (eg, property damage, controlling access to education or work).[4]
  Technology-facilitated IPV refers to controlling or violent behaviors through the use of technology[4] and is exceedingly common with a recent systematic review highlighting that nearly three-quarters of young Canadians experience technology-facilitated IPV.[5] Examples of this include online stalking, harassment, identity theft, or nonconsensual release of private information or images.
- Sexual violence: Any forms of abuse forcing or coercing a partner to take part in a sex act.[6] This includes sexual assault, threats for refusing sex, and nonphysical sexual events (eg, use of sexually degrading language).
  Nonconsensual distribution of pornography ("revenge porn") refers to the sharing of sexually explicit material without a person's consent.[7] This form of IPV may be used to blackmail, control, humiliate, or ostracize a partner, and may threaten their reputation and livelihood. This is not a rare occurrence, with nearly 1 in 10 participants of a recent American study describing previous nonconsensual pornography distribution.[7]
  Reproductive coercion refers to behavior interfering with reproductive health and choices.[8] This includes sabotaging contraception, blocking access to prenatal care, contraception, abortions, or deliberately removing a condom during sex ("stealthing").

INTIMATE PARTNER VIOLENCE: WHY EMERGENCY PROVIDERS SHOULD CARE

IPV impacts people of all ages, sexual orientations, gender identities, socioeconomic, racial, ethnic, religious, and cultural backgrounds. More than half of Canadian IPV survivors are college or university educated and only 5% report having no income.[9] Although IPV is experienced by all genders, women sustain higher IPV-related morbidity and mortality, most frequently at the hands of men.[10] Many groups lack representation within IPV-related research despite encountering increased risk and barriers to care. They include women aged 15 to 24; indigenous patients;

2SLGBTQ + patients; patients living with a disability; patients from rural, remote, and northern communities; and immigrant and refugee patients.[2,11–14]

Three in 10 women and 1 in 10 men have experienced IPV in their lifetime.[15] A woman is murdered by her intimate partner every 5 days in Canada[16] and every 3 days in the United States.[17] These rates have increased during 2022,[18] likely caused by COVID-19-related restrictions.[19] Despite reports demonstrating frequent presentations to the ED, one study found that physicians only identified 5% of IPV cases and just over 10% asked about IPV.[20] The ED is seen as society's safety net. Although ED physicians frequently fail to ask about IPV, 89% of individuals surveyed stated they would have been comfortable disclosing if someone had asked.[21,22] Within this context, ED physicians have an important opportunity and role in preventing morbidity and mortality from IPV.

HUMAN TRAFFICKING: BREAKING DOWN THE MYTHS

Case 2: The trauma team receives an alert that a man is being transported for a limb-threatening injury; his arm was caught in machinery at work. On arrival, paramedics relay additional information that the patient is concerned about seeking medical attention because his temporary foreign worker permit expired and he is no longer formally employed. As the team prepares to address the limb-threatening injury, the trauma physician identifies that after critical limb care is provided, efforts should be made to screen for HT and connect the patient to supports during his admission.

The term HT may trigger images of two girls traveling to Europe, getting kidnapped, and a memorable speech from the protagonist talking about his particular set of skills. Although there are many accurate depictions of HT in the media, they often portray a narrow spectrum of presentations, propagate common myths, and create bias in who is determined to be at risk.

So what are the truths and what are the myths behind this human rights violation? HT is defined by the United Nations using three components[23]:

1. Act: recruitment process (eg, invitation to work at a nightclub)
2. Means: coercion, deception, abduction, fraud, or force
3. Purpose: sexual or labor exploitation

In North America, a common example is termed "grooming."[24] Grooming is when the individual is manipulated or "groomed" into a relationship resulting in dependence and willingness to engage in certain situations in which they would otherwise not have become involved.[24] These individuals are coerced into working in the sex trade under the pretense that they are helping to pay back the support from the trafficker.[24] In Case 1, that of a young female desperate to contact her partner after she was in a motor vehicle collision, this may be an example of a patient in a groomed relationship. Grooming creates complex barriers including an individual not being aware that they are being trafficked.[24] Furthermore grooming creates challenges when trying to leave an exploitative situation because there is great dependence on the trafficker for a multitude of supports including social, occupational, shelter, and financial.[24]

Not all sex trade work is sexual exploitation.[25] Individuals choosing to work in the sex trade should not be persecuted and the role of the medical team should be to ensure that they are supported to work in the safest manner possible. They should, however, still be screened for HT.[25]

Not all HT is sexual exploitation. This is illustrated by the example in Case 2, a man presenting to the trauma bay following a workplace injury. Maybe this was just an accident. Or maybe it was caused by fatigue from breaching safe work-hour policies, inadequate training, or a generally unsafe working environment. What makes this case potentially HT, and in this case labor trafficking, comes back to the definition of act, means, and purpose. Labor trafficking is generally described as working in unsafe conditions, receiving inappropriate payment, or working hours that breach labor laws.[26]

Is human smuggling the same as trafficking? Human smuggling is a transnational crime involving the illegal entry of an individual into a country that they are not permitted to enter.[27] HT may include cases of smuggling, but under the definition of trafficking, no border crossing is required.[26] In fact, in Canada, most HT cases are domestic, meaning that they have not involved migrating across an international border.[28]

Anyone can be a victim/survivor. Similar to IPV, although marginalized populations are at increased risk of HT, it is important to remember that trafficking does not discriminate to particular patient demographics.[29] That being said, Statistics Canada published that out of reported cases in 2019, 95% of individuals were female and 21% were minors.[29] Furthermore, only 11% experienced trafficking by someone they did not know.[29]

In any encounter where you suspect you have identified HT, keep in mind that the patient may not have yet identified themselves as someone experiencing exploitation.[25,30] This can make it all the more challenging to offer resources and support. The previous definitions are challenging and a lack of full comprehension of the legal definitions should not be a barrier to providing care. The role of health care providers is not to determine if HT has occurred, but rather to identify red flags to then make connections to interdisciplinary team members and community resources.[25,30]

PLENTY OF NEEDLES IN THE HAYSTACK: HOW DO WE FIND THESE PATIENTS ON OUR NEXT SHIFT?

In North America, 44% of women murdered by their intimate partner had visited an ED in the last year; 93% of these survivors visited specifically for IPV-related injury.[31] Similar misses are occurring with HT despite knowing that it presents in the ED; one study identified that more than 85% of interviewed trafficked persons reported having contact with a health care provider while they were being trafficked.[32] These patients are in our EDs, our trauma bays, and they may even be the person working next to you. Studies highlighted between 20% and 27% of nurses, physicians, and paramedics having experienced IPV themselves.[20] The 2016 murder of Canadian family physician Elana Fric by neurosurgeon Mohammed Shamji and the 2018 murder of American emergency physician Tamara O'Neal by her fiancé outside of the hospital are reminders to regularly check on colleagues.[22,33]

It is time we learned the red flags (**Boxes 1** and **2**) that can help identify an individual experiencing or at risk of IPV/HT.

The concept of universal screening is controversial, with differing interpretations of the literature, and multiple screening tools, which are cumbersome to implement in a trauma setting. This controversy arises from studies that electronically screened patients in a variety of health care settings and those screening positive receiving a printed list of IPV resources. The health care providers were not alerted to their positive screen, nor did they intervene to help facilitate any further IPV care. With just more than a third of the patients accessing services, these studies have been interpreted as positive and negative by various medical societies. Emergency medicine recommends universal screening within the ED as supported in position statements from the Society of Academic Emergency Physicians (SAEM) and the Canadian Association of Emergency Physicians (CAEP).

> **Box 1**
> **Common red flags of individuals experiencing intimate partner violence[34]**
>
> Delay in seeking care
>
> Long-standing untreated medical conditions
>
> Unwilling to disclose history
>
> History that changes over time
>
> Unexplained injuries
>
> Injuries incongruent with mechanism
>
> Multiple injuries at various stages of healing
>
> Posterior rib fractures
>
> Defensive injuries
>
> Restraint injuries
>
> Strangulation injury/facial petechiae
>
> Multiple visits for same presentation, chronic pain, mental health

BARRIERS TO SCREENING
Why Are We Not Asking?

1. Time
2. Training
3. Access to resources
4. Lack of privacy
5. Sentiment that care cannot be provided in the ED
6. Belief that patients can leave a violent/exploitative situation at any time

> **Box 2**
> **Red flags signifying risk of human trafficking, to be used in addition to list of red flags seen in IPV[25,26,28]**
>
> Lack of access to personal identification documents
>
> No health insurance
>
> Unable to speak local language despite living in area for a long time
>
> Unfamiliar with local surroundings
>
> Minor patient presenting with older partner or presenting alone
>
> Person accompanying patient is answering all the questions
>
> Patient or accompanying person are frequently asking when they can leave
>
> Branding with tattoos
>
> Employer controlling access to food and housing
>
> Dangerous living/work conditions
>
> Controlled or limited access to pay
>
> Working long hours or unable to leave the workplace

7. Challenges understanding factors resulting in behaviors termed "uncooperative" patients: cycle of abuse results in mistrust and possible aggressive behavior, declining investigations or treatment because of barriers of needing to return to partner/trafficker[22,35]

What to Ask

The simplest statements to ask with a high yield for picking up IPV are[34]:

1. Do you feel safe at home? This can also highlight other issues relevant to their care and discharge.
2. Has someone hurt you? This uses accessible language, and does not label the patient as abused/victim, because they may not see themselves this way.
3. Summarizing what you have observed and heard from the patient followed by expressing your concern for safety and how you may be able to help.

There are several screening tools (**Boxes 3** and **4**) being developed for HT. We recommend the newly published Rapid Appraisal for Trafficking (RAFT) tool, which was validated in the ED to screen for sex and labor trafficking.[36] This tool was developed from an extensive screening assessment tool from the Vera Institute of Justice,[37] not validated in the ED, but a highly valuable tool that is used in addition to RAFT. There is additionally a short screening tool for Child Sex Trafficking[38] published by Dr Jordan Greenbaum and her team, which is found on the Health, Education, Advocacy, Linkage (HEAL) Trafficking Web page.

Where to Ask

Triaging is a nearly universal experience for those who seek urgent care and is the perfectly imperfect location for this brief screening to occur. However, trauma patients often bypass triage. So, where do we screen them? Identifying red flags is a process that should occur longitudinally throughout all levels of the patient's care. Trauma and ED physicians should ask police and medical first responders about possible red flags that may have been present on scene. It is difficult to screen in the trauma bay given the need for rapid resuscitation and disposition to either imaging, the operating room, or the ED. It is, however, a place where red flags are recognized, as demonstrated in Cases 1 and 2, and used to activate the need for screening at a later time in the patient's care.

Some centers additionally use the method of self-screening. This may include:

- Virtual or paper questionnaires
- Posters in washroom with contact information (**Fig. 1**)
- Placing a sticker on urine collection container lid to alert health care provider (see **Fig. 1**)

Perhaps it is time to design a poster for your washrooms, trauma bay, or CT scanner.

How to Ask

Before getting into the details of trauma-informed care, let us talk about interpretation.

- Resist the urge to use family, partners, or friends as your interpreter. Remember, most trafficked persons know their traffickers as family members, partners, friends, and employers.[29]
- If you do not have access to an interpretation line, many HT resources may be able to assist, including the National Human Trafficking Hotline or Canadian

---

Box 3
The Rapid Appraisal for Trafficking (RAFT) tool to screen for sex and labour trafficking[36]

1. It is not uncommon for people to stay in work situations that are risky or even dangerous, simply because they have no other options. Have you ever worked, or done other things, in a place that made you feel scared or unsafe?

2. In thinking back over your past experience, have you ever been tricked or forced into doing any kind of work that you did not want to do?

3. Sometimes people are prevented from leaving an unfair or unsafe work situation by their employers. Have you ever been afraid to leave or quit a work situation because of fears of violence or threats of harm to yourself or your family?

4. Have you ever received anything in exchange for sex (eg, a place to stay, gifts, or food)?

Human Trafficking Hotline, which provide free 24/7 access to interpretation by telephone.

- If you have no other access, using your telephone or other electronic device not owned by the patient/family to translate can also work.

Trauma-informed care is not the care provided as part of trauma resuscitation. It is defined as an approach that emphasizes educating patients about violence, normalizing the conversation, and supporting them to share their own experience.[25] As Dignity Health and HEAL Trafficking explain, the encounter "is not for [the] patient to disclose victimization, but for providers to treat, educate, and empower the patient."[25] This is a method of patient care that is implemented the moment a patient enters the trauma bay because it does not take away from the ability to address the immediate resuscitation steps.

It is important to ask for permission to screen and to limit the number of questions to avoid retraumatization.[25,30] Additionally, you should inform your patient before discussion on circumstances that mandate reporting. Reminding your patient of what remains confidential may aid in disclosure because there is often misunderstanding and fear surrounding the role of police and child and family services. Introducing this conversation may include such statements as:

1. I would like to ask you some personal questions about your safety that can help me care for you better. Is it ok that I ask you a few questions now?
2. It is my practice to ask all my patients about violence because we know that violence is common in our society. Is it safe for me to ask you a few questions?

Box 4
Advocates for human rights labor trafficking self-screening tool

1. Is someone holding your personal documents for you?

2. Does someone else control the decisions you make about your life?

3. Do you owe money to your boss, the person who hired you, or the person who helped you find the job?

4. Are you receiving your pay?

5. Are you afraid something bad will happen to you or someone else if you leave your work?

The Advocates for Human Rights published a self-screening card available in multiple languages to screen for labor trafficking.[39] This has not yet been validated in a health care setting.

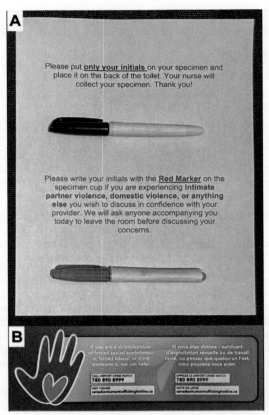

Fig. 1. (*A*) Sample poster for urine collection container self-screening. Photo credit: LGBTQ Nation. (*B*) Example of self-screening posters in washrooms. Picture taken with permission of Edmonton International Airport.

A trauma-informed approach using the brief screening tools previously mentioned has a major impact on the morbidity of the patient, with a supportive response to disclosure having a six-fold reduction in mental illness (eg, posttraumatic stress disorder) and substance use in the year following the disclosure.[40] Do not interpret a patient declining resources or reporting as a sign of treatment failure.[25] The stages of change model describes how survivors move through a series of progressions before reaching a point of feeling prepared to leave their abusive or exploitative situation.[30] Although it may seem discouraging as the provider, know that implementing trauma-informed care plants a seed that not only fosters a feeling of safety in returning for support in the future, but importantly helps progress an individual through the stages of change model.[25,30] Even one brief conversation demonstrating kindness can ultimately be lifesaving.[25,30]

POLICE: WHEN SHOULD THEY BE INVOLVED?
Minors

- Familiarize yourself with local mandatory reporting requirements[41]
  - Suspected violence, abuse, or neglect

- ○ Sexual activity with partner outside of permitted age difference
  - ○ Sexual activity with partner who is in position of authority
  - ○ Sexual activity for profit
- Your closest pediatric hospital can also serve as an invaluable resource for specific questions or unique situations

Adults

Check your local jurisdiction for guidelines because they may include mandatory reporting for adult patients. Engagement with the justice system is not wanted by many survivors.[42] Many violence survivors have had poor interactions with law enforcement previously and may fear criminalization (eg, if they engage in sex work as employment, or for deportation if they have not established a permanent residency).[42] IPV cases often have poor outcomes for the survivor, even when pursued to the fullest extent of the law.[43] Additionally, survivors may fear retaliation toward themselves or their families if law enforcement is notified.[42]

WHAT ABOUT THE MEDICINE: CARE AT THE INTERSECTION OF THE MEDICAL AND LEGAL SYSTEMS

The short answer is, it is the same. Use the same clinical tools and rules to provide care for the patient's injuries, no matter what the cause. Do not get distracted or intimidated just because this involves IPV/HT. **Table 1** highlights specific considerations in these populations. The current recommendation for patients of 23 weeks or greater gestation is a minimum of 4 hours of fetal heart rate monitoring posttrauma.[44] Of particular note, survivors who are strangled have a six-fold increased risk of being murdered in the upcoming year.[45]

WRITER'S BLOCK: HOW TO DOCUMENT THIS EMERGENCY DEPARTMENT VISIT

A recent retrospective chart review of Canadian ED physicians' screening and documentation practices revealed that just over half of patients with IPV-related injuries had no documentation of assailant identity.[46] Recording verbatim "spontaneous exclamations," which are statements made by someone immediately after an event, is considered by the court to be exceptionally credible because of the proximity in time to the event and their decreased likelihood to be premeditated.[27] **Box 5** expands on forensic documentation.

GIMME SHELTER: HOW TO KEEP YOUR HUMAN TRAFFICKING/INTIMATE PARTNER VIOLENCE PATIENT AND TEAM SAFE WITHIN THE EMERGENCY DEPARTMENT

There is an increased risk of homicide after separation; leaving is the riskiest action patients take.[48] At the time of leaving, the risk of homicide increases four-fold, thus the survivor of IPV needs to be able to make a clean escape, often cutting ties completely with their abuser.[48] This also means that we need to keep this patient safe within our EDs and trauma units.

- Chart and tracking board deidentification
- Patient in visible secure location
- Limiting visitors to only patient-approved
- If patient wants a visitor present, do not make efforts to separate them
- If the abuser/trafficker is also a patient, keeping them separate and informing security

Table 1
Special considerations in medical management of IPV and HT

Antibiotic Coverage	Strangulation Injuries[45]	Forensic Considerations[42]
Consider broadened antibiotic coverage for sexually transmitted infections Follow guidelines based on local resistance patterns	Be sure to ask about strangulation including: What was used Loss of consciousness, including proxy signs, such as tongue biting and incontinence Were they suspended Pain Vocal changes Head and neck examination: Vascular Neurologic Airway/phonation Petechiae Bruising CT angiogram: Airway, vascular, or neurologic compromise Petechiae or bruising Loss of consciousness or altered mental status	Always wear gloves when examining or performing procedures to prevent contamination with your own DNA Medical care always comes before forensic considerations If IPV/HT specialty care program available, can work to provide medical and forensic care concurrently Specialty teams can assist with documentation, trauma-sensitive photographs Wounds are washed and repaired as per standard care

All efforts should be made to maintain safety of patients by escalated chart security, such as having systems to "lock" chart access for IPV-related visits. This may include hiding names from electronic medical record trackers, blocking the automatic online publication of IPV-related documentation, and flagging any attempt to access charts.

Remember, patients may be hesitant to seek medical attention because of their immigration status (eg, Case 2, the patient with an expired temporary foreign worker permit). The HT hotlines listed in **Fig. 2** are an excellent resource that can direct your team and the patient to immigration supports. For example, in Canada, trafficked persons are eligible for a Temporary Resident Permit of up to 180 days and in the United States a T nonimmigrant status visa for up to 4 years, both of which are extended to additional family members and during the allotted time frame additional supports are provided to aid in securing further work and residency permits.[49,50]

There is unfortunately no perfect answer on how to best manage the many competing needs of a busy department with those of a vulnerable patient in need of screening that may have lifesaving outcomes. Identifying nonphysician team members who are able to assist in screening is vital to this time management.[25] If available, it is also helpful to identify a safe location for screening that does not disrupt flow of access to resuscitation rooms. **Fig. 2** demonstrates several considerations that can be implemented in developing an IPV/HT screening and care pathway in the ED.

WHO YOU GONNA CALL?

- Canadian Human Trafficking Hotline: 1-833-900-1010, https://www.canadianhumantraffickinghotline.ca
- National Human Trafficking Hotline: 1-888-373-7888, Text 233733, https://humantraffickinghotline.org

---

Box 5
Documentation strategies for IPV/HT

Documentation Do's and Don'ts[47]

- Be detailed, objective, and complete ("if it was not charted, it was not done").

- Write clearly and legibly.

- Record the time you meet the patient and the time the patient states the injuries/events occurred.

- Write descriptive clinical facts and observations (record all the same information you would put in for a bar fight or motor-vehicle collision).

- Record appearance and range of emotional responses (eg, tearful, anxious, fearful, shaking, calm, or indifferent).

- Use quotations around patient statements.

- Avoid any of: "patient in no acute distress" (has different meaning in legal system than use for clinical stability), and "patient alleges/claims" (this is a legal term implying skepticism from physician).

- We do not say "alleged ankle sprain" or "alleged chest pain"; the same should apply for not using "alleged" for IPV. Instead, use "patient states" or "patient reports."

- Use a ruler to measure injuries and a body chart to draw injury locations.

- Involve specialized teams to collect evidence (photographs, DNA) with patient's consent.

- Document assessments for children and if reported to local child protective team.

- Discharge diagnosis: label this as IPV/HT; no euphemisms, such as "social crisis" or "neck pain." Proper recorded discharge diagnosis is key for hospital coding, implications for funding, research, and advocacy.[47]

- Sexual assault and domestic violence specialized care programs: https://www.forensicnurses.org/
- Child, youth, and family services
- Social work
- Other local organizations with peer support staff, forensic nurses

HOW TO SAVE A LIFE
Risk Evaluation

Clinicians should always ask their patients about prior strangulation and access to firearms. Prior nonfatal strangulation is associated with a nearly 800% increased risk of being killed by an intimate partner[51] and access to a gun increases the risk of intimate-partner homicide by 500%.[52] In the United States, increased access to firearms generates particular lethality with an average of 70 women killed per month by their partners.[32]

The Ontario Domestic Assault Risk Assessment and the Danger Assessment are two well-validated tools that estimate the risk of repeated assault and future lethality.[53] The higher the score, the more likely that the patient's violent partner will commit more assaults, commit them sooner, and cause more serious injuries.[53] Key questions clinicians should remember to ask their patients from these tools include[53]:

1. Has he/she/they choked you?
2. Does he/she/they own a gun?
3. Have you left him/her/them after living together during the past year?

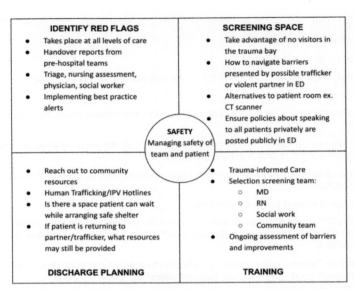

Fig. 2. Considerations in development of IPV/HT screening and care pathway in the ED.

4. Has he/she/them threatened to harm or kill anyone?
5. Do you believe he/she/they is capable of killing you?
6. Has he/she/they had a prior correctional sentence?

Approach to Safety Planning

Clinicians should have a clear approach to safety planning for any patient who discloses IPV/HT, especially in the case where a specialized team may not be available. Safety planning refers to a patient-centered, trauma-informed approach in helping patients set actions to reduce harm and increase preparedness once they are discharged from the ED.[25] Safety planning should take into account the patient's children, and safety at home, at work, online, and during separation. Many online resources are available to this effect, most of which can be printed and given to patients to read in the ED. General counseling from clinicians should include the following:

- Identify trustworthy individuals (eg, friends, family, neighbors, coworkers), and set up a code word to identify immediate danger.
- Store a "go-bag" at their house (cash, keys, clothes, medications, and original or copies of important documents and identification).
- During violence episodes, avoid being cornered in small spaces and avoid rooms with potential weapons. Try to remove yourself before the situation escalates if possible.
- Call 911 for immediate danger.

SUMMARY

IPV and HT are extremely common experiences within ED patients. Although these presentations can occur in any patient, ED providers should be aware of groups at increased risk of experiencing violence and exploitation, particularly watching for red flags. Use of evidence-based screening tools, practice of trauma-informed care, and multidisciplinary approaches to management should be prioritized to decrease IPV and HT-related morbidity and mortality.

Screening for IPV and HT may not seem like an acute medical emergency, but it is important to remember that although the initial presentation may falsely seem benign, if that first opportunity to offer help is missed, the next presentation may be accompanied by serious health consequences or even death.[13,25] The ED is the port in the storm for these patients, and a supportive, positive patient experience, even if the patient chooses to return to a violent situation, illuminates the path back to safety in a future visit.[13,25,30]

CLINICS CARE POINTS

- A patient choosing to return to an abusive partner or trafficker is not a failure of care; survivors often reflect on initial visits that connected them to resources and started the stages of change that ultimately led to lifesaving outcomes.

- An absence of life-threatening conditions at initial presentation does not predict absence of fatal outcomes in the future.

- Take strangulation seriously. Always ask about it, remember indications for imaging, and recognize strangulation as a critical risk factor for future mortality.

- Anyone accompanying the patient can be an abusive partner or trafficker; always find a way to speak to your patient one on one, even if it is in the CT scanner.

- Screening is completed in many ways; consider how self-screening and referral tools may work best in your department if staff screening is not yet practical.

- Anyone can be a victim and everyone deserves to be a survivor.

ACKNOWLEDGMENTS

The authors thank Rifaa Carter. All of the authors work directly with individuals experiencing IPV and HT and have partnered with organizations providing community care to these populations. Although they recognize that many unique perspectives exist based on individual experiences, this paper was additionally reviewed by an individual experiencing IPV to foster a person-centered approach.

DISCLOSURE

The authors have nothing to disclose.

REFERENCES

1. Understanding and addressing violence against women [Fact sheet]. World Health Organization. Available at: http://apps.who.int/iris/bitstream/handle/10665/77432/WHO_RHR_12.36_eng.pdf?sequence=1. Accessed March 15, 2022.
2. Cotter A. Intimate partner violence in Canada, 2018: an overview. In: Juristat, editor. Statistics Canada catalogue no. 85-002-X ed 2018.
3. What is Spiritual Abuse? Domestic Violence Hotline. Available at: https://www.thehotline.org/resources/what-is-spiritual-abuse/. Accessed March 15, 2022.
4. About Family Violence. Government of Canada. Available at: https://www.justice.gc.ca/eng/cj-jp/fv-vf/about-apropos.html. Accessed March 15, 2022.
5. Dragiewicz M., Harris B., Woodlock D., et al., Domestic violence and communication technology: survivor experiences of intrusion, surveillance, and identity crime. The Australian Communications Consumer Action Network. Available at: http://accan.org.au/grants/completed-grants/1429-domestic-violence-and-

communication-technology-victim-experiences-of-intrusion-surveillance-and-identity-theft.

6. Violence prevention – intimate partner violence [fast facts]. Center for Disease Control and Prevention. 2021. Available at: https://www.cdc.gov/violenceprevention/intimatepartnerviolence/fastfact.html. Accessed March 15, 2022.

7. Ruvalcaba Y, Eaton A. Nonconsensual pornography among U.S. adults: a sexual scripts framework on victimization, perpetration, and health correlates for women and men. Psychol Violence 2019. https://doi.org/10.1037/vio0000233.

8. Silverman J, Raj A. Intimate partner violence and reproductive coercion: global barriers to women's reproductive control. PLoS Med 2014;11(9):e1001723.

9. General Social Survey: An overview. Canada: Statistics Canada; 2022.

10. Section 2: police-reported intimate partner violence in Canada. Canada: Juristat; 2019.

11. CDC. Violence against American Indian and Alaska Native People [Fact Sheet]. Center for Disease Control and Prevention. Available at: https://www.cdc.gov/injury/pdfs/tribal/Violence-Against-Native-Peoples-Fact-Sheet.pdf. Accessed March 15, 2022.

12. Harland K, Peek-Asa C, Saftlas A. Intimate partner violence and controlling behaviors experienced by emergency department patients: differences by sexual orientation and gender identification. J interpersonal violence 2021;36(11–12):6125–43.

13. Breiding M, Armour B. The association between disability and intimate partner violence in the United States. Ann Epidemiol 2015;25(6):455–7.

14. Moffitt P, Aujla W, Giesbrecht C, et al. Intimate partner violence and COVID-19 in rural, remote, and Northern Canada: relationship, vulnerability and risk. J Fam Viol 2020;37(5):775–86.

15. Black M., Basile K., Breiding M., et al., The National Intimate Partner and Sexual Violence Survey (NISVS): 2010 Summary Report, 2011. Available at: https://www.cdc.gov/violenceprevention/pdf/nisvs_report2010-a.pdf.

16. Roy J, Marcellus S. Homicide in Canada – 2018. Statistics Canada catalogue no 85-002-X. Canada: Juristat; 2019.

17. Intimate Partner Homicide *in* 2019. National Violent Death Reporting System Reports. Available at: https://wisqars.cdc.gov/nvdrs/nvdrsController.jsp. Accessed March 15, 2022.

18. Incident-based crime statistics, by detailed violation. 2016. Available at: http://www23.statcan.gc.ca/imdb/p2SV.pl?Function=getSurvey&lang=en&db=imdb&adm=8&dis=2&SDDS=3302. Accessed March 1, 2022.

19. Muldoon K, Denize K, Talarico R, et al. COVID-19 pandemic and violence: rising risks and decreasing urgent care-seeking for sexual assault and domestic violence survivors. BMC Med 2021;19(1):20.

20. Director T, Linden J. Domestic violence: an approach to identification and intervention. Emerg Med Clin North America 2004;22:1117–32.

21. Ansara D, Hindin M. Exploring gender differences in the patterns of intimate partner violence in Canada: a latent class approach. J Epidemiol Community Health 2010;64(10):849–54.

22. Ansara D, Hindin M. Formal and informal help-seeking associated with women's and men's experiences of intimate partner violence in Canada. Soc Sci Med 2010;70(7):1011–8.

23. Human Trafficking FAQs. United Nations. Available at: https://www.unodc.org/unodc/en/human-trafficking/faqs.html. [Accessed 20 March 2022]. Accessed.
24. Love and trafficking: how traffickers groom & control their victims. https://polarisproject.org/blog/2021/02/love-and-trafficking-how-traffickers-groom-control-their-victims/. [Accessed 20 March 2022].
25. Protocol Toolkit: for developing a response to victims of human trafficking in health care settings. 2019. Available at: https://healtrafficking.org. Accessed March 28, 2022.
26. Labour trafficking. Government of Canada. Available at: https://www.canada.ca/en/public-safety-canada/campaigns/human-trafficking/labour-trafficking.html. Accessed March 18, 2022.
27. Fact Sheet #2: Trafficking in persons and human smuggling. Government of Canada. Available at: https://www.justice.gc.ca/eng/rp-pr/cj-jp/tp/hcjpotp-gtpupjp/fs-fi/fs2-fi2.html. Accessed March 23, 2022.
28. National action plan to combat human trafficking. Government of Canada. Available at: https://www.publicsafety.gc.ca/cnt/rsrcs/pblctns/ntnl-ctn-pln-cmbt/index-en.aspx. Accessed March 23, 2022.
29. Ibrahim D. Trafficking in persons in Canada. 2021. Available at: https://www150.statcan.gc.ca/n1/pub/85-005-x/2021001/article/00001-eng.htm.   Accessed March 20, 2022.
30. Understanding victim mindset & the stages of change model. Kristen French Child Advocacy Centre Niagara. Available at: https://www.kristenfrenchcacn.org/human-trafficking/victim-mindset-stages-of-change/. Accessed March 9, 2022.
31. Daugherty JDHDE. Intimate partner violence screening in the emergency department. J Postgrad Med 2008;54:301–5.
32. Lederer L, Wetzel C. The health consequences of sex trafficking and their implications for identifying victims in healthcare facilities. Ann Health L 2014;23(1):61–91.
33. Brice-Saddler M. The devastating loss of the doctor killed at a Chicago hospital by her former fiancé. Wash Post. Available at: https://www.washingtonpost.com/nation/2018/11/20/greatest-hands-possible-doctor-killed-chicago-hospital-remembered-her-compassion/. Accessed March 15, 2022.
34. Bakes K, Buchanan J, Moirera M, et al. Chapter 99: intimate partner violence. 7th edition. Emergency medicine secrets. United States: Elsevier; 2021.
35. Intimate partner violence screening in the emergency department: U.S. medical residents' perspectives. International quarterly of community health education. journals.sagepub.com/doi/abs/10.2190/IQ.30.1.c. [Accessed 15 March 2022].
36. Chisolm-Straker M, Singer E, Strong D, et al. Validation of a screening tool for labor and sex trafficking among emergency department patients. J Am Coll Emerg Physicians Open 2021;2(5):e12558.
37. Screening for human trafficking: guidelines for administering the Trafficking Victim Identification Tool (TVIT). 2014. Available at: https://www.vera.org/downloads/publications/human-trafficking-identification-tool-and-user-guidelines.pdf. Accessed March 25, 2022.
38. Greenbaum J, Dodd M, McCracken C. A short screening tool to identify victims of child sex trafficking in the health care setting. Pediatr Emerg Care 2018;34(1):33–7.
39. Labour Trafficking Self-Assessment Card. The advocates for human rights. Available at: https://www.theadvocatesforhumanrights.org/Publications/Index?id=374. Accessed March 25, 2022.

40. Ansara D, Hindin M. Psychosocial consequences of intimate partner violence for women and men in Canada. J Interpers Violence 2011;26(8):1628–45.

41. Child Abuse is Wrong: What can I do? Government of Canada. Updated December 6, 2021. Available at: https://www.justice.gc.ca/eng/rp-pr/cj-jp/fv-vf/caw-mei/index.html. Accessed March 28, 2022.

42. Muldoon K, Drumm A, Leach T, et al. Achieving just outcomes: forensic evidence collection in sexual assault cases. J Emerg Med 2018;35(12):746–52.

43. Foord J. Why do we continue to blame victims of sexual assault? YWCA Saskatoon. Available at: https://www.ywcasaskatoon.com/why-do-we-continue-to-blame-victims-of-sexual-assault/. Accessed March 28, 2022.

44. Jain V, Chari R, Maslovitz S, et al. Guidelines for the management of a pregnant patient. J Obstet Gynecol Can 2015;37(6):553–71.

45. MacDonald Z, Eagles D, Yadav K, et al. Surviving strangulation: evaluation of non-fatal strangulation in patients presenting to a tertiary care sexual assault and partner abuse care program. Can J Emerg Med 2021;23:762–6.

46. Vonkeman J, Atkinson P, Fraser J, et al. Intimate partner violence documentation and awareness in an urban emergency department. Cureus 2019;11(12):e6493.

47. Hoang R. Where is the love? Intimate partner violence in the emergency department. Available at: https://emottawablog.com/2018/01/where-is-the-love-intimate-partner-violence-in-the-emergency-department/. Accessed March 15, 2022.

48. Johnson H. Limits of a criminal justice response: trends in police and court processing of sexual assault. Sex assault Canada law. Canada: Leg Pract Women's Act; 2012. p. 613–34.

49. Temporary resident permits (TRPs): considerations specific to victims of trafficking in persons. Government of Canada. 2016. Available at: https://www.canada.ca/en/immigration-refugees-citizenship/corporate/publications-manuals/operational-bulletins-manuals/temporary-residents/permits/considerations-specific-victims-human-trafficking.html#sec2. Accessed May 20, 2022.

50. Victims of human trafficking: T Nonimmigrant Status. U.S. Citizenship and Immigration Services. 2021. Available at:https://www.uscis.gov/humanitarian/victims-of-human-trafficking-and-other-crimes/victims-of-human-trafficking-t-nonimmigrant-status. . Accessed May 20, 2022.

51. Glass N, Laughon K, Campbell J, et al. Non-fatal strangulation is an important risk factor for homicide of women. J Emerg Med 2008;35(3):329–35.

52. Campbell J, Webster D, Koziol-McLain J, et al. Risk factors for femicide in abusive relationships: results from a multisite case control study. Am J Public Health 2003;93(7):1089–97.

53. Ontario Domestic Assault Risk Assessment. 2005. Available at: https://grcounseling.com/wp-content/uploads/2016/08/domestic-violence-risk-assessment.pdf. Accessed March 28, 2022.

Management of Pain and Agitation in Trauma

Reuben J. Strayer, MD

KEYWORDS

- Trauma • Polytrauma • Analgesia • Sedation • Agitation • Procedural sedation
- Pain

KEY POINTS

- Non-pharmacologic measures to improve pain management in polytrauma include clearing the cervical spine and splinting fractures as early as feasible.
- Agitated polytrauma patients who demonstrate critical resuscitative urgency or severe agitation are best managed with dissociative-dose ketamine, administered at the outset of care by the intramuscular route.
- Dissociated patients may be managed with vigilant procedure sedation-level monitoring and airway readiness and allowed to emerge from dissociation after initial resuscitative maneuvers, or if strong indications for intubation are present, paralyzed and intubated once control has been established and preparations made for intubation.
- Non-critical agitated polytrauma patients should be treated for pain and then a titratable sedative such as midazolam or droperidol, based on the cause of agitation.
- Polytrauma patients requiring procedural sedation to facilitate painful procedures should be evaluated for appropriateness of emergency department (ED)-based PSA based on anesthetic risk and procedural urgency, and carried out with continuous attention to ventilation. When hypoventilation is detected, it is treated according to a measured, stepwise approach.

INTRODUCTION: I DO NOT HEAR BREATH SOUNDS ON THE RIGHT

A trauma team has assembled in the trauma bay after notification that a man in his 20s is en route with basic life support (BLS) medics and police after having been assaulted with a baseball bat and a knife. The patient arrives being held down screaming *I need something for pain! Get off me and get me something for pain!* The team leader cannot yet see the patient, who is surrounded by personnel trying to move him to the ED stretcher but can hear that at least the airway is intact. The clinician at the head of the bed attempts to engage the patient verbally without success so commences the primary survey, announcing *multiple contusions to the right side of the head and face. Pupils reactive bilaterally. Stab wound to the right flank. Good breath sounds*

Maimonides Medical Center, 4821 Fort Hamilton Parkway, Brooklyn, NY 11219, USA
E-mail address: emupdates@gmail.com

Emerg Med Clin N Am 41 (2023) 117–129
https://doi.org/10.1016/j.emc.2022.09.003
0733-8627/23/© 2022 Elsevier Inc. All rights reserved.

emed.theclinics.com

on the left. I do not hear breath sounds on the right. The patient is struggling against attempts to restrain him and loudly reminds the team that he is in pain. The nurse tells the team leader that he cannot get a line because the patient is too agitated. The monitor shows a heart rate (HR) of 140, BP 100/60, and an oxygen saturation of 87%.

This polytrauma patient is in pain, agitated, may soon require tube thoracostomy—an intensely painful procedure—and may have one or more life-threatening injuries needing prompt diagnosis and treatment. These life threats include a traumatic brain injury, which requires transfer and cooperation for computed tomographic (CT) imaging, and if traumatic brain injury (TBI) is identified, management may rely, in part, on an accurate neurological examination. Moreover, effective management of pain may forestall the urgent use of potentially dangerous sedatives, or, effective management of agitation may forestall the urgent use of potentially dangerous analgesics. However, it is uncertain, at the outset of care, which is the more urgent priority, how urgently the patient may require a painful life-saving procedure such as chest decompression, and whether endotracheal intubation (ETI)—which would simultaneously manage pain, agitation, and upcoming painful procedures—is safe, appropriate, or worth obscuring downstream neurological assessments.

Managing Pain in the Polytrauma Patient

The multiple injured patient often arrives in severe pain that is routinely undertreated in many centers. Because the initial focus of protocolized trauma care is accomplishing a set of specific assessments and maneuvers that does not include addressing pain or distress, symptom control is subordinated to a secondary priority. It may be appropriate in patients with serious injuries for trauma teams to proceed down an algorithmic series of steps designed to rapidly diagnose and treat immediate life threats; however, undertreated pain is itself a threat, as dangerous injuries are more difficult to diagnose in the patient distracted and agitated by severe pain. Clinicians may be reluctant to provide effective analgesia in the undifferentiated or hypotensive trauma patient for concerns around the potential for opioids to worsen hemodynamic status. However, poorly managed traumatic pain is also associated with a variety of downstream harms including chronic pain, posttraumatic stress disorder, and longer intensive care unit (ICU) and hospital stays. Most importantly, failure to treat pain promptly and effectively, especially severe pain as is often caused by trauma, is a failure to attend to a core mission of medicine, the relief of suffering. It is therefore essential that clinicians who care for injured patients have an analgesic strategy that is safe and effective for patients across the spectrum of trauma severity.

Early intubation of the polytrauma patient in severe pain who is clearly headed for the operating room accomplishes a variety of goals simultaneously: in addition to securing the airway, the properly induced and intubated patient is unconscious and therefore free of pain and emotional distress, still to facilitate imaging, and easily anesthetized for painful procedures or surgery, if indicated. It is therefore appropriate, compassionate care to intubate patients with intractable pain from, for example, traumatic amputation, or multiple severe orthopedic injuries, during the initial phase of management, once the team is cognitively and materially ready, and the procedure can be performed safely. Ketamine is usually the appropriate induction agent when rapid sequence intubation (RSI) is performed in trauma because it offers a variety of advantages over alternatives, including potent analgesia. In patients who do not have clear indications for intubation such as critical compromise of airway or breathing, and who do not have definitively operative findings, the decision to intubate in trauma is based on a nuanced evaluation of benefits, harms, and timing, as discussed below.

Many nonpharmacologic measures can greatly improve the analgesic management of injured patients (**Box 1**). Backboards are for extrication and transport and should be removed on arrival. Cervical spine immobilization collars offer questionable benefit and are associated with a variety of harms,[1] including significant discomfort. Immediate removal when their prehospital placement was not indicated (eg, in penetrating trauma) or clinical clearance using a validated decision tool should be performed as early as feasible, and in stable patients who do not meet such criteria, clearance based on imaging should be a high priority. Unsplinted fractures can cause severe pain that is often ameliorated by immobilization. Painful procedures such as nasogastric tube and foley catheter insertion are appropriately no longer part of a standard trauma assessment; however, in many centers the rectal examination is still routine. This painful and humiliating practice should only be performed for specific, limited indications such as a concern for penetrating rectal injury. Logrolling is of limited value and can be very painful and even dangerous; this maneuver should often be deferred or limited to a quick visual inspection, especially in patients who will receive whole-body CT.[2–4] If a painful procedure is indicated in an awake patient, the clinician should explain the procedure, set expectations, and describe steps to be taken to minimize pain. This preprocedural briefing alleviates anxiety, which strongly contributes to pain and distress.

Most injured patients in pain are stable and without concern for an immediate life threat. The major barrier to timely and effective analgesia in stable trauma patients is clinician inattention or deprioritization. Using departmental pain management protocols, incorporating pain medications into trauma order sets and including pain control in trauma checklists nudges providers to consider the treatment of pain at the outset of care. Although pain scales are often incorporated into nursing assessments, the optimal method for determining if a patient will benefit from being treated with a pain medication is to ask the patient if they wish to be treated with a pain medication.

Most polytrauma patients who are not hemodynamically compromised but are in moderate or severe pain should be treated with a parenteral opioid as first-line therapy. Morphine has slightly longer time to onset compared with fentanyl; however, its much longer duration of action confers a significant advantage, especially in a busy ED where timely pain reassessment is difficult and redosing may be delayed. Nonelderly, nonfrail, normally perfused adults should be treated with an initial dose of morphine at 0.1 to 0.15 mg/kg by the intravenous, intramuscular, or subcutaneous route. If vascular access is delayed in a patient in severe pain, it is appropriate to administer the initial dose intramuscular (IM) or subcutaneous (SC). Further doses should be administered at 0.1 mg/kg as needed. Fentanyl is frequently used in trauma

---

Box 1
Nonpharmacologic approaches to pain in trauma

Remove backboard as early as feasible

Remove cervical spine collar clinically or as soon as imaging allows

Splint/immobilize fractures

Only perform painful procedures/maneuvers such as rectal examination, nasogastric tube, foley catheter, and log roll when specifically indicated, not routinely

Utilize smallest chest drainage catheters possible

Preprocedural patient briefing

and is an excellent analgesic option if the patient will be frequently reassessed for pain. Fentanyl is administered at 1 to 1.5 mcg/kg IV and may also be delivered by intranasal atomizer at 2 mcg/kg.

Analgesic-dose ketamine is safe and very effective for pain; however, the use of ketamine in subdissociative doses is burdened by psychoperceptual effects that are usually perceived as odd or even enjoyable but sometimes as uncomfortable or frightening. The incidence of bothersome psychoperceptual effects is diminished by slowing its distribution to the brain[5]; this is most commonly done by administering ketamine over 10 to 30 minutes using an intravenous drip such as 0.25 mg/kg IV over 20 minutes. Ketamine may also be effectively delivered intranasally at 0.75 to 1 mg/kg,[6] or via nebulization (ideally with a breath-actuated nebulizer) at 0.75 to 1.5 mg/kg.[7,8] The window between effective analgesia and intrusive psychoperceptual effects is in some patients very narrow but is likely widened by calming medications such as benzodiazepines, butyrophenone antipsychotics, or opioids; for this reason, ketamine is in most circumstances best used as a second-line agent for opioid-refractory pain.

Nitrous oxide (N_2O) is a volatile anesthetic gas administered in combination with oxygen via inhalation as an analgesic, anxiolytic, and sedative. N_2O can be self-administered using a demand-valve scavenger system, which allows for rapid, effective relief of pain and anxiety, both of which are common in injured patients.[9] N_2O has a long record of safety and has few adverse effects; however, it may not be used until pneumothorax has been excluded and its contraindications also include first or second trimester pregnancy.[10] Although N_2O requires specialized equipment that limits its availability in emergency settings, it is an excellent analgesic modality for patients in moderate-to-severe pain who are able to use one hand for self-administration.[11]

With the increase of point-of-care ultrasound, regional anesthesia performed by emergency clinicians has emerged as a powerful technique that is often highly effective for relieving traumatic pain of any severity. When bupivacaine or (preferably) ropivacaine is used, nerve blocks provide long-lasting analgesia without exposing the patient to the harms of systemic analgesics. Although most often used to treat extremity pain, several truncal blocks are available to treat pain from thoracic injuries; the serratus anterior plane block effectively relieves pain from rib fractures, which can interfere with breathing and are particularly dangerous in the elderly, who are also more likely to be harmed by opioids.

Trauma patients in shock present an analgesic challenge. For patients in profound or refractory shock, poorly perfused with systolic blood pressure less than 70, all efforts must be focused on identifying and treating the cause of shock. Any potent analgesic will act as a sympatholytic in this context and could worsen hemodynamics; therefore, treatment of pain is appropriately deferred until central perfusion is restored. Fortunately, these patients usually have a diminished level of consciousness and diminished memory of their resuscitation. However, when perfusion and mental status are improved, prompt assessment and treatment of pain returns to high priority.

In between stable injured patients and decompensated polytrauma patients in shock are patients who are bleeding with the potential to deteriorate but who are centrally perfused, with good mentation. These patients may be most at risk for under-treatment of pain as resuscitation is ongoing but the level of consciousness and potential to suffer with pain is preserved. For tenuous but mentating patients, fentanyl is preferred over morphine for its relative hemodynamic neutrality. The dose is reduced to 0.5 mcg/kg IV, which can be repeated every 10 to 15 minutes as needed for pain, as perfusion status allows. Analgesic-dose ketamine is well-supported by prehospital and military experience,[12,13] at a slightly reduced dose versus stable patients.

Finally, many stable polytrauma patients have prolonged stays in the emergency department, which may hinder appropriate reassessment (by both physicians and nurses) and redosing of pain medications. Patient-controlled anesthesia drips of morphine, fentanyl, hydromorphone, or ketamine provide highly effective, long-lasting relief of pain, are empowering to patients, and liberate nursing resources. Analgesia strategy in polytrauma is summarized in **Fig. 1**.

Managing Agitation in the Polytrauma Patient

Polytrauma patients often arrive agitated or develop agitation during their initial assessment. Agitation may be the result of intoxication (which commonly accompanies trauma), pain, brain injury, malperfusion or hypoxia, psychiatric disease, delirium, or emotional distress related to being injured, the circumstances that led to their injury, or how they are treated by medical providers. Apart from possibly being caused by a dangerous condition, agitation itself is a danger to the badly injured patient, by interfering with the identification and treatment of traumatic life threats.

The management of agitation at the outset of trauma care depends primarily on the severity of injury and the severity of agitation but also on the underlying cause of agitation as well as the nature and urgency of the indicated medical or surgical therapies. However, because determining the severity of injury and indicated therapies may be

Primary Trauma Survey/ Identification of immediate life threats

Consider intubation & general anesthesia:
Airway or respiratory compromise
Early or ongoing hemodynamic instability
Anticipated early operative intervention
Injury causing uncontrollable pain or distress
Severe agitation

Multiple Injuries or Severely Painful Injuries

Profound/Refractory Shock
Loss of central pulses
Systolic BP < 70 mmHg

All efforts focused on identification and treatment of shock

Decreased level of consciousness/obtundation is the rule
Consider withholding analgesia until hemodynamics improved

Shock/Occult Shock
Poorly perfused extremities
Loss of peripheral pulses
Isolated or persistent SBP < 105 mmHg
Shock index > 0.9
Base deficit ≤ -6.0

Fentanyl 0.5 mcg/kg IV
Ketamine 0.1–0.3 mg/kg IV over 10–20 min

Stable

Fentanyl 1–1.5 mcg/kg IV
Morphine 0.1–0.15 mg/kg IV
Ketamine 0.2–0.3 mg/kg IV over 10–20 min

Throughout Resuscitation
Reassess hemodynamics, analgesia q10-15 min
Repeat bolus analgesia to effect
Consider non-pharmacological adjuncts to alleviate pain

Consider Maintenance Infusions
Titrate to effect
If intubated, add sedative drip as needed

Fentanyl 2 mcg/kg bolus then 1 mcg/kg/hour IV
Morphine 0.1 mg/kg bolus then 0.1 mg/kg/hour IV
Ketamine Non-intubated (analgesia) 0.3 mg/kg/h IV
Ketamine Post-intubation (dissociation) 1 mg/kg/h IV

Non-pharmacological adjuncts

Early discontinuation of spinal immobilization (long board, rigid collar) when clinically appropriate

Reduce and splint/immobilize injuries, including open fractures/ dislocations, bony pelvic injuries (stable or unstable) and significant soft tissue/burn injuries

Foley catheter to decompress bladder

Pre-procedure patient briefing for anticipated painful procedures

Fig. 1. Analgesia in polytrauma.

hindered by the patient's agitation, a complex interplay between agitation, pain, and resuscitative priorities can confound development of a therapeutic plan.

It is common practice in many centers to move quickly to ETI in agitated polytrauma patients, which allows the treating team to take immediate control of the patient and pivot to resuscitation. However, this strategy exposes patients who would not otherwise require ETI to its risks and may not allow for appropriate preparation and physiologic optimization before the procedure. The rise of ketamine as a treatment of agitation offers the capability to immediately calm and control the patient, without assuming the risks of RSI or the harms of ETI.

Ketamine was developed in the 1960s as an alternative to phencyclidine to provide dissociative anesthesia, where the patient is isolated from external stimuli and therefore perceives no pain. Although nystagmus and reflexive movements are common, the dissociated patient is incapable of volitional action and is generally still. However, unlike with conventional sedatives and anesthetics, airway reflexes and cardiorespiratory function are usually preserved: the ketamine-dissociated patient is *awake but unconscious.* Because ketamine reliably produces dissociation with a wide therapeutic window when administered by either the intravenous or intramuscular route, it is of particular value in treating agitation that poses an immediate threat to either patient or provider, and has been extensively studied in the management of injured and agitated patients in emergency, prehospital, and military settings.[14–16]

Trauma patients who present agitated but with no concern for a dangerous injury or medical condition can be managed similarly to the nontrauma agitated patient, with the caveat that the less assessable the patient by history and physical examination, the more likely that patient has an occult injury, concealed from recognition by their altered mentation.

Many agitated polytrauma patients either have evidence of a dangerous injury or their presentation indicates the prompt exclusion of such injuries by expeditious evaluation and imaging, which requires a cooperative or still patient. The initial management of the agitated polytrauma patient is summarized in **Fig. 2**. The injured patient with evidence of an immediate life threat, such as a penetrating chest wound with hypoxia and hypotension, whose agitation obstructs assessment and treatment, requires immediate calming and control. Additionally, patients without signs of critical resuscitative urgency may be sufficiently agitated that immediate danger to self or staff arises from the behavioral disturbance itself. Agitation hindering treatment of an immediate life threat and agitation that is uncontrollably violent both represent *dangerously severe agitation*.

The management of dangerously severe agitation begins by assembling adequate force to safely subdue the patient, which is one person for each limb and one for the head, which does not include the clinical team leader or the nurse administering medications. Face mask oxygen covering the mouth and nose is then applied to the patient, with the strings tightened so that the mask is closely affixed to the face. Early use of face mask oxygen empirically treats hypoxia, a critical cause of agitation, as well as controlling spit. The clinician should deliberately identify and relieve dangerous restraint holds such as compression of the neck or chest/back. Unless the patient has an intravenous line that is known to be functional, dangerously severe agitation should be treated with medications delivered intramuscularly, through the clothes unless an appropriate injection site is already exposed. Attempting IV access on a severely agitated patient is a needlestick risk and delays the onset of sedation, which is a critical pitfall in this context.

Although ketamine dissociation requires resuscitation-level monitoring and is more likely to result in intubation than conventional titratable sedatives, it is the treatment of

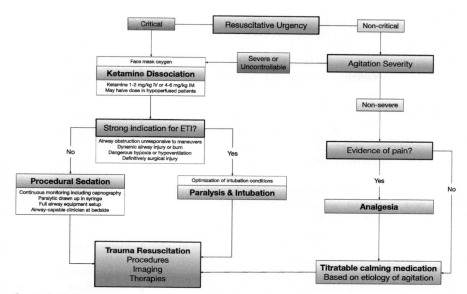

Fig. 2. Agitation management in the trauma patient.

choice for dangerously severe agitation because establishing immediate control of the patient is such an urgent priority. Although the use of dissociative-dose ketamine in nonintubated patients to facilitate painful procedures has an extensive record of safety,[17] hypoventilation may occur from a variety of mechanisms including airway malpositioning, excess secretions, laryngospasm, and central apnea; all dissociated patients who are not intubated must therefore be managed as in procedural sedation with continuous cardiorespiratory monitoring including capnography, paralytic and full airway equipment setup at bedside, and an airway-capable clinician immediately available.

The standard dissociative dose of ketamine is 1 to 2 mg/kg IV or 4 to 6 mg/kg IM. Although existing data are conflicting,[18] hypotensive patients may be at greater risk for adverse events when higher ketamine doses are used, and this risk must be weighed against the urgency of achieving a still patient to facilitate resuscitation. The effect of subdissociative ketamine is unpredictable; some patients will be calmed but others will require additional doses, introducing a potentially dangerous delay in their trauma assessment. It is reasonable to reduce the ketamine dose by up to half in hypoperfused patients; however, when the concern for critical injury is high, it is likely prudent to err toward a dose that will certainly dissociate the patient, so that needed tests and treatments can be expeditiously performed.

Once dissociation has calmed the dangerously agitated trauma patient, trauma resuscitation may commence in parallel with preparations to intubate, which include equipment readiness, optimization of the patient's physiology, and development of a team-based airway strategy. ETI should then be pursued if the patient demonstrates a strong intubation indication: airway obstruction not relieved by repositioning, suction, or simple airway adjuncts, dynamic airway injuries such as a penetrating wound to the neck or airway burns, dangerous hypoventilation or hypoxemia unresponsive to supplemental oxygen, definitively surgical injury such as bowel evisceration, or uncontrollably severe traumatic pain, as discussed above.

Absent a clear indication, intubation can be deferred in favor of procedural sedation monitoring including continuous capnography and readiness for airway management with paralytic and resuscitationist clinician immediately available. Nonintubated dissociated patients may be taken for CT imaging provided that the capability to intubate (in the CT suite, if necessary) is continued. Additional doses of ketamine may be required to maintain dissociation and should be quickly available. Many agitated trauma patients managed initially with dissociative-dose ketamine, once imaging demonstrates no dangerous injuries, can be allowed to emerge from dissociation. A conventional sedative such as midazolam or droperidol/haloperidol may be required to manage further agitation or psychiatric distress that can occur on emergence.

Agitated polytrauma patients who do not demonstrate critical resuscitative urgency or uncontrollable violence can be managed in a stepwise fashion that prioritizes sedation safety over speed and efficacy. Pain often drives or contributes to agitation in this group, and analgesia should be a high treatment priority as described above. Morphine, fentanyl, and analgesic-dose ketamine effectively treat pain and may have a salutary effect on agitation apart from their analgesic effect. N_2O is an excellent treatment of the moderately agitated trauma patient in pain, owing to its complementary sedating and anxiolysis effects.

Many agitated trauma patients will require treatment with calming medications after appropriate analgesia. The commonly used agitation cocktail, haloperidol 5 mg and lorazepam 2 mg, combined in the same syringe and injected intramuscularly, is very safe, and will be effective in most patients, eventually. However, sedation after "5 and 2" often takes 15 to 20 minutes, because haloperidol is relatively slow-acting, and lorazepam is erratically absorbed intramuscularly. Droperidol and midazolam are modestly more effective than haloperidol and lorazepam, but significantly faster, with a similar safety profile, and are therefore preferred.

Droperidol has been repeatedly demonstrated to be safe and effective in the management of agitation and because it is associated with less respiratory depression than benzodiazepines and is particularly well suited to manage agitation associated with alcohol intoxication, which commonly complicates trauma presentations. The use of droperidol has been curtailed by concerns around QT prolongation; however, these concerns have been allayed by large case series demonstrating a very high degree of safety,[19–21] and The American College of Emergency Physicians recommends that clinicians use droperidol at 5 to 10 mg intramuscular (IM) or intravenous (IV) "given studied doses up to 20 mg, regardless of initial monitoring capability or electrocardiogram (EKG)."[22] Antipsychotics are the preferred treatment of agitation thought to be due to psychiatric disease, medical delirium, or dementia. Haloperidol or olanzapine may be substituted for droperidol, with dose increased by ~50%.

Midazolam is far more reliably effective when given intramuscularly than alternatives and is therefore the IM benzodiazepine of choice for any indication. The dose of IM midazolam when used as monotherapy in the treatment of agitation is 2 to 10 mg; however, doses greater than 2 mg and especially 5 mg or greater can cause respiratory depression, especially in the presence of other risk factors for respiratory depression such as alcohol intoxication, obesity, or obstructive sleep apnea. Midazolam should be used cautiously by the intravenous route, at half the IM dose, with close attention to respiration; lorazepam 1 to 2 mg IV is an appropriate substitute for midazolam when the patient has intravenous access. Benzodiazepines are the first-line treatment of agitation thought to be due to alcohol (or benzodiazepine) withdrawal or stimulant toxicity.

A combination of droperidol and midazolam will provide safe, effective, rapid sedation of nearly all agitated patients. For undifferentiated agitation, excellent results will usually be achieved with 5 to 10 mg droperidol, depending on patient size and degree of agitation, mixed with 2 to 5 mg midazolam. It is common at many centers to add 25 to 50 mg diphenhydramine to sedation cocktails; however, this does not improve efficacy and is associated with significantly increased the length of stay, oxygen desaturation, and use of physical restraints.[23] An antimuscarinic should be administered when indicated for extrapyramidal symptoms but not added routinely to calming medications. The treatment of nonsevere agitation is summarized in **Fig. 3**.

Procedural Sedation in the Polytrauma Patient

Procedural sedation and analgesia (PSA) is the use of drugs delivered systemically to facilitate procedures that are painful and/or anxiety provoking. PSA occurs on the spectrum of analgesia and agitation management but is distinguished from the more routine use of analgesic and calming agents by the higher risk of cardiorespiratory compromise, which mandates continuous resuscitation-level monitoring and readiness for airway management. PSA is being performed when, in a nonintubated patient, benzodiazepines and opioids are used in combination in sufficient doses to depress level of consciousness, when ketamine is used in dissociative dose ($\geq$1 mg/kg IV or $\geq$4 mg/kg IM), or when propofol or etomidate is used in any dose. PSA is routinely used in polytrauma to facilitate fracture reduction, tube thoracostomy, and wound or burn management. PSA may also be performed to enable rapid assessment and imaging in the agitated patient, as described above.

PSA entails important risks, especially in a seriously injured patient, and a crucial step in the performance of PSA is an explicit consideration of the appropriateness of ED-based PSA for a given patient. A checklist is recommended to prompt clinicians to this concern, as well as for decision support around the elements of PSA preparation and execution. The less cardiorespiratory reserve, the more difficult airway features, and the less procedural urgency, the more likely the patient should not receive PSA in the emergency department; other options include regional or local anesthetic, PSA or general anesthesia in the operating room, or ETI in the ED. Because many polytrauma patients will require surgery early in their care, for patients with risk factors for PSA adverse events, strong consideration should be given to either ETI or deferral of the procedure until theater.

Once a preprocedural assessment has confirmed that the patient is an appropriate candidate for ED-based PSA, the PSA medication is chosen based on the

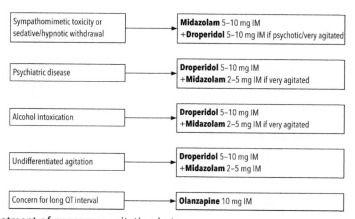

Fig. 3. Treatment of nonsevere agitation in trauma.

characteristics of the patient, procedure, and setting (**Table 1**). Brief procedures that require muscle relaxation, such as joint reduction, are often best managed with propofol. Although propofol can cause a drop in blood pressure as a sympatholytic and vasodilator, hypotension in the trauma patient should be assumed to be due to hemorrhage or circulatory obstruction unless these dangerous causes have been confidently excluded. Ketamine PSA is preferred for longer procedures such as fracture reduction or chest drainage. When dissociative-dose ketamine is used for PSA, rigidity, concerning hypertension, and emergence psychiatric distress can be treated with small aliquots of propofol or midazolam.

Oxygenation should be maximized before and during PSA with a nasal cannula underneath a high-flow oxygen face mask. Optimal oxygenation prolongs safe apnea time, allowing a measured, safe response to hypoventilation, as described below.

Although blood pressure and circulation remain a focus of care during PSA in the polytrauma patient, procedural sedation is most likely to cause harm by hypoventilation. Once PSA induction has occurred, ventilation should be continuously monitored by a member of the team who is not performing the procedure being facilitated. When hypoventilation occurs, the response should not be assertive bag-mask ventilation, which introduces the risk of stomach insufflation and dangerous regurgitation, especially when performed hastily. The management of PSA-induced hypoventilation should proceed deliberately down a series of steps, as slowly and cautiously as patient physiology allows (**Box 2**). Procedural sedation concludes when the patient responds to questions and maintains a normal oxygen saturation on room air. For

Table 1		
Procedural sedation and analgesia medications		
Agent	**Dose**	**Comments**
Propofol	0.5–1 mg/kg IV, then 0.5 mg/kg q1–2 min prn	Preferred for shorter procedures and where muscle relaxation is of benefit; avoid if hypotension is a concern. Egg and soy allergy *not* a contraindication
Ketamine	1–2 mg/kg IV over 30–60 sec or 4–5 mg/kg IM, repeat half dose prn	Preferred for longer procedures; avoid if hypertension/tachycardia is a concern; have midazolam or propofol available to manage emergence distress; muscle tone is preserved or increased; postprocedure emesis may be mitigated by prophylactic ondansetron
Etomidate	0.1–0.15 mg/kg IV, then .05 mg/kg q2–3 min prn	Intraprocedure myoclonus or hypertonicity, as well as postprocedure emesis, are common
Fentanyl	1–2 mcg/kg IV, then 1 mcg/kg q3–5 min prn	Comparatively delayed onset of action; do not redose too quickly
Midazolam	.05 mg/kg IV, then .05 mg/kg q3–5 min prn	Comparatively delayed onset of action; do not redose too quickly
Naloxone	0.01–0.1 mg/kg IV or IM (typical adult dose 0.4 mg)	Will precipitate withdrawal in opioid-dependent patients
Flumazenil	0.01 mg/kg IV (typical adult dose 0.2 mg) over 20 s, max 1 mg	Only use in patients known to be benzodiazepine-naïve (eg, pediatrics)

Box 2
Procedural sedation and analgesia intervention sequence

Detect hypoventilation early (capnography, chest rise, breath sounds, mask fogging)

Position the patient (torso upright, head and neck well aligned with chin lift)

Jaw thrust

Suction if secretions present

Laryngospasm notch pressure: bilateral, firm pressure medially and cephalad (up and in)

Nasal airways

Consider reversal agents if opioids or benzodiazepines have been used

Bag mask ventilation or, if deeply unconscious, laryngeal mask ventilation

Endotracheal intubation

---

polytrauma patients who may have underlying insults to oxygenation or circulation and may have received psychotropic medications that interfere with assessment of mental status, a longer period of PSA-level monitoring may be required to verify postprocedural safety.

SUMMARY: CASE RESOLUTION

Polytrauma patients usually require analgesia, commonly require medications to treat agitation, and often require procedural sedation to facilitate painful procedures. The introductory case describes a young man arriving very agitated, screaming in pain after being assaulted with blunt and penetrating force, and the initial assessment raises concern for several life-threatening injuries including tension pneumothorax. This patient must be calmed promptly so that resuscitation can occur, including the immediate need to establish vascular access and likely to decompress the chest. Conventional management might call for RSI and intubation; however, the patient has no intravenous line for medication administration and transitioning to positive pressure ventilation with an untreated pneumothorax could precipitate cardiovascular collapse. Alternatively, the patient might be treated with "5 and 2," intramuscular haloperidol and lorazepam, which is likely insufficient dosing to calm the patient and will take much longer than desired, given the acuity of illness. Instead, 5 team members are deployed to hold down the patient while the team leader applies face mask oxygen, and the nurse administers 400 mg of intramuscular ketamine. Two minutes later, nystagmus is noted and the patient is still. As intravenous vascular access is established, ultrasound confirms right-sided pneumothorax, and a finger thoracostomy is performed to a rush of air and improvement of vital signs. The primary survey is completed as a chest tube is placed, and the team leader requests preparations for intubation, although for now the plan is procedural sedation. The patient is placed on a transport monitor with continuous capnography and taken to CT with airway equipment and medications, accompanied by the airway physician. CT shows a well-placed chest tube with resolution of pneumothorax, a small traumatic subarachnoid hemorrhage, and low-grade splenic laceration. Twenty minutes later, the patient starts to emerge from dissociation with mild agitation but calms with 8 mg IV morphine and 2.5 mg IV droperidol. One hour later, he is cooperative and answering questions. He is admitted to surgical intensive care unit (SICU) on a morphine patient-controlled analgesia (PCA) pump and discharged 3 days later in good condition.

CLINICS CARE POINTS

- Incorporate analgesia into departmental trauma order sets and checklists to nudge clinicians to provide early, effective analgesia.
- Regional nerve blocks, analgesic-dose ketamine and nitrous oxide are complementary modalities that can be used very effectively in injured patients.
- The use of dissociative-dose ketamine at the outset of management of polytrauma patients who are either uncontrollably violent, or are likely to have an immediately dangerous condition, can preclude the need for intubation.

DISCLOSURE

The author reports no conflicts of interest or funding relevant to the preparation of this article.

REFERENCES

1. Serigano O, Riscinti M. cervical spine motion restriction after blunt trauma. Acad Emerg Med 2021;28(4):472–4.
2. Leech C, Porter K, Bosanko C. Log-rolling a blunt major trauma patient is inappropriate in the primary survey. Emerg Med J 2014;31(1):86.
3. Rodrigues IFDC. To log-roll or not to log-roll - That is the question! A review of the use of the log-roll for patients with pelvic fractures. Int J Orthop Trauma Nurs 2017;27:36–40.
4. Singh Tveit M, Singh E, Olaussen A, et al. What is the purpose of log roll examination in the unconscious adult trauma patient during trauma reception? Emerg Med J 2016;33(9):632–5.
5. Motov S, Mai M, Pushkar I, et al. A prospective randomized, double-dummy trial comparing IV push low dose ketamine to short infusion of low dose ketamine for treatment of pain in the ED. Am J Emerg Med 2017;35(8):1095–100.
6. Shimonovich S, Gigi R, Shapira A, et al. Intranasal ketamine for acute traumatic pain in the Emergency Department: a prospective, randomized clinical trial of efficacy and safety. BMC Emerg Med 2016;16(1):43.
7. Dove D, Fassassi C, Davis A, et al. comparison of nebulized ketamine at three different dosing regimens for treating painful conditions in the emergency department: a prospective, randomized, double-blind clinical trial. Ann Emerg Med 2021;78(6):779–87.
8. Fassassi C, Dove D, Davis AR, et al. nebulized ketamine used for pain management of orthopedic trauma. J Emerg Med 2021;60(3):365–7.
9. Herres J, Chudnofsky CR, Manur R, et al. The use of inhaled nitrous oxide for analgesia in adult ED patients: a pilot study. Am J Emerg Med 2016;34(2):269–73.
10. Ducassé JL, Siksik G, Durand-Béchu M, et al. Nitrous oxide for early analgesia in the emergency setting: a randomized, double-blind multicenter prehospital trial. Acad Emerg Med 2013;20(2):178–84.
11. Kariman H, Majidi A, Amini A, et al. Nitrous oxide/oxygen compared with fentanyl in reducing pain among adults with isolated extremity trauma: a randomized trial. Emerg Med Australas 2011;23(6):761–8.
12. Morgan MM, Perina DG, Acquisto NM, et al. Ketamine use in prehospital and hospital treatment of the acute trauma patient: a joint position statement. Prehosp Emerg Care 2021;25(4):588–92.

13. Moy R, Wright C. Ketamine for military prehospital analgesia and sedation in combat casualties. J R Army Med Corps 2018;164(6):436–7.

14. Barbic D, Andolfatto G, Grunau B, et al. rapid agitation control with ketamine in the emergency department: a blinded, randomized controlled trial. Ann Emerg Med 2021;78(6):788–95.

15. Bernard S, Roggenkamp R, Delorenzo A, et al. Ketamine in Severely Agitated Patients Study Investigators. Use of intramuscular ketamine by paramedics in the management of severely agitated patients. Emerg Med Australas 2021;33(5): 875–82.

16. Melamed E, Oron Y, Ben-Avraham R, et al. The combative multitrauma patient: a protocol for prehospital management. Eur J Emerg Med 2007;14(5):265–8.

17. Godwin SA, Burton JH, Gerardo CJ, et al. Clinical policy: procedural sedation and analgesia in the emergency department. Ann Emerg Med 2014;63(2): 247–58.e18, published correction appears in Ann Emerg Med. 2017 Nov;70(5):758.

18. Colorado Department of Public Health & Environment. Ketamine investigatory review panel final report. 2021. https://cdphe.colorado.gov/ketamine-investigatory-review-panel-report-overview. Accessed June 30, 2022.

19. Cole JB, Lee SC, Martel ML, et al. The incidence of QT prolongation and torsades des pointes in patients receiving droperidol in an urban emergency department. West J Emerg Med 2020;21(4):728–36.

20. Gaw CM, Cabrera D, Bellolio F, et al. Effectiveness and safety of droperidol in a United States emergency department. Am J Emerg Med 2020;38(7):1310–4.

21. Calver L, Page CB, Downes MA, et al. the safety and effectiveness of droperidol for sedation of acute behavioral disturbance in the emergency department. Ann Emerg Med 2015;66(3):230–8.e1.

22. American College of Emergency Physicians. Policy statements. Ann Emerg Med 2021;77(6):e127–33.

23. Jeffers T, Darling B, Edwards C, et al. Efficacy of combination haloperidol, lorazepam, and diphenhydramine vs. combination haloperidol and lorazepam in the treatment of acute agitation: a multicenter retrospective cohort study. J Emerg Med 2022;62(4):516–23.

Advances in Trauma Ultrasound

Samuel Austin, DO[a],*, Daniel Haase, MD, RDMS, RDCS[b], Joseph Hamera, MD[b]

KEYWORDS

- Ultrasound • Trauma • Resuscitation • FAST • Critical care • FREE • RUSH • TEE

KEY POINTS

- New uses for ultrasound are continuing to be incorporated in trauma and resuscitation.
- The extended focused assessment with sonography for trauma can have utility in both blunt and penetrating trauma.
- The Rapid Ultrasound in Shock and Hypotension examination is useful in determining the etiologies of undifferentiated shock.
- The Focused Rapid Echocardiographic Examination is an accurate rapid assessment of quantitative and qualitative cardiac function.
- Transesophageal echocardiogram may be a useful adjunct for hemodynamic monitoring, but more research is needed.

THE EXTENDED FOCUSED ASSESSMENT WITH SONOGRAPHY IN TRAUMA

In the acutely injured patient, the Focused Assessment with Sonography in Trauma (FAST) examination has become a staple in initial trauma management. Traditionally, the purpose of the FAST examination was to rapidly identify hemoperitoneum and/ or hemopericardium. In the experienced operator, this bedside assessment can typically be done in 3 to 4 minutes[1] and consists of four primary views: the right upper quadrant (RUQ), the left upper quadrant (LUQ), the pelvis or pouch of Douglas in women, and a subxiphoid cardiac view.

Review of Basic Focused Assessment with Sonography in Trauma Technique

During the RUQ assessment, a low-frequency curvilinear or phased array transducer is placed along the right mid-axillary line with the indicator-oriented cephalad. Care is

[a] Department of Surgery, Program in Trauma, R Adams Cowley Shock Trauma Center, University of Maryland School of Medicine, 22 South Greene Street, Baltimore, MD 21201, USA;
[b] Department of Emergency Medicine, University of Maryland School of Medicine, The R. Adams Cowley Shock Trauma Center, Program in Trauma, University of Maryland School of Medicine, 110 S Paca St, Baltimore, MD 21201, USA
* Corresponding author.
E-mail address: samuel.austin@umm.edu

Emerg Med Clin N Am 41 (2023) 131–142
https://doi.org/10.1016/j.emc.2022.09.004
0733-8627/23/© 2022 Elsevier Inc. All rights reserved.

made to identify the hepatorenal space (Morison's pouch) and image down to the caudal tip of the liver, which maximizes the sensitivity for the identification of free fluid.

The operator then proceeds to the LUQ, where the transducer is placed on the left posterior axillary line and indicator pointing cephalad. Using the spleen as an acoustic window, the sonographer should then identify the splenorenal space and the space between the spleen and the diaphragm with an anterior to posterior sweep.

The transducer is then placed in the abdominal midline immediately superior to the pubic symphysis, held longitudinally with the probe indicator pointing towards the patient's head. A right-left sweep is performed to visualize the whole bladder. As the pelvis depends mostly on the location of the peritoneum, this view holds important significance in the FAST examination.[2] In males, the most common location for the identification of free fluid is in the rectovesical pouch, superior to the bladder. In females, free fluid most commonly initially accumulates in the pouch of Douglas, located between the bladder and the uterus.

Lastly, the operator performs a cardiac assessment using the subxiphoid view. The transducer is placed immediately inferior and to the patient's right of the xiphoid process, oriented toward the patient's left shoulder. Placing the transducer to the patient's right allows the operator to use the liver as an acoustic window. This view often requires added depth for adequate cardiac visualization. The subxiphoid view is focused on the identification of hemopericardium. A pericardial effusion is seen as an anechoic space between the visceral and parietal pericardium. For the purposes of the FAST examination, any free fluid identified in the pericardial space is assumed to represent blood until proven otherwise.

Depending on the mechanism of injury, the order to the FAST examination is not a hard and fast rule. For example, in patients with penetrating chest injuries, the subxiphoid view should be obtained first to assess for hemopericardium and cardiac tamponade. In the assessment for hemoperitoneum, the most sensitive location for the identification of free fluid is around the caudal tip of the liver and Morison's pouch. Sensitivities and specificities vary but have previously been reported approximately 80% and 100%, respectively.[3]

Ultrasound for the Detection of Pneumothorax

An extended FAST (E-FAST) has been implemented to broaden the assessment for potential sources of hemodynamic instability in the traumatically injured patient. The ability of ultrasound to identify lung pleura abnormalities has added a quick and simple method to identify a traumatic pneumothorax. E-FAST has shown potentially greater accuracy in the detection of an occult pneumothorax missed on chest X-ray, particularly in the patient laying supine in the trauma bay.[4]

The lung pleura can be best identified using a high-frequency linear probe along the anterior chest wall in the sagittal plane. The view should include a superior and inferior rib with a hyperechoic pleural line connecting the two ribs. A pneumothorax can be diagnosed by assessing *lung sliding*, *lung pulse*, *lung point*, and M-mode.

Lung sliding is visualized while a patient is breathing and is a product of the dynamic visceral pleura moving along the static parietal pleura along the chest wall.[5] However, when air is introduced into this potential space, the scattering of sound waves through air (attenuation) prevents the visualization of the "sliding" of the visceral pleura.

Lung pulse is the appearance of pulsations of the pleural line and is more frequently identified in the left hemithorax. This occurs from transmitted cardiac pulsations, displacing the pleural surfaces. This is considered a normal finding in an intact lung, and thus is expected to be absent in a pneumothorax. The presence of a lung pulse can essentially rule out a pneumothorax.[6]

M-mode can be a useful adjunct in pneumothorax assessment but is not considered necessary for diagnosis. When M-mode is applied in a normal lung, the minimal motion of the chest wall produces straight lines with an appearance like waves of an ocean. The hyperechoic pleura appears like a shoreline, and the lung parenchyma, which sits deepest in the image, produces a sand-like appearance. This forms an image like a seashore; hence, the term *Seashore sign* when referring to normal lung sliding. When air is present in a pneumothorax, thereby abolishing lung sliding, the stagnant appearance of lung parenchyma mirrors the appearance of soft tissue in the near field, generating the *barcode* (or *stratosphere*) *sign* (**Fig. 1**).

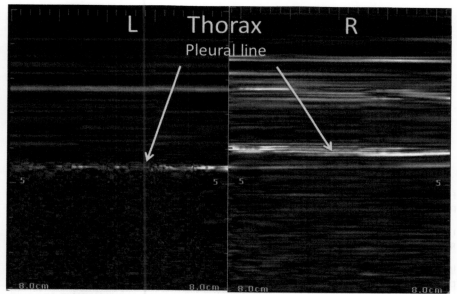

Fig. 1. Left: *Seashore sign* seen in normal lung sliding. Right: *Barcode sign* seen in absent lung sliding.

The most specific sign seen on pneumothorax assessment is the *lung point*. This appears as a transition point from normal lung sliding to the absence of lung sliding when visualizing the pleura. Visualization of the lung point is 100% accurate in the detection of a pneumothorax.[7]

Owing to its rapidity in performance, and the ability to make diagnoses at the bedside during either the primary or secondary survey, sonographic identification of a pneumothorax in the critically ill trauma patient can expedite the performance of potentially life-saving tube thoracostomy.

Ultrasound for the Detection of Hemothorax

With only a slight modification made to the E-FAST and minimal time added, thoracic views can be obtained to assess for hemothorax. While evaluating the RUQ and LUQ, the examiner can use the posterolateral approach to find the posterior diaphragmatic recess. This technique involves scanning slightly cephalad to the RUQ and LUQ until the hyperechoic diaphragm is visualized. Immediately above is the supradiaphragmatic space. This space can be challenging to image but sliding the transducer inferiorly and rocking superiorly can better use the liver or spleen as an acoustic window.

In a normal assessment, the lung will appear hazy, gray due to the attenuation of sound as it travels through a well-aerated lung. If a hemothorax is present, it will appear as an anechoic or hypoechoic area above the diaphragm, accumulating posteriorly. The fluid can act as an acoustic window to allow for the visualization of lung pleura, which may appear as floating in the lung space.[8] In addition, due to fluid's exceptional ability to transmit sound, the thoracic spine can be visualized above the diaphragm when fluid in the lung is present. This represents a finding called *spine sign* (**Fig. 2**). Point-of-care ultrasound (POCUS) has shown both a sensitivity and specificity of approximately 93% in detecting pleural effusions.

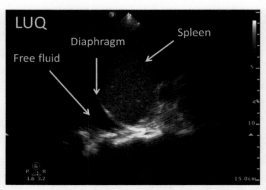

Fig. 2. Pleural effusion on LUQ ultrasound seen as an anechoic area superior to the diaphragm. The spine sign is seen at the bottommost aspect of image.

ULTRASOUND APPLICATION IN CRITICAL CARE MANAGEMENT AND RESUSCITATION

In the management of critically ill polytrauma patients, identifying sources of shock is paramount for appropriate management. Ultrasound has become a useful resource in trauma and critical care both in the identification of sources of hypotension and guiding resuscitation. Although the FAST examination has become an integral part of advanced trauma life support (ATLS) for the rapid identification of intraperitoneal or intrathoracic fluid and pneumothorax, critically ill patients can often present with multiple comorbidities that can complicate potential etiologies of their hypotension and continued resuscitation. As outcomes in shock depend on severity and duration, timely diagnosis can play a key role in improving patient outcomes.[9]

The Rapid Ultrasound in Shock and Hypotension Examination

When the critically ill patient has continued hypotension despite the absence of obvious hemorrhage, identification of the source is paramount. The Rapid Ultrasound in Shock and Hypotension (RUSH) has been described as an adjunctive modality for bedside evaluation for etiologies of shock. In addition to the standard E-FAST, the RUSH examination includes a qualitative echocardiographic assessment, the inferior vena cava (IVC) and aorta, along with a possible additional assessment for ectopic pregnancy and deep venous thrombosis (DVT). Findings of this examination can potentially help to differentiate among different etiologies of shock (**Table 1**).

Cardiac examination includes the parasternal long and short, apical-4 chamber, and subxiphoid views using a curvilinear and/or phased-array probe. A thorough "pump" assessment should include evaluations for pericardial effusions or cardiac

Table 1
Views of the rapid ultrasound in shock and hypotension examination and how findings correspond to different etiologies of shock[10]

Assessment	Hypovolemic Shock	Cardiogenic Shock	Obstructive Shock	Distributive Shock
Pump	Hypercontractility Small chamber appearance	Hypocontractility Dilated chamber appearance	Hypercontractility Pericardial effusion Cardiac tamponade Evidence of right Ventricular strain Visualized cardiac thrombus	Hyper- or hypocontractility (early vs late sepsis)
Tank	Flat/collapsible IVC Flat jugular veins Intraperitoneal or intrathoracic free fluid	Distended/non-collapsible IVC Distended jugular veins Lung comet-tail artifact Intraperitoneal or Intrathoracic free fluid	Distended/non-collapsible IVC Distended jugular veins Absent lung sliding	Normal vs flat/collapsible IVC Intraperitoneal or Intrathoracic free fluid
Pipes	Abdominal aortic aneurysm (AAA) Aortic dissection	N/a	DVT	N/a

tamponade, left ventricular (LV) contractility, and right ventricular (RV) dilation. Pericardial effusion or cardiac tamponade can be visualized using a subxiphoid approach and will appear as an anechoic area within the pericardial space. Clotted blood or complex fluid can take on a heterogenous or isoechoic appearance. It is important to distinguish pericardial fluid from pleural fluid, which can easily be confused. If a pericardial effusion is identified, it is important to assess for evidence of tamponade. This can be done by primarily assessing the right atrium and right ventricle. The right heart is a lower pressure system; thus, it is more susceptible to collapse when exposed to increased inward pressures. Thus, cardiac tamponade may rapidly be identified by abnormal inward deflections of the right atrium and/or right ventricle (representing collapse) during diastole (**Fig. 3**).

From the subxiphoid view, the IVC can rapidly be identified by rotating the probe so that the indicator is directed toward the head of the patient. The size and degree of collapsibility of the IVC has been shown to correlate with central venous pressure (CVP) in spontaneously breathing patients.[11–13] Measurement of IVC diameter and degree of collapsibility should be taken approximately 2 cm caudal to where the IVC enters the right atrium or 2 to 3 cm caudal to the IVC-hepatic vein confluence. In M-mode, the caval index can be determined by the following equation:

$$CI = \frac{D_{IVC-MAX} - D_{IVC-MIN}}{D_{IVC-MAX}}$$

where CI is the caval index, $D_{IVC-Max}$ is the maximum IVC diameter during expiration, and $D_{IVC-Min}$ is the minimum IVC diameter during inspiration.

A static IVC diameter <1.5 cm and CI > 50% can be indicative of a low CVP (<5–8 mm Hg), whereas a static IVC diameter >2.5 cm and CI < 50% can be indicative of an elevated CVP (>15 mm Hg). A CI < 20% is considered highly specific for elevated CVP.[14] In the assessment of the critically ill patient, correlating the IVC assessment with echocardiographic findings can aid in determining the etiology of shock.

The parasternal long and short views are useful for estimating LV ejection fraction and chamber size. On the basis of the amount of estimated change in the LV chamber size, the contractility can be categorized as normal, hyperdynamic, mild, moderately, or severely reduced.[15] In addition, the interventricular septum can be visualized with its relation to the left and right ventricles. Bowing of the septum toward the left ventricle could be representative of a dilated right ventricle and possible elevated right heart pressures.

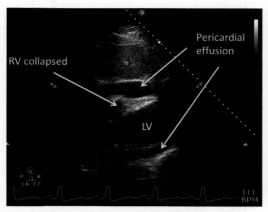

Fig. 3. RV collapse during systole seen in cardiac tamponade.

In certain patient populations, adequate IVC views can be difficult to obtain and preclude volume assessment, particularly in surgical patients. Visualizing the internal jugular (IJ) veins has been shown to be a useful adjunctive, and potentially more accurate, measure of CVP.[16] The patient's head of the bed should be elevated to 30° to 45°. The IJ veins can be examined for their distention and height in the neck, along with their collapsibility between exhalation to inspiration. With a normal CVP, the IJ should appear to close with inspiration at a level near the clavicles. However, in elevated CVP, the IJ may remain distended nearer to the angle of the jaw with a reduced degree of respiratory collapse. Measuring the level of the neck at which the IJ appears to collapse to the angle of Louis can allow the operator to more accurately estimate the CVP.[17]

The aorta is viewed to assess for major vascular emergencies, such as abdominal aortic aneurysm (AAA) or aortic dissection. Evaluation for AAA should be done throughout the whole length of the abdominal aorta until the aortic bifurcation to the common iliac arteries. Measurements of >3.0 cm from outer wall to outer wall in the transverse orientation, including the presence of any thrombi, are diagnostic for an AAA. Risk of aneurysmal rupture occurs when the aorta measures >5.0 cm.[18] As a ruptured AAA will likely result in retroperitoneal bleeding, which can be difficult to identify on ultrasound, identification of AAA in a patient with clinical signs and symptoms of rupture and/or hemodynamic instability should raise concern for the AAA as the source of their instability.

An aortic dissection may be recognized by either aortic root dilation or the presence of an intimal flap within the aorta. To assess for aortic root dilation, the heart is assessed in the parasternal long axis (PSLX). This permits visualization of the aortic outflow tract. A normal aortic root measures less than 4.0 cm when measuring from the outer wall to the inner wall. An aortic root wider than this should raise concern for an ascending aortic dissection. Simultaneously, the presence of a pericardial effusion and/or color flow-visualization of aortic regurgitation would further raise suspicion of an ascending aortic dissection. In both the assessment for an ascending or descending aortic dissection, direct visualization of an intimal flap can be diagnostic. Early identification of an AAA or aortic dissection, which can often be mistaken for more common diagnoses based on physical examination, can facilitate appropriate consultation and/or definitive management.

The Focused Rapid Echocardiographic Examination

The Focused Rapid Echocardiographic Examination (FREE) was developed to be a bedside cardiac assessment that places a larger emphasis on quantitative function. Although more formal assessment has traditionally been reserved for either an invasive approach with a transesophageal echocardiogram (TEE) or a cardiology consult for a formal transthoracic echocardiogram (TTE), the FREE offers an additional bedside assessment to expeditiously assess cardiac function in critically ill patients.[19] In the critically injured trauma patient, accurate assessment of cardiac function and fluid status is a key aspect of their care.

The FREE consists of the same standard four views as TTE and the IVC. The advantage of the FREE is that it allows the operator to assess more accurately left and RV function. Specifically, it categorizes patients based on cardiac function, preload, afterload, and cardiac anatomy to make clinical decisions regarding use of fluids, vasopressors, and inotropes.[19,20] These quantitative measurements are feasible but can be time-consuming, particularly in the critically ill patient. In this setting, rapid assessments of the left ventricular outflow tract velocity time integral (LVOT VTI) and tricuspid annular plane systolic excursion (TAPSE) can quickly quantify LV and RV function. In all views of the FREE the qualitative ventricular function can be evaluated along with the assessment of the valvular integrity, such as insufficiency or stenosis.

EMERGING AND ADVANCED CONCEPTS IN TRAUMA AND CRITICAL CARE ULTRASOUND

Ultrasound in Penetrating Trauma

The use of ultrasound and the FAST examination was traditionally reserved for the detection of intra-abdominal free fluid in blunt trauma or hemopericardium. However, its role in penetrating trauma has not been reviewed as extensively.

In hemodynamically stable patients, there is more time for additional diagnostic tests. The FAST in penetrating trauma has shown varying sensitivity (28.1% to 100%) with high specificity (94.1% to 100%).[21–28] Although its sensitivity has consistently been lower than other diagnostic modalities, such as local wound exploration, diagnostic peritoneal lavage, or computed tomography (CT) scan, it continues to show utility as an extremely specific test. A positive FAST should facilitate prompt exploratory laparotomy. A negative FAST does not preclude the need for further diagnostic imaging or further operating room (OR) management. However, patients with a negative FAST have also been associated with low mortality rates.[28,29]

The patient with penetrating trauma to the torso and unstable vital signs requires immediate transfer to the OR for exploratory surgery regardless of a negative or positive FAST result. However, the E-FAST examination can help to identify which surgical incision or approach will most likely reveal the source of life-threatening injury. In contrast to its role in penetrating abdominal trauma, ultrasound is of particular use in penetrating injury to the chest. It is a rapid assessment for the identification of pericardial effusion and a positive pericardial FAST has been shown to be highly sensitive and specific for hemopericardium, facilitating prompt intervention.[30]

Identification of Diaphragmatic Injury

Without extension to the traditional E-FAST, during the RUQ and LUQ evaluations the diaphragm can simultaneously be assessed for injury. As it is becoming more commonplace to routinely assess for hemothorax, the diaphragm is routinely identified. In approximately 5% of blunt abdominal traumas, the diaphragm is concomitantly injured. Findings on supine chest radiography can be innocuous and may be missed on CT scan as well. By maintaining a high index of suspicion in trauma, ultrasound can be a useful adjunct for identifying injuries to the diaphragm. Sonographic findings can include visualization of the diaphragm appearing as a flap in the pleural fluid or herniation of the spleen into the hemithorax. In addition, M-mode can be placed over the free edge of the diaphragm to evaluate its motion during respirations.[31]

Use of Transesophageal Echocardiography in Trauma Resuscitation

The use of POCUS is continuing to become an essential aspect of acute and continued resuscitation. Despite its increased invasiveness compared with TTE, TEE offers the advantage of enhanced cardiac visualization and improved diagnostic accuracy. In addition, there are multiple factors that may limit the feasibility of TTE, such as body habitus, mechanical ventilation limiting image quality, use in the operative/postoperative setting, and chest or abdominal trauma. Applying TEE to the critically ill surgical patient can ultimately lead to improved hemodynamic monitoring.

Like TTE, TEE has four primary views: mid-esophageal four-chamber, transgastric short axis, bicaval, and the mid-esophageal long axis (**Fig. 4**). The bicaval view also allows for visualization of the superior vena cava (SVC) and IVC. Even with limited prior TEE exposure, it has been shown that correct probe placement and obtaining

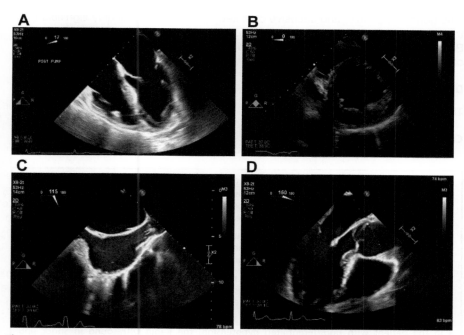

Fig. 4. Four main TEE views: (*A*) mid-esophageal four-chamber, (*B*) transgastric short axis, (*C*) bicaval, and (*D*) mid-esophageal long axis.

adequate images is easily teachable and can have a major influence on critical decision-making.[32] Obtaining these major views can play a key role in guiding ongoing resuscitation by identifying key pathologies, such as hypovolemia, ventricular hypokinesis, pericardial effusion or tamponade, or pleural effusions.

In the intraoperative setting, TEE serves the role of accessible, continuous hemodynamic monitoring when more invasive means are unable to be established (via arterial line or pulmonary artery catheterization). While simultaneously assessing LV and RV anatomy and function, it can aid in real-time decision-making regarding the need for volume resuscitation versus inotropic support. For the patient presenting with acute chest trauma, TEE can be used as an adjunct in the assessment of underlying cardiac or aortic injury. As CT imaging may be precluded due to hemodynamic instability, TEE has shown significant accuracy in the diagnosis of traumatic cardiac injury, pericardial effusion, valvular injury, and acute proximal aortic injury. In the assessment of cardiac injury, TEE has shown accuracy in identifying myocardial contusions and lacerations, pericarditis, aneurysms, and chordae tendinae injury. As opposed to some traditional markers of myocardial injury, such as electrocardiogram (ECG) changes and cardiac enzyme elevation, TEE has shown significantly increased sensitivity and specificity.[33,34] This is clinically relevant as patients with myocardial contusions are associated with increased mortality.

Overall, TEE has shown significant utility in hemodynamic monitoring and resuscitation. The extent of its role in acute trauma resuscitation needs to be more formally studied.

SUMMARY

Implementation of bedside ultrasound has become an integral component of acute care and continued resuscitation in the critically ill trauma patient. Physicians in the emergency, operative, and intensive care settings can readily identify significant pathologies with relatively low invasiveness, cost to the patient, and radiation exposure. Both TTE and TEE should be considered in all patients requiring ongoing resuscitative care.

DISCLOSURE

The authors have nothing to disclose.

CLINICS CARE POINTS

- The E-FAST is a highly specific exam that can provide rapid information on the presence of intraperitoneal injury in acute trauma. A positive FAST in blunt or penetrating trauma should lead the provider to consider early operative intervention. A negative FAST, however, does not definitely rule out an intraperitoneal injury

- A positive FAST in penetrating abdominal trauma warrants prompt transfer to the operating room for exploratory laparotomy. The presence of a pericardial effusion on ultrasound in penetrating torso trauma is hemopericardium until proven otherwise.

- For the acute trauma patient laying supine, point-of-care ultrasound of the lungs assessing for lung sliding and/or a lung point is a rapid and accurate test for the identification of pneumothorax. Hemothorax can be identified on the FAST by the presence of free fluid cephalad to the diaphragm.

- In the patient with undifferentiated hypotension, the Rapid Ultrasound in Shock and Hypotension (RUSH) is a useful adjunct to the initial work-up. The Focused Rapid Echocardiographic Examination (FREE) can provide quantitative data of cardiac function to help predict response to fluid resuscitation versus the need for vasopressors or inotropic support.

- The diaphragm on ultrasound is a hyperechoic structure and can be rapidly identified to assess for diaphragmatic injury.

- The use of Transesophageal echocardiography (TEE) in trauma is expanding to include early identification of traumatic cardiac injury and intraoperative hemodynamic monitoring.

REFERENCES

1. Haase DJ, Murthi SB. Ultrasound for point-of-care imaging: performing the various exams with technical tips. Shock Trauma Man Oper Tech 2020;149–83. https://doi.org/10.1007/978-3-030-275969.
2. Manson WC, Kirksey M, Boublik J, et al. Focused assessment with sonography in trauma (FAST) for the regional anesthesiologist and pain specialist. Reg Anesth Pain Med 2019;44(5):540–8.
3. Stengel D, Bauwens D, Rademacher G, et al. Association between compliance with methodological standards of diagnostic research and reported test accuracy: meta-analysis of focused assessment of us for trauma. Radiology 2005; 236(1):102–11.
4. Kirkpatrick AW, Sirois M, Laupland KB, et al. Hand-held thoracic sonography for detecting post-traumatic pneumothoraces: the extended focused assessment with sonography for trauma (EFAST). J Trauma Inj Infect Crit Care 2004;57(2): 288–95.
5. Haskins SC, Tsui BC, Nejim JA, et al. Lung ultrasound for the regional anesthesiologist and acute pain specialist. Reg Anesth Pain Med 2017;42(3):289–98.

6. Copetti R. Lung pulse with pneumothorax. Anesthesiology 2019;131(3):666.
7. Lichtenstein D, Meziere G, Biderman P, et al. The 'lung point': an ultrasound sign specific to pneumothorax. Intensive Care Med 2000;26(10):1434–40.
8. Montoya J, Stawicki SP, Evans DC, et al. From fast to E-FAST: an overview of the evolution of ultrasound-based traumatic injury assessment. Eur J Trauma Emerg Surg 2015;42(2):119–26.
9. Rahulkumar HH, Bhavin PR, Shreyas KP, et al. Utility of point-of-care ultrasound in differentiating causes of shock in resource-limited setup. J Emerg Trauma Shock 2019;12(1):10–7.
10. Perera P, Mailhot T, Riley D, et al. The rush exam 2012: rapid ultrasound in shock in the evaluation of the critically ill patient. Ultrasound Clin 2012;7(2):255–78.
11. Wiwatworapan W, Ratanajaratroj N, Sookananchai B. Correlation between inferior vena cava diameter and central venous pressure in critically ill patients. J Med Assoc Thai 2012;95(3):320–4.
12. Kircher BJ, Himelman RB, Schiller NB. Noninvasive estimation of right atrial pressure from the inspiratory collapse of the inferior vena cava. Am J Cardiol 1990; 66(4):493–6.
13. Jue J, Chung W, Schiller NB. Does inferior vena cava size predict right atrial pressures in patients receiving mechanical ventilation? J Am Soc Echocardiogr 1992; 5(6):613–9.
14. Mayse ML. Chapter 8. Ultrasound of the inferior vena cava. In: Carmody KA, Moore CL, Feller-Kopman D, et al, editors. Handbook of Critical Care and Emergency Ultrasound. New York, NY: McGraw Hill; 2011. p. 83–90.
15. Seif D, Perera P, Mailhot T, et al. Bedside ultrasound in resuscitation and the rapid ultrasound in shock protocol. Crit Care Res Pract 2012;2012:1–14.
16. Murthi SB, Fatima S, Menne AR. Ultrasound assessment of volume responsiveness in critically ill surgical patients. J Trauma Acute Care Surg 2017;82(3): 505–11.
17. Lipton B. Estimation of central venous pressure by ultrasound of the internal jugular vein. Am J Emerg Med 2000;18(4):432–4.
18. Barkin AZ, Rosen CL. Ultrasound detection of abdominal aortic aneurysm. Emerg Med Clin North Am 2004;22(3):675–82.
19. Ferrada P, Murthi S, Anand RJ, et al. Transthoracic focused rapid echocardiographic examination: real-time evaluation of fluid status in critically ill trauma patients. J Trauma Inj Infect Crit Care 2011;70(1):56–64.
20. Glaser JJ, Carderelli C, Galvagno S, et al. Bridging the gap: Hybrid Cardiac Echo in the Critically Ill. J Trauma Acute Care Surg 2016;81(5).
21. Boulanger BR, Kearney PA, Tsuei B, et al. The routine use of sonography in penetrating torso injury is beneficial. J Trauma 2001;51:320–5.
22. Biffl WL, Kaups KL, Cothren CC, et al. Management of patients with anterior abdominal stab wounds: a Western Trauma Association multicenter trial. J Trauma 2009;66:1294–301.
23. Brooks A, Davies B, Smethhurst M, et al. Prospective evaluation of nonradiologist performed emergency abdominal ultrasound for haemoperitoneum. Emerg Med 2004;21:e5.
24. Kirkpatrick AW, Sirois M, Ball CG, et al. The hand-held ultrasound examination for penetrating abdominal trauma. Am J Surg 2004;187:660–5.
25. Soffer D, McKenney MG, Cohn S, et al. A prospective evaluation of ultrasonography for the diagnosis of penetrating torso injury. J Trauma 2004;56:953–7 [discussion: 7–9].

26. Soto JA, Morales C, Munera F, et al. Penetrating stab wounds to the abdomen: use of serial US and contrast-enhanced CT in stable patients. Radiology 2001; 220:365–71.
27. Tayal VS, Beatty MA, Marx JA, et al. FAST (focused assessment with sonography in trauma) accurate for cardiac and intraperitoneal injury in penetrating anterior chest trauma. J Ultrasound Med 2004;23:467–72.
28. Udobi KF, Rodriguez A, Chiu WC, et al. Role of ultrasonography in penetrating abdominal trauma: a prospective clinical study. J Trauma 2001;50:475–9.
29. Quinn AC, Richard S. What is the utility of the focused assessment with sonography in trauma (fast) exam in penetrating torso trauma? Injury 2011;42(5):482–7.
30. Matsushima K, Khor D, Berona K, et al. Double jeopardy in penetrating trauma: get fast, get it right. World J Surg 2017;42(1):99–106.
31. Blaivas M, Brannam L, Hawkins M, et al. Bedside emergency ultrasonographic diagnosis of diaphragmatic rupture in blunt abdominal trauma. Am J Emerg Med 2004;22(7):601–4.
32. Arntfield R, Pace J, Hewak M, et al. Focused transesophageal echocardiography by emergency physicians is feasible and clinically influential: observational results from a novel ultrasound program. J Emerg Med 2016;50(2):286–94.
33. Garcia-Fernandez MA, Lopez-Perez JM, Perez-Castellano N, et al. Role of transesophageal echocardiography in the assessment of patients with blunt chest trauma: correlation of echocardiographic findings with the electrocardiogram and creatine kinase monoclonal antibody measurements. Am Heart J 1998; 135(3):476–81.
34. Leichtle SW, Singleton A, Singh M, et al. Transesophageal echocardiography in the evaluation of the trauma patient: a trauma resuscitation transesophageal echocardiography exam. J Crit Care 2017;40:202–6.

Minor Procedures in Trauma

Jesse Shriki, DO, MS[a],*, Sagar B. Dave, DO[b,c]

KEYWORDS

- Trauma • Central venous access • Thoracostomy • Hemothorax • Pneumothorax
- Regional anesthesia

KEY POINTS

- Knowledge of the anatomy and physiology is crucial to procedural skill.
- Use the ultrasound before, during, and after, respectively, to plan/map anatomy, perform, and confirm your procedure.
- It is no longer sufficient to just walk through the steps of a procedure; one must also understand the best approach for the patient that minimizes pain and discomfort.
- Never put in a device that is just handed to you without considering the downstream effects (eg, has the patient had multiple central lines there? Will I need a computed tomography with contrast?).
- Know the individual steps of each procedure and practice them with intent.

Procedures in medicine, whether they be performed under the auspices of trauma, critical care, or emergency medicine, are a cornerstone in the care of the ill patient. The difference between being a proceduralist and being expert, lies in the knowledge of not only knowing all aspects of that procedure but tailoring that procedure to the needs of the patient in front of you and then, incorporating their care into it. With the rampant availability of ultrasound (US) and a wide arsenal of anesthetics and sedatives, it is no longer acceptable to "just" do the procedure. Emphasis should be placed, equally, on ensuring that a procedure is carried out as accurately and as painlessly as possible while keeping in mind the rapidity under which it should be undertaken.

[a] Department of Critical Care, Banner-University Medical Center, 1111 East McDowell Road, Phoenix, AZ 85006, USA; [b] Department of Emergency Medicine, Emory University School of Medicine, Grady Memorial Hospital, 1750 Gambrell Drive Northeast, Hospital Tower, Suite T5L41, Atlanta, GA 30322, USA; [c] Department of Anesthesiology, Emory University School of Medicine, Grady Memorial Hospital, Emory University Department of Anesthesiology, 1750 Gambrell Drive Northeast, Hospital Tower, Suite T5L41, Atlanta, GA 30322, USA
* Corresponding author.
E-mail address: shrikido@gmail.com

Emerg Med Clin N Am 41 (2023) 143–159
https://doi.org/10.1016/j.emc.2022.09.008
0733-8627/23/© 2022 Elsevier Inc. All rights reserved.

CENTRAL VENOUS CATHETER

The central venous catheter (CVC) is synonymous with critical care. Despite the prevalence of US-guided peripheral catheters and intraosseous lines, central lines still find a use in trauma and intensive care. Overuse, however, can lead to a wide array of morbidity and mortality and should only be done when absolutely necessary.

History

In 1929 a German surgical resident passed a 4-French (Fr), 35-cm ureteric catheter from his own left antecubital vein and then took a radiograph that showed it in the right atrium. Weeks later this new technique was used on a woman with peritonitis to deliver epinephrine and glucose directly to the heart. Although she did temporarily improve, nevertheless, she ultimately died. Subsequent to this he injected contrast into his own right heart to demonstrate the ability of imaging of the coronary and pulmonary arteries.[1] Thus, the central venous catheter was borne. In 1952 in Acta Radiologica Dr Sven Ivar Seldinger published his new technique of catheter replacement of the needle in percutaneous angiography. This technique was modified and went on to revolutionize CVC placement, which at the time required exposure of the artery or trocar punctured.[2]

Rapid Resuscitation

When rapid resuscitation is needed, and permissive hypotension is not the priority currently, there exist many options for resuscitation: intraosseous, rapid infusion cannulae, and a multitude of central access cannulae. Thus, one should know the general flow rates for these devices. Mathematically, the Poiseuille (pronounced PWAA-Z-A) equation predicts flow (see Equation 1), and therefore, a large diameter (via the radius) is the most important factor, as it increases exponentially. Another important factor is a short length, as a shorter length will increase flow. Through this we can also understand why a more viscous product (ie, blood) will decrease flow and a pressure bag will increase flow.

Variable	Parameter
Q	Flow
P	Pressure
r	radius
n	viscosity
l	length

$$Q = \frac{\pi P r^4}{8nl}$$

Equation 1: The Poiseuille equation. The flow (Q) is proportional to the pressure and the fourth power of the radius and inversely proportional to the length and viscosity.

The Multilumen Access Catheter (aka MAC, Arrow/Teleflex, PN, USA) is a dual lumen introducer (**Fig. 1**). The term "introducer" implies that along with the one large lumen and one smaller lumen, there is a third port through which other catheters (eg, right heart catheter or pacemaker wires) can be placed. Catheter sizing can be measured in terms of French size or gauge (g) size; however, it is common to measure single lumen catheters (and needles) by gauge system and multilumen catheters by French size. For comparison, 1 Fr = 0.3 mm (mm) and gauge, originally used initially for use in wire manufacture thus roughly correlates to multiples of 1/1000 of an inch.[3]

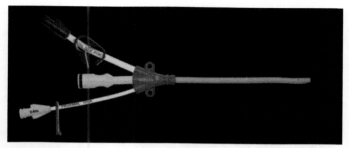

Fig. 1. The Multilumen Access Catheter (aka MAC, Arrow/Teleflex, PN, USA). One of many options for a resuscitation line that has multiple ports. Brown port is a large-bore lumen; the middle acts as an introducer for a PA catheter. PA, pulmonary artery.

When comparing flows as was done by Milne and colleagues, it was found that both a 9-Fr MAC and a 9-Fr introducer (aka Cordis, FL, USA) could both attain up to flows of 1 L/min with the MAC slightly faster than the Cordis. They found, by way of comparison, a 14-g dual lumen catheter flows 4 times slower than a 9-Fr MAC.[4] In a separate trial Traylor and colleagues showed that a 14-g PVC and 8.5-Fr CVC had statistically significant faster flow rates than a triple lumen catheter even with a pressure bag.[5] All these findings can be predicted by the Poiseuille equation.

Probably the most important concept in resuscitation was said by the Chinese general Sun Tzu: "Know thy enemy and know yourself; in a hundred battles, you will never be defeated."[6] The enemy of vascular access is not just the line that is placed but the vasculature itself. Successful vascular access of an elderly end-stage renal patient with superior vena cava stenosis[7] from multiple central lines is vastly different than vascular access in a young patient with no vascular disease. If you know what lines you are best at and what lines work in what types of patients, you will never be defeated. As a final pearl, the single biggest mistake I see in the resuscitation room is when the physician does not pay attention to the label on the vascular access device and places whatever is handed to them. Resuscitation lines should be stored separately from vascular delivery lines in order to avoid placing the wrong line.

Analgesia for Central Venous Catheters

In addition to rapid resuscitation, central lines are placed for other reasons including medication administration as in pressors, hemodynamic monitoring as in the case of a right heart catheterization, or therapy as in the case of extracorporeal membrane oxygenation cannulae. In cases where the internal jugular vein is used, an excellent adjunct to the pain of central line placement is the superior cervical plexus block. This is a simple-to-perform plane block where lidocaine is infiltrated along the posterior surface (plane) of the sternocleidomastoid (SCM) muscle at the midpoint of neck and can be easily found by US (**Fig. 2**) just lateral to the location where one would place an US-guided internal jugular line. A 5 mL of 2% lidocaine and 5 mL of normal saline can then be administered directly posterior to the SCM. This plane block anesthetizes the superior cervical plexus that essentially supplies sensation on the ipsilateral side of the neck from the ear lobe to the clavicle; this will effectively anesthetize all steps including dilation of the central line. In my opinion, patient comfort is improved greatly when a central line is performed on the awake patient and uses little to no rescue lidocaine. This plane block works very well for transvenous pacemaker placement, right heart catheterization, and, especially, placement of venovenous extracorporeal membrane oxygenation cannula in the right internal jugular location.

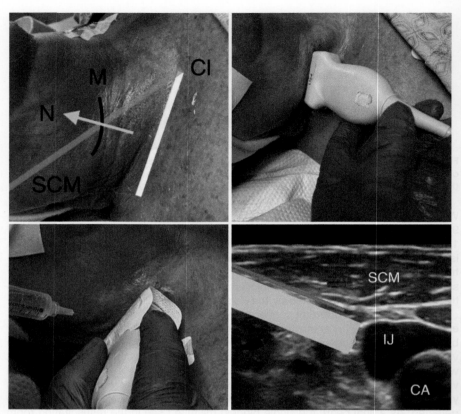

Fig. 2. Steps of the superior cervical plane block (SCP). (*Top left*) Surface anatomy of SCP block. Cl, clavicle; SCM, sternocleidomastoid muscle; M, midpoint of the SCM; N (*yellow arrow*), nerve exiting from the SCM muscle. (*Top right*) Placement of ultrasound probe for SCM block. (*Bottom left*) Needle placement relative to US probe. Note this block can be done in the plane of the US probe (not pictured) or perpendicular to the plane of the US probe (picture). It is logistically easier to do the block perpendicular to the probe as in pictures. (*Bottom right*) Sonographic anatomy. SCM, sternocleidomastoid muscle; IJ, internal jugular vein; CA, carotid artery. Red line is deep border of SCM muscle; yellow rectangle is plane of injection of local anesthetic.

Central Line Anatomy and Cannulation

There are 4 main locations amenable to central access. Two subclavian locations (infra- and supraclavicular), the internal jugular location and the femoral location.

The subclavian central line has 2 approaches, the commonly known infraclavicular and the less known supraclavicular. In the infraclavicular approach, the patient should be supine. Some investigators advocate for a towel under the patient's spine, lengthwise, to arch the shoulders[8,9]; however, too much arching or turning the head away from side of cannulation can inhibit access. The shoulders should be either neutral or depressed with gentle traction on the arms. The needle insertion point has been described at the midline (original description) of the clavicle and at the junction of the medial and proximal third of the clavicle and even lateral to this.[9] Likely the optimal needle insertion site is at midline of the clavicle or lateral to this and 1 to 2 m inferior to the bottom edge of the clavicle.[8] US can be used for the infraclavicular approach but if the vein is cannulated lateral to the clavicle it will be considered technically an axillary vein line and the needle angle will be much steeper than without US guidance (**Fig. 3**).

The supraclavicular approach to the subclavian is best identified with US to locate the junction of the internal jugular and subclavian vein where they join (**Fig. 4**). The needle is directed 15° below the coronal plane and 45° to the sagittal plane such that the confluence is met at a relatively stable depth of about 1.5 cm[9]; this was formerly known as the pocket shot in the vernacular.[10]

The internal jugular is easily found with US guidance (**Fig. 5**). It is cannulated at the apex of the triangle formed by the meeting of both heads of the SCM. In this era of prevalent US, and under specific recommendations from the Agency for Healthcare Research and Quality (AHRQ), it should, without exception, be cannulated under US guidance.[11] Knowledge of the landmark anatomy is still helpful, as the needle should be directed toward the ipsilateral nipple.[12] The internal jugular is always in close approximation to the ipsilateral common carotid, and thus special care should be

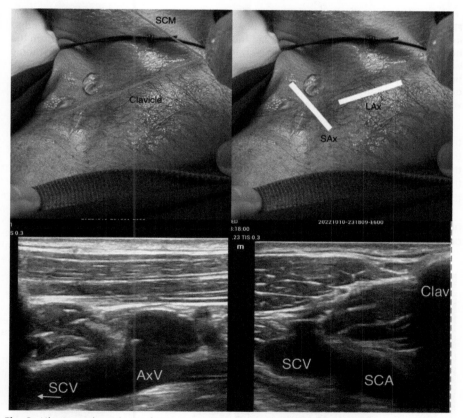

Fig. 3. Ultrasound guidance for the infraclavicular approach to the subclavian vein (SCV). (*Top left*) Surface anatomy shown with the clavicle and sternocleidomastoid muscle (SCM). The axillary vein (this becomes the SCV under the clavicle). (*Top right*) White bar represents placement of US probe in either the short axis (SAx) or long axis (LAx) position. (*Bottom left*) Sonoanatomy from the LAx view. (*Bottom right*) Sonoanatomy from the LAx view.

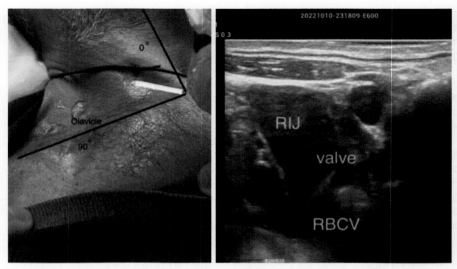

Fig. 4. The supraclavicular approach to the subclavian is best identified with ultrasound to locate the junction of the internal jugular and subclavian vein where they join to form the brachiocephalic vein. Picture above is the positioning. The clavicle makes a 90-degree angle with the midline of the neck. The ultrasound probe (*white block on left panel*) is positioned between these 2 landmarks at 45°. It is at this point on the right that the right internal jugular (RIJ) is accessible for direct access. Seen in panel B is the RIJ, the right brachiocephalic vein (RBCV), and a valve separating the two.

taken not to puncture the posterior wall of the internal jugular out of concern for having the wire mistakenly traverse the ipsilateral common carotid. It should be remembered that when placing a central venous catheter in the left internal jugular as opposed to the right internal jugular, a catheter 4 cm longer (20 cm vs 16 cm) should be used given the extra distance.

Lastly, the common femoral vein can be found medial to the common femoral artery and ends at the inguinal ligament where it then becomes the external iliac vein. The correct site of access then is below the inguinal ligament in the common femoral

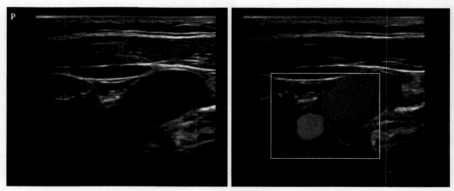

Fig. 5. The internal jugular (IJ) is easily found with ultrasound guidance. Notice the oblong shape and relatively thinner walls of the IJ (*blue*) compared with carotid (*red*).

vein next to the common femoral artery. This location of central venous access should always be performed under US guidance as marker of quality per the AHRQ.[11]

Technique

- The vessel of choice PRIOR TO CANNULATION should be mapped out by US for vascular abnormalities (course, thrombosis, and so forth), then prepped and draped
  - Pro tip: place a "Chux" under the head, shoulder, or leg where the central line will be placed, especially in the case of a large-bore catheter
- Using US guidance, the vein will be identified
  - Pro tip: anesthetize the area under US guidance to find your angle of entry, gauge the depth of entry, and ensure you are exactly centered on the vessel
  - Pro tip: use the M-mode marker (not actual M-mode) as a midline screen marker
  - Pro tip (for the advanced proceduralist only): once you know your angle of entry and have confirmed location of needle insertion, you can instead first incise the area using a scalpel incise instead of a needle (modified technique); this will obviate the need to make a scalpel incision later and prevent the formation of a skin bridge. Caution should be advised as to not make too large an incision.
- Using a needle enter the skin and the vein in question
  - Pro tip: point the J of the wire in the direction you want the wire to go
  - Pro tip: in the SCV location point the bevel down to prevent going cephalad into the internal jugular vein
- While ensuring to keep the needle absolutely still, remove the syringe and advance the wire through the needle
- Rail the wire intermittently while advancing
  - Railing is the process of sliding the wire back and forth to ensure it moves EASILY in the vessel
  - Any resistance to wire entry should constitute a new stick, as you are not in the lumen of the vessel or there may be clot blocking the wire movement
- The wire should advance very easily and should be able to traverse up to 30 cm (the black marker) without meeting resistance.
  - Any resistance along the way should signal an incorrect course (eg, into a branch vessel) and the wire should be mostly withdrawn and readvanced
- Remove the needle
- Confirm wire position with US again and follow wire down the course of vein
  - Pro tip: one may at this point want to confirm placement with a short vascular catheter (blue and white catheter in most CVC kits) and see blood flow from the vessel
- Load the dilator
- If not already done, a small nick in the skin should be made to prevent kinking of the wire
- The dilator should go in easily with minimal resistance and follow the course of the wire
  - Resistance should signal incorrect course of the wire
- You should gently rail the wire while dilating
- Dilate 3 times to ensure appropriate dilation rail with each dilation
- Remove dilator and you should now see blood flow
- Place the catheter over the wire and advance to the appropriate position just outside the heart at the vena cava and right atrial junction

- Ensure ability to draw back on all ports. Inability to do this may signal entry into a branch vein and incorrect placement
- Secure the central line directly to the skin; there is no need for the included clip to be secured
- Cover the CVC with a chlorhexidine (CHG)-impregnated gauze

Complications

Although searching the literature for comparison of central line–associated blood stream infections (CLABSI) will yield conflicting meta-analyses, in the largest multi-center trial published to date, the 3Sites trial, subclavian vein placement was associated with reduced infectious risk relative to internal jugular or femoral vein sites. As such, the internal jugular and femoral vein sites had a similar incidence of CLABSI. Femoral lines did have a statistically high rate of symptomatic deep venous thrombosis. Furthermore, as one would imagine, the subclavian vein had the higher pneumothorax (pnx) rate as having a significant decrease in mechanical complications compared with subclavian vein access.[13] Although the rate of arterial injury is likely unknown and underreported, these injuries should be kept in mind. A dilated artery in any location can cause a fistula and a subsequent pseudoaneurysm that may require vascular surgery intervention. Once an artery is dilated, the dilator should not be removed if possible and a vascular surgery consult should be called. Any growing hematoma in the area of a current or prior central line should be investigated with a formal arterial and possible venous doppler US by radiology. The wire should be checked to ensure it is in the vessel. Both US and railing are excellent techniques to confirmation wire position; this will prevent an ectopic location of a central line, as at any location the CVC may be placed into a false passage (**Fig. 6**). Lastly, the wire should always be accounted for in a checklist format after the procedure to ensure it does not become a retained foreign body in a vessel (**Fig. 7**).

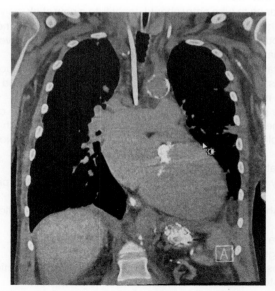

Fig. 6. Ectopic location of a central line (hemodialysis catheter) placed into a false passage in the mediastinum.

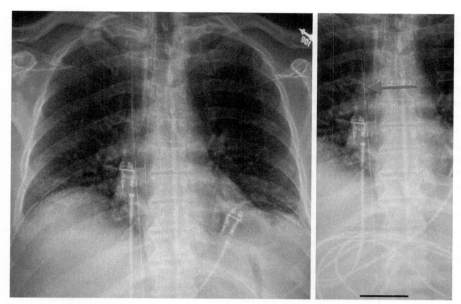

Fig. 7. The wire should always be accounted for in a checklist format after the procedure to ensure it does not become a retained foreign body in a vessel as seen in superior vena cava (SVC) in this image. (*Left*) Wire in SVC. (*Right*) Zoomed image of left; red arrow shows wire placement.

TUBE THORACOSTOMY

The drainage of chest pathology can be traced all the way back to Hippocrates; however, it was John Vigo of Rome in 1514 who attempted to publish the first guidelines for the management of penetrating chest trauma.[14] It only took another 60 years for Ambrose Pare to realize that "...if blood remains in the chest, mischief will follow."[15] It is on this long history that we have knowledge of draining the chest. Thus, we should approach the placement of chest tubes with a thorough understanding of the surgical anatomy, physiology, and pathology of the chest, along with the mechanics of drains.

Anatomy and Definitions

Anatomically, the lung is surrounded by a serous membrane, the pleura, that folds back on itself to form a fluid filled, potential space of the pleural cavity. The part of the membrane that abuts the chest wall is the parietal pleura and the visceral pleura abuts the lung. In the uninjured lung, the pressure in pleural cavity is negative (less than atmospheric pressure) with respect to the alveolar pressure. This negative pressure is created by an inward force by the elastic lungs that want to collapse and an outward stable force of the chest wall that opposes this elasticity.[16] When measured (in terms of weight of a column of water) these pressures are −8 cm during inspiration and −3.5 cm during expiration. However, if there is obstruction, as in coughing, then forced inspiration can be as high as −54 cm and forced expiration can be as high as +70 cm $H2O$.[17]

A pnx is a disruption of the pleura and negative pressure; this forms a gradient that preferentially collects air until there is no longer a pressure difference or until the communication is sealed. A tension pnx develops when that disruption is so great that the collected air displaces the ipsilateral lung and shifts the mediastinum shift toward the contralateral side. This leads to worsening hypoxia and mechanical compression of the heart and vascular structures of the chest.[16]

Indications

Indications for tube thoracostomy depend on the pathology as there are slight differences for hemothorax (htx) andpnx. For this discussion we will limit the scope to traumatic pathology and not include medical or spontaneous causes. In the setting of an unstable trauma patient the decision to insert a tube thoracostomy (TT) becomes somewhat straight forward. Those who cannot make it past "C" of the A-B-C evaluation by Advanced Trauma Life Support (ALTS) standard should often get a chest tube as a suspicion of tension pnx or massive hemothorax demands immediate placement.[18] There is likely a cut-off amount of hemothorax that is safe to be observed,[19] however, there is no agreement and even less data to suggest what that amount is or how to measure it. At this time however, the rate of empyema in those with undrained hemothorax is approximately 33% based on small studies.[20] It is this specter that drives current guidelines that recommend for every hemothorax, regardless of size, drainage should be considered with initial attempt by tube thoracostomy.[21]

It is known that a small pnx can be managed with observation only but a large pnx is at increased risk of failing conservative treatment and will require a chest tube. Determining at what point an intervention should occur has remained somewhat controversial. There are only retrospective and no large randomized controlled trials to base decisions on and a myriad of methods to measure remaining lung volume. The American College of Chest Physicians defines a small pnx as one that on chest radiograph (CXR) the distance from the collapsed lung apex to the cupula (apical part of the costal pleura) measured is less than 2 cm. Using this definition, a trial in South Africa of 125 patients with a small traumatic pnx found a failure of observation in only 1 of 125 patients with less than 1.5 cm on CXR and 3/125 with less than 2 cm on CXR.[22] With computed tomography (CT) becoming more prevalent, one study looked at measuring the size of PTX on CT by measuring the radial distance between the parietal and visceral pleura in a line perpendicular to the chest wall on axial imaging of the largest air pocket (**Fig. 8**). Using a cutoff of 35 mm to determine a small pnx, this study found 89% of 832 patients with a pnx were successfully managed conservatively.[23] Thus,

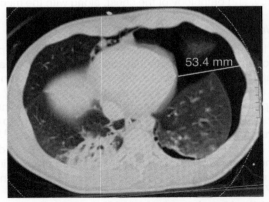

53.4 mm

Fig. 8. Example of measuring the size of PTX on CT by measuring the radial distance between the parietal and visceral pleura in a line perpendicular to the chest wall on axial imaging of the largest air pocket.

best evidence at this time suggests that patients with normal vital signs and a traumatic pnx less than 1.5 cm on CXR or less than 35 mm radial distance on CT or less than 10% thoracic volume on CT can be managed with conservative treatment and observation.[24]

Occult pnx is generally defined as one that is not detected by radiography or physical examination but found on subsequent CT[25] and/or lung US. For an occult pnx, guidelines recommend observation on positive pressure.[21] The 2021 OPTICC trial of occult pnx and positive pressure randomized 75 patients to observation and 69 patients to drainage. Statistically, they found no difference in the rate of patients requiring (as determined by clinician) the need for a chest tube in 38% of observed and 25% of drained ($P = .14$); however, this 13% difference would seem clinically significant, thus shared decision-making is encouraged in these situations. They also found that after 5 days 40% of the observation group did require a chest drain.[26]

Preoperative Management

Once it has been determined that intervention is required, some preprocedural management is required. A systematic review of the literature on the use of antibiotics in traumatic chest tube management found approximately a 6% absolute risk reduction in the incidence of both empyema and pneumonia.[27] As such, there seems to be trend to benefit in antibiotics around the time of insertion chest tube placement in both blunt and penetrating trauma. However, more than a single dose does not seem necessary.[28]

Tube Size Selection

Chest tubes come in a variety of sizes. Historically larger tubes, greater than 36 Fr, were recommended for drainage of blood from the chest with minimal evidence. In 2012, Inaba and colleagues showed 28 to 32 Fr chest tubes were comparable in amount of blood drained in hemothorax and complications.[29] Of interest, Peter Rhee and colleagues conducted both a retrospective 7-year review and a randomized controlled trial of 14 Fr pigtail catheters versus 32 to 40 Fr chest tubes and in both trials found a trend to larger output in the pigtail catheter and no statistical difference in failure rate.[30,31] For now, consensus tends toward larger tubes (28 Fr) but as data grow this may change. Along with sizing of chest tube comes insertion technique. Smaller pigtail catheters are usually placed over a wire whereas, larger bore tubes are placed by an open method using the operator finger to sweep inside the pleural cavity. There is an alternative method referred to as trocar-guided placement where a sharp object is thrust into the cavity. This technique has no built-in safety check such as a finger sweep nor the ability to aspirate back abnormal pleural cavity contents. Therefore, the trocar method should be avoided because of its higher incidence of complication rate and injury to surrounding structures.[32,33]

Analgesia and Sedation

It is of critical importance to appropriately sedate and treat pain of a patient before performing a tube thoracostomy, as it is an extremely painful procedure. At minimum, intravenous sedation with ketamine and/or propofol along with intermittently dosing of opioids should be considered, depending on the hemodynamics of the patient. Even if the patient is intubated and sedated one should administer local anesthesia if hemodynamics permit. If this is not an emergent procedure, one might also consider a nerve plane block such as the serratus anterior plane block (SAPB). Although the detailed description is beyond the scope of this article, the SAPB has been associated with decreased pain and decreased opioid consumption in the postprocedure phase.[34–36]

Positioning

Positioning is essential to success. Having the bed at the appropriate height, all tools available organized in the order of use, and the patient supine with the arm abducted from the body are all critical. One should also place the US, if being used, on the contralateral side for obvious ergonomic reasons. This investigator encourages the use of a soft restrain to keep the ipsilateral arm in the appropriate position abducted and above the head. Needle decompression at the second intercostal approach (Monaldi approach) is no longer encouraged by ATLS guidelines because of incorrect estimation of the position of the clavicle.[37] In fact, in the setting of an experienced traumatologist given the complication rate of needle thoracostomy[38] skipping the needle and going straight to chest tube is usually best. Lastly, and to exhibit procedural forethought, included in positioning should be the placement of one absorbable (aka "Chux") pad under the patient on the affected side and one on the floor for the inevitable drainage that will collect there.

Ideal placement of the chest tube position is just above the diaphragm for drainage and no lower than the midaxillary line for the patient's comfort. Although dogma teaches that a pnx should be placed in the apex and a hemothorax should be placed low in the pleural space, the literature would suggest otherwise.[39] Even TT placement in an intrapleural fissure does not seem to be a reason for the need to replace a chest tube.[39] Therefore, as long as the chest tube is in the pleural cavity and not kinked nor intraparenchymal or some other ectopic placement, the literature suggests not to remove the tube nor place a second chest tube.[40,41]

Open chest tube technique

- Appropriately sterilize, prepare, and drape the selected location.
- After having the selected chest tube at the ready, place a clamp on the dital end of the chest tube at the ready place on clamp on the distal end of the chest tube.
- A 2 to 3 cm incision through skin and subcutaneous fascia is made at the fourth intercostal space or inframammary fold.
- A curved hemostat is then used to bluntly dissect the muscle layer just above the top (cranial) part of the rib.
- Place one of the prongs of the curved hemostat through the sentinel eye of the chest tube, thus clamping only one side.
- To control puncture depth, hold the curved hemostat with the thumb on top of the hemostat with only 2 to 3 cm of the curved clamp free.
- Puncture through the pleura into the rib space.
- Keeping the hemostat in place pass the small finger into the chest sweeping 360° to ensure no other structures are involved.
- Slide the tube off the clamp with a clockwise twisting motion in a downward and cranial direction.
- Secure the chest tube in place then cover with Vaseline gauze, 4x4 gauze, and foam tape.

Pigtail chest tube via Seldinger technique

- Appropriately sterilize, prepare, and drape the selected location[a]
- Have a "double setup" on the US, placing both the linear probe and the phased array "cardiac" probe in probe covers and placing on the field sterilely

---

[a] There are a variety of such tubes and you should make yourself familiar ahead of time with the ones available at your institution.

- Use the phased array probe to get an overview of the area to perform the procedure
- Use the linear probe thereafter to locate arterial structures with color Doppler
- Place 3 mL of lidocaine into a 5 mL syringe and connect an 18-g introducer needle with or without a sheath to the syringe.
- Once the ideal location has been selected by US, use the 18-g introducer needle to enter the pleural space while aspirating (this may be done under dynamic US guidance or static US guidance). You should see bubbles in the syringe or fluid in the syringe confirming placement.
- Place a 0.035' wire through the needle into the space in a Seldinger fashion
- Place a dilator over the wire and make an incision over the wire in front of the dilator
- The pigtail chest tube (PCT) should have a rigid plastic introducer (not a metal trocar) to remove the pigtail shape and straighten it.
- Dilate the tissue 3 times to ensure appropriate dilation
- Remove the dilator and place the chest tube with rigid introducer over the wire into the chest cavity to the chest wall marker on the tube
- Remove wire and introducer, leaving only the PCT
- Place a 3-way stopcock at the end of the chest tube for easy sampling or instillation of enzymes in the future
- Some PCTs have a string that is used to hold the pigtail shape[a]
- Secure the PCT to the skin
- Place a CHG-impregnated gauze over the chest tube insertion site
- Secure the PCT to the chest wall with a urinary catheter stabilization device (eg, Stat-Lock from a urinary catheter)

Complications

Although positioning does not seem to be a complication of TT placement, other serious complications can occur, including bleeding, skin breakdown, subcutaneous placement, dislodgement, empyema, and organ damage. Bleeding, although likely the most common complication, can be minimized with US guidance especially using the linear probe to identify the intercostal artery. For study purposes it has been assumed that thoracentesis has an analogous complication rate to a 14-Fr chest tube placement.[42] Then extrapolating from a study by Ault and colleagues, that looked at 9320 thoracentesis, they found a 0.5% bleeding risk and no relationship to coagulation-related laboratory values.[43] There are less data on patients taking clopidogrel; however, only a small increase in bleeding was seen in those patients.[44] In a UK survey among several hospital systems many complications were seen such as lung or chest wall injury, wrong side, lost wire, and ectopic locations. Ectopic locations had a high mortality and included intraabdominal location, heart, subclavian vessels, colon, inferior vena cava, and esophagus.[45] Bronchopleural and bronchoalveolar fistulas, abnormal communications between bronchi or parenchymal lung tissue, respectively, may occur. Retained hemothorax can lead to empyema with a high rate if not drained or managed properly.[20] Unfortunately, at this time risk factors for retained hemothorax are not well understood but likely relate to larger initial hemothorax volumes, worse injury, and mechanical ventilation. Likely, video-assisted thoracoscopy by a surgeon should be performed instead of a second chest tube; alternatively, administration of enzymatic and lytic therapy can be performed, which may have similar efficacy.[28]

Aftercare

Aftercare of the chest tube should include a thorough understanding and inspection of the thoracic drain vacuum systems, daily CXR, and your institution's policies and practices of how to advance the chest tube care. Thoracic drainage systems in current use are based around what is known as the 3-bottle system. The first system was a single bottle connected to a chest drain and then to a vacuum; however, these would fail (as can be imagined) when increased resistance to drainage would occur the more the bottle is filled; this was improved when a water seal bottle was added to act as a one-way valve so that air does not go back in. Both oscillation of fluid level and bubbling can be seen in the water seal bottle. The oscillation is referred to as tidaling and is directly proportional to the amount of empty space (lung reexpansion[17]). It should be monitored daily and will signal either complete reexpansion or kinking of the tube in incomplete reexpansion. The bubbling in the chamber will continue as long as there is air in the empty pleural space to drain out or if there is a connection to the bronchi, as in a bronchopleural fistula.

Tube thoracostomy removal varies between different specialties and physicians. It will perform a graduated removal process. Usually there is some form of graduated removal process where removal process starts with going from suction to water seal and possibly to a clamping trial before removal. The evidence for this is sparse and is all centered around the harm/benefit relationship of having to reinsert a chest tube for an incompletely expanded lung. TT should be removed too early versus longer length of stay and increased patient discomfort should the tube be left in too long. Most of the data on graduated tube removal are more applicable to pnx than hemothorax. One should be familiar with the practice patterns of the hospital, as there is incomplete evidence supporting this.

Lastly, the idea that a chest tube removal should be timed with the respiratory cycle has not been proved definitely as of yet. Evidence to the contrary was shown in a trial of 102 chest tube removals where the number of recurrent pneumothoraces was the same ($\sim 7\%$) in exhalation and inhalation.[46] Likely a large breath or cough in either direction could potentially be problematic but specific respiratory pattern timing is probably unnecessary.

As with any medical practice that has been around for a long time, chest tubes still have more dogmatic principles it would seem than evidence-based ones. We should keep in mind that evidence-based medicine, however, involves not just the data but the patient experience as well. We must understand the harms and benefits of all practices related to chest tubes so that we may explain them to the patient so that they can be involved in and understand the reasoning for chest drainage as a therapy for traumatic disease of the chest.

CLINICS CARE POINTS

Central Venous Access
- The Poiseuille equation predicts that a large diameter increases flow exponentially and pressure increases flow proportionally, whereas length and fluid viscosity are inversely proportional (hinder) to flow.
- Key to successful procedural skill is knowledge of anatomy and the complications that occur along the way.
- Knowledge of plane blocks, specifically the superior cervical plexus block, when performing the internal jugular lines is critical to a successful procedure.

- Preprocedural setup of Chux and towels will help minimize soiling hospital sheets and prevent patients from sitting in blood.
- The Agency for Healthcare Research and Quality stated, the Internal Jugular line should be, without exception, cannulated under US guidance.
- Wires to guide catheters should be used carefully with the technique of railing, which means that the wire moves freely and flawlessly through the vessel.
- Wires should be placed carefully in the vessels only when you are sure your cannula is as close to the center of the vessel to not bend or kink the wire.
- According to recent literature, femoral lines do have a statistically high rate of symptomatic deep venous thrombosis but not line of infections, and the subclavian vein has a higher pneumothorax rate.

Chest Tubes

- The rate of empyema in those with undrained hemothorax is approximately 33% based on small studies.
- Best evidence at this time suggests that patients with normal vital signs and a traumatic pneumothorax less than 1.5 cm on CXR or less than 35 mm radial distance on CT or less than 10% thoracic volume on CT can be managed with conservative treatment and observation.
- With periprocedural antibiotics, there is an approximate 6% absolute risk reduction in the incidence of both empyema and pneumonia.
- Currently, consensus tends toward larger tubes (28F) for hemothorax; however, data are accumulating that may change this.
- Aftercare of the chest tube should include a thorough understanding and inspection of the thoracic drain vacuum systems, daily CXR, and your institution's policies and practices of how to advance the chest tube care.

DISCLOSURE

The authors have nothing to disclose.

REFERENCES

1. Beheshti MV. A concise history of central venous access. Tech Vasc Interv Radiol 2011;14:184–5.
2. Seldinger SI. Catheter replacement of the needle in percutaneous arteriography; a new technique. Acta Radiol 1953;39:368–76.
3. Iserson KV. The origins of the gauge system for medical equipment. The J Emerg Med 1987;5:45–8.
4. Milne A, Teng JJ, Vargas A, et al. Performance assessment of intravenous catheters for massive transfusion: A pragmatic in vitro study. Transfusion 2021;61:1721–8.
5. Traylor S, Bastani A, Butris-Daut N, et al. Are three ports better than one? An evaluation of flow rates using all ports of a triple lumen central venous catheter in volume resuscitation. Am J Emerg Med 2018;36:739–40.
6. Ratcliffe S. Oxford essential quotations. Oxford, UK: Oxford University Press; 2017.
7. Labriola L, Seront B, Crott R, et al. Superior vena cava stenosis in haemodialysis patients with a tunnelled cuffed catheter: prevalence and risk factors. Nephrol Dial Transpl 2018;33:2227–33.
8. Kitagawa N, Oda M, Totoki T, et al. Proper shoulder position for subclavian venipuncture: a prospective randomized clinical trial and anatomical perspectives using multislice computed tomography. Anesthesiology 2004;101:1306–12.
9. Tan BK, Hong SW, Huang MH, et al. Anatomic basis of safe percutaneous subclavian venous catheterization. J Trauma 2000;48:82–6.

10. Williams MF, Eisele DW, Wyatt SH. Neck needle foreign bodies in intravenous drug abusers. Laryngoscope 1993;103:59–63.
11. Shojania KG, Duncan BW, McDonald KM, et al. Making health care safer: a critical analysis of patient safety practices. Evid Rep Technol Assess (Summ) 2001; i-x:1.
12. Ahn S, Ryu HG, Koo CH, et al. Validation of the ipsilateral nipple as the needle directional guide during right internal jugular vein catheterization: A prospective observational study. Asian J Surg 2019;42:362–6.
13. Parienti JJ, Mongardon N, Mégarbane B, et al. Intravascular Complications of Central Venous Catheterization by Insertion Site. N Engl J Med 2015;373:1220–9.
14. Lindskog GE. Some historical aspects of thoracic trauma. J Thorac Cardiovasc Surg 1961;42:1–11.
15. Churchill ED. Wound surgery encounters a dilemma. J Thorac Surg 1958;35: 279–90.
16. Charalampidis C, Youroukou A, Lazaridis G, et al. Pleura space anatomy. J Thorac Dis 2015;7:S27–32.
17. Munnell ER. Thoracic drainage. Ann Thorac Surg 1997;63:1497–502.
18. Molnar TF. Thoracic Trauma: Which Chest Tube When and Where. Thorac Surg Clin 2017;27:13–23.
19. Demetri L, Martinez Aguilar MM, Bohnen JD, et al. Is observation for traumatic hemothorax safe. J Trauma Acute Care Surg 2018;84:454–8.
20. Karmy-Jones R, Holevar M, Sullivan RJ, et al. Residual hemothorax after chest tube placement correlates with increased risk of empyema following traumatic injury. Can Respir J 2008;15:255–8.
21. Mowery NT, Gunter OL, Collier BR, et al. Practice management guidelines for management of hemothorax and occult pneumothorax. J Trauma 2011;70:510–8.
22. Kong VY, Oosthuizen GV, Clarke DL. The selective conservative management of small traumatic pneumothoraces following stab injuries is safe: experience from a high-volume trauma service in South Africa. Eur J Trauma Emerg Surg 2015; 41:75–9.
23. Bou Zein Eddine S, Boyle KA, Dodgion CM, et al. Observing pneumothoraces: The 35-millimeter rule is safe for both blunt and penetrating chest trauma. J Trauma Acute Care Surg 2019;86:557–64.
24. Williams D, Penn M. Can patients with traumatic pneumothorax be managed without insertion of an intercostal drain? Trauma 2021;23:74–9.
25. Wall SD, Federle MP, Jeffrey RB, et al. CT diagnosis of unsuspected pneumothorax after blunt abdominal trauma. AJR Am J Roentgenol 1983;141:919–21.
26. Clements TW, Sirois M, Parry N, et al. OPTICC: A multicentre trial of Occult Pneumothoraces subjected to mechanical ventilation: The final report. Am J Surg 2021;221:1252–8.
27. Ayoub F, Quirke M, Frith D. Use of prophylactic antibiotic in preventing complications for blunt and penetrating chest trauma requiring chest drain insertion: a systematic review and meta-analysis. Trauma Surg Acute Care Open 2019;4: e000246.
28. Choi J, Villarreal J, Andersen W, et al. Scoping review of traumatic hemothorax: Evidence and knowledge gaps, from diagnosis to chest tube removal. Surgery 2021;170:1260–7.
29. Inaba K, Lustenberger T, Recinos G, et al. Does size matter? A prospective analysis of 28-32 versus 36-40 French chest tube size in trauma. J Trauma Acute Care Surg 2012;72:422–7.

30. Bauman ZM, Kulvatunyou N, Joseph B, et al. A Prospective Study of 7-Year Experience Using Percutaneous 14-French Pigtail Catheters for Traumatic Hemothorax/Hemopneumothorax at a Level-1 Trauma Center: Size Still Does Not Matter. World J Surg 2018;42:107–13.
31. Bauman ZM, Kulvatunyou N, Joseph B, et al. Randomized Clinical Trial of 14-French (14F) Pigtail Catheters versus 28-32F Chest Tubes in the Management of Patients with Traumatic Hemothorax and Hemopneumothorax. World J Surg 2021;45:880–6.
32. Osinowo O, Softah AL, Eid Zahrani M. Ectopic chest tube insertions: diagnosis and strategies for prevention. Afr J Med Med Sci 2002;31:67–70.
33. John M, Razi S, Sainathan S, et al. Is the trocar technique for tube thoracostomy safe in the current era. Interact Cardiovasc Thorac Surg 2014;19:125–8.
34. Chu GM, Jarvis GC. Serratus Anterior Plane Block to Address Postthoracotomy and Chest Tube-Related Pain: A Report on 3 Cases. A A Case Rep 2017;8:322–5.
35. Lin J, Hoffman T, Badashova K, et al. Serratus Anterior Plane Block in the Emergency Department: A Case Series. Clin Pract Cases Emerg Med 2020;4:21–5.
36. Liu X, Song T, Xu HY, et al. The serratus anterior plane block for analgesia after thoracic surgery: A meta-analysis of randomized controlled trails. Medicine (Baltimore) 2020;99:e20286.
37. Hohenberger GM, Schwarz A, Hohenberger F, et al. Evaluation of Monaldi's approach with regard to needle decompression of the tension pneumothorax-A cadaver study. Injury 2017;48:1888–94.
38. Kaserer A, Stein P, Simmen HP, et al. Failure rate of prehospital chest decompression after severe thoracic trauma. Am J Emerg Med 2017;35:469–74.
39. Benns MV, Egger ME, Harbrecht BG, et al. Does chest tube location matter? An analysis of chest tube position and the need for secondary interventions. J Trauma Acute Care Surg 2015;78:386–90.
40. El-Faramawy A, Jabbour G, Afifi I, et al. Complications following chest tube insertion pre-and post-implementation of guidelines in patients with chest trauma: A retrospective, observational study. Int J Crit Illn Inj Sci 2020;10:189–94.
41. Huber-Wagner S, Körner M, Ehrt A, et al. Emergency chest tube placement in trauma care - which approach is preferable. Resuscitation 2007;72:226–33.
42. Linder K, Epelbaum O. Percutaneous pleural drainage in patients taking clopidogrel: real danger or phantom fear. J Thorac Dis 2018;10:5162–9.
43. Ault MJ, Rosen BT, Scher J, et al. Thoracentesis outcomes: a 12-year experience. Thorax 2015;70:127–32.
44. Abouzgheib W, Shweihat YR, Meena N, et al. Is chest tube insertion with ultrasound guidance safe in patients using clopidogrel. Respirology 2012;17:1222–4.
45. Harris A, O'Driscoll BR, Turkington PM. Survey of major complications of intercostal chest drain insertion in the UK. Postgrad Med J 2010;86:68–72.
46. Bell RL, Ovadia P, Abdullah F, et al. Chest tube removal: end-inspiration or end-expiration. J Trauma 2001;50:674–7.

The Big Five—Lifesaving Procedures in the Trauma Bay

Sagar B. Dave, DO[a,b,*], Jesse Shriki, DO[c]

KEYWORDS

- Trauma • Thoracotomy • Perimortem C-Section • Resuscitative hysterotomy
- Circothyroidtomy • Burr hole • Trephination • Lateral canthotomy

KEY POINTS

- The biggest mistake in regard to a cricothyroidotomy is not performing the procedure soon enough. The only equipment needed is scalpel, bougie, and an endotracheal tube.
- When performing a resuscitative thoracotomy, consider a clamshell thoracotomy as it allows greater access, assists in intervention, and does not increase mortality.
- Burr hole craniotomy should be performed in patients with deteriorating neurologic status, a Glasgow Coma Scale < 8, lateralizing signs, and evidence of epidural or subdural hematoma in the absence of timely neurosurgical intervention.
- Resuscitative hysterotomy should be considered in all women in the third trimester of pregnancy who present in the extremis after traumatic injury. Outcomes for both the fetus and mother improve the sooner the procedure is performed.
- The most common pitfall when performing a lateral canthotomy is an incomplete dissection of the inferior crus and should be interrogated after the procedure.

INTRODUCTION

"The Big Five" a term that refers to the elephant, leopard, lion, buffalo, and rhinoceros—which are considered the most dangerous animals in Africa. Similar to the Safari, through the vast wilderness of trauma, one may come across the Big Five procedures that are elusive, demand preparation, and are difficult to master. Although resuscitation in trauma requires a multidisciplinary and multifaceted approach, one of the Big Five procedures may need to be performed as lifesaving and improving

[a] Department of Emergency Medicine, Emory University School of Medicine, Grady Memorial Hospital, 1750 Gambrell Drive Northeast, Hospital Tower, Suite T5L41, Atlanta, GA 30322, USA; [b] Department of Anesthesiology, Emory University School of Medicine, Emory Critical Care Center, Emory University, 1750 Gambrell Drive Northeast, Hospital Tower, Suite T5L41, Atlanta, GA 30322, USA; [c] Department of Emergency Medicine, Banner University Hospital, Banner-University Medical Center, 1111 East McDowell Road, Phoenix, AZ 85006, USA
* Corresponding author.
E-mail address: sbdave2@emory.edu

Emerg Med Clin N Am 41 (2023) 161–182
https://doi.org/10.1016/j.emc.2022.09.009
0733-8627/23/© 2022 Elsevier Inc. All rights reserved.

emed.theclinics.com

intervention. This article focuses on and reviews these five critical procedures: crico-thyroidotomy, burr holes, resuscitative thoracotomy, emergent hysterotomy, and lateral canthotomy.

CRICOTHYROIDOTOMY

> **Key points**
>
> - The biggest mistake in regard to a cricothyroidotomy is not performing the procedure soon enough.
> - Key equipment: scalpel, bougie, and endotracheal tube.
> - Laryngeal handshake will keep you midline and assist in maintaining landmarks.
> - There will be more bleeding than you expect.

Introduction

Hypoxia and airway obstruction are potentially preventable causes of acute traumatic death. A compromised airway leads to 34% of prehospital deaths in trauma.[1] Approximately 7% to 28% of all trauma patients require airway management.[2,3] Outside of increasing mortality, incidence of hypoxia and hypercapnia also worsened morbidity with other traumatic injuries, most notably traumatic brain injury. Definitive airway management is most frequently performed as endotracheal intubation with a low failure rate of 1%.[4] The most commonly used emergency surgical airway management is the cricothyroidotomy, a procedure where a tube is placed through an incision in the cricothyroid membrane. Although this procedure is known to be associated with complications, avoiding it results in high morbidity and mortality.[5] Though performed less than 1% of the time and despite a decrease in training, success rates for cricothyroidotomy range from 89% to 100%.[6–9]

Nature of the Problem

"Can't oxygenate, Can't Ventilate"—an adage used to describe a dangerous scenario where oral, nasopharyngeal demands emergent definitive airway management that requires cricothyroidotomy. In trauma, this occurs due to airway obstruction or compromise from injuries such as:

1. Displacement of the skull and facial bones blocking the nasopharyngeal airway,
2. Obscured supraglottic space with bone fragments, vomitus, or blood,
3. Soft-tissue swelling or edema,
4. Penetrating or blunt trauma displacing structures such as the epiglottis, arytenoids, or tracheal rings leading to cervical airway compromise.

As this procedure is indicated in emergent situations, there are no absolute contraindications for an emergent cricothyroidotomy. Relative contraindications include previous tracheal surgery, laryngotracheal disruption, and children under the age of 6.[10,11]

Anatomy

When evaluating a patient in potential need of a surgical airway, it is important to note the anatomic structures involved in a cricothyroidotomy. The cricothyroid membrane is inferior to the thyroid cartilage, superior to the cricoid cartilage, and bordered laterally by the bilateral cricothyroideus muscles. This can be located by palpating the laryngeal prominence (also known as the "Adam's Apple"), then moving inferiorly approximately 2 cm to a slight depression before the round signet ring of the cricoid cartilage.

Pre-procedure Planning

There are multiple kits and prepackaged instruments available for performing percutaneous cricothyroidotomy. This approach uses the Seldinger technique with a needle through the cricothyroid membrane. It is preferable in children up to 10 to 12 years because it is anatomically easier to perform with less potential damage to the larynx and surrounding structures. The superior aspect of the pediatric trachea is not well developed in children, and surgical incisions through the cricothyroid membrane are associated with a higher incidence of subglottic stenosis.

In traumatic injuries, open cricothyroidotomy is superior to the percutaneous technique due to speed and preference in emergent situations.[12] The essential equipment needed for an open cricothyroidotomy is a scalpel, bougie, and tracheostomy tube or a 6.0 endotracheal tube. Ready the room by standing on the side of the patient that is your dominant hand and the respiratory therapist, ventilator, and assistant if available to the opposite side. Position the bed to a height at your elbow level and position the patient with a roll under the shoulder to extend the neck. Attempt to mitigate the potential for infection and bleeding—prepare the neck with antiseptic coating, have suction on the side you are standing, and mark the cricothyroid membrane as time and patient stability allows.

Procedural Approach

1. Begin with the "laryngeal handshake"—taking your nondominant hand, grasp the patient's larynx with your thumb and middle finger, stabilizing your hand with your hypothenar prominence. Identify the cricothyroid membrane with your index finger. This is crucial as it will provide continuous landmark guidance and midline reference (**Fig. 1**).
2. Using your dominant hand, make vertical incision from the mid-thyroid cartilage to the mid-cricoid cartilage. Having a larger incision can be beneficial to identify structures and facilitate placement particularly in larger individuals.
3. Orient the scalpel horizontally and insert the blade horizontally through the membrane penetrating less than 0.5 cm. Incise laterally to the margins tethered to the thyroid cartilage.
4. Dilate the incision with your finger or the handle of the scalpel.
5. Maintaining this track, place the bougie into the opening.
6. Place the airway using the Seldinger technique.

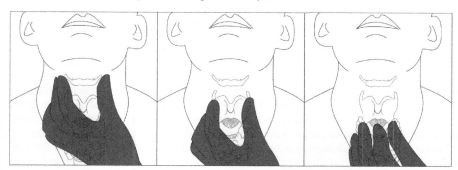

Fig. 1. Laryngeal handshake. (https://www.clinicalkey.com/#!/search/laryngeal%20hand shake?scrollTo=1-s2.0-S1932227520300756-gr1.)

Post-Procedure

- If an endotracheal tube was used, be mindful that mainstem intubation commonly occurs. Ideal placement should be assessed with a portable X-ray or fiberoptic bronchoscopy.
- Securing an endotracheal tube can be difficult with modern holsters. Consider using a tracheal tie or umbilical tape.

Outcomes

Complication rates for cricothyroidotomy differ based on clinical scenarios, location, and performers ranging from 0% to 54%.[13] The worst outcome and most significant complication associated with cricothyroidotomy is failure to place the airway in the trachea. Confirm placement with end-tidal CO_2 detection and optimize placement based on radiographs or fiberoptic bronchoscopy. There will undoubtedly be more bleeding than anticipated during the procedure and similarly this will be true after the procedure. Using "Figure 8" or horizontal mattress hemostatic suturing can help slow or stop small vessel bleeding. Infection and subglottic stenosis are later complications. Though not all patients need to have conversion to tracheostomy (one study showing 7 of 15 surviving patients did not require conversions) conversion in a controlled environment within 3 days is recommended.[14]

Summary

Cricothyroidotomy is an infrequently done procedure though one that can be life-saving. Consider this procedure for every patient who requires a definitive airway. The only equipment needed is a scalpel, bougie, and endotracheal tube. The biggest mistake most people make with cricothyroidotomy is not performing it soon enough.

RESUSCITATIVE THORACOTOMY

Key points

- Prepare the team, system, and yourself as soon as possible in the setting of thoracotomy.
- Deprioritize chest compressions.
- Clamshell thoracotomy allows greater access, assists in intervention, and does not increase mortality.
- Always perform the pericardiotomy.
- Detach the inferior pulmonary ligament to mobilize the left lung.
- Cross-clamping the aorta has variable benefits.

Introduction

The resuscitative thoracotomy in the emergency department or the trauma bay is perhaps the most dramatic, invasive, and controversial procedure that can be performed on an injured patient. Even with great interest and effort in attaining the skills necessary to perform it, resuscitative thoracotomy carries a survival far less than 50%. It requires rapid decision-making, skilled performance, readily available equipment, and a system in place to perform this procedure effectively to maximize survival.

Thoracotomy for resuscitation began being used in the United States in the late 1800s by Dr Schiff as a way to perform open cardiac massage.[15] The most common reason for thoracotomy was resuscitation for medical cardiac arrest for the majority of the twentieth century. In the second half of the 1900s, with the demonstrated efficacy of closed chest compressions, the advent of external defibrillation, and protocolization of cardiopulmonary resuscitation, the need for open cardiac massage was essentially eliminated.[16–18] Yet the use for thoracotomy for open cardiac massage and open repair of thoracic injuries was renewed by Beall and colleagues[19] and swung the pendulum supporting its use in traumatic patients in the extremis.[20]

Since then, there have been various investigations on the efficacy, ethics, and indications for resuscitative thoracotomy.[21–27] One must balance the ability to perform a lifesaving bedside intervention to the risk of iatrogenic injuries to the team and the ethics of performing a procedure on a potentially nonsurvivable patient.

Nature of the Problem

Traumatic cardiac arrest is different from medical cardiac arrest. The primary problem in medical cardiac arrest is often arrhythmia, pulmonary embolism, myocardial infarction, sepsis, or toxins; however, in trauma, hemorrhagic shock, pneumothorax, and cardiac tamponade are the primary insults. Hemostasis, decompression, and optimizing physiology are the primary goals in patients who are in extremis due to traumatic injuries. With this in mind, the resuscitation of a trauma patient (to maximize survival) varies from advanced cardiac life support (ACLS) in the following ways:

- De-prioritize chest compressions: In most settings, chest compressions are the priority in cardiac arrest. Focus of recent studies and versions of the ACLS algorithm minimizes interruptions in chest compressions as this is associated with improved survival.[28–30] In trauma, chest compressions seem to worsen tamponade physiology, do not increase cardiac output in the setting of hemorrhagic shock, and impede the team from performing procedures.[31] For this reason, de-prioritizing chest compressions and focusing on administering blood volume and decompression is key.
- Fix the injury and compression: Controlling hemorrhage is a key portion in the resuscitation of a traumatic arrest. To this point, the resuscitative thoracotomy allows for access to the intrathoracic space. Here physicians can intervene to perform temporizing maneuvers to control bleeding and decompress the pericardium to allow for effective cardiac output.
- Assist the physiology of resuscitation: Access to the thoracic cavity also allows for interventions to increase cardiac output, increase coronary and cerebral blood flow, and continue resuscitation. Maneuvers such as open cardiac massage, direct defibrillation, aortic cross-clamp, and intracardiac epinephrine can be done, yet their efficacy is debatable.

Indications

Three questions to ask when considering thoracotomy are as follows:

1. Are there signs of life?
2. Duration of arrest?
3. What are the goals of the procedure?

Defining signs of life would include cardiac electrical activity, spontaneous respiratory effort, pupillary response, palpable pulse, measurable blood pressure, sonographic cardiac activity, or end-tidal CO_2. The duration of arrest from prehospital teams can be difficult to acquire but it is important to attempt to be as detailed as possible. Helpful points can include time of emergency medical services call, time of prehospital team arrival, and time of hospital arrival. The last question maybe the most important in terms of defining what the goal of the procedure is. Generally, the goals are evacuation of pericardial blood, direct hemostatic control, and attempts to optimize coronary and cerebral blood flow. Other interventions include abdominal vascular control or bronchovenous air embolism.

With these questions and considerations in mind, the past 2 decades have seen multiple studies and guidelines for the indication of resuscitative thoracotomy. A review of 25 years of resuscitative thoracotomies, brought forth indications and contraindications in 2000. The following year, the American College of Surgeons – Committee on Trauma established guidelines and recommendations for penetrating cardiac, noncardiac thoracic, and abdominal vascular injuries for the resuscitative thoracotomy. This was furthered in 2006, when a retrospective review of resuscitative thoracotomies outlined indications and contraindications separated by penetrating versus blunt trauma. Subsequently, guidelines were stratified by presence or absence of signs of life and duration of arrest before arrival.

The most recent guidelines from the Eastern Association for the Surgery of Trauma and the Western Trauma Association give guidance for decisions in these matters[32,33]:

- Strongly recommend resuscitative thoracotomy with:
  - Presenting pulseless with signs of life after penetrating thoracic injury
- Conditionally recommend resuscitative thoracotomy with:
  - Presenting pulseless to the emergency department without signs of life after penetrating thoracic injury if cardiopulmonary resuscitation (CPR) is less than 15 min
  - Presenting pulseless to the emergency department with or without signs of life after penetrating extrathoracic injury, if CPR is less than 5 min.
  - Presenting pulseless to the emergency department with signs of life after blunt injury, if CPR is less than 10 min.
- *Conditionally recommend against resuscitative thoracotomy with:
  - Presenting pulseless to the emergency department without signs of life after blunt injury

*Other indications for thoracotomy include massive hemothorax defined by greater than 1500 mL out of the chest tube initially or 250 per hour for 3 hours. With this in mind, in blunt traumatic arrest, without signs of life and cardiac arrest less than 10 minutes, I suggest bilateral chest tubes and sonographic evaluation of the heart. If there is evidence of massive hemothorax or pericardial blood I would consider performing resuscitative thoracotomy.

Pre-procedure Planning

Preparation is crucial in resuscitative thoracotomies as they are infrequently performed with less than 1000 per year mostly in urban, large-volume trauma centers.[34] Preparing the system, team, and equipment before patient arrival can help maximize survival and minimize adverse events.

The clinician should notify the operating room, anesthesia staff, appropriate surgical teams (such as trauma or cardiothoracic), and blood bank before beginning an emergency department thoracotomy. This will assist in minimizing time to definitive repair in the operating room and availability for massive transfusion protocols.

The initial resuscitation should begin and continue as a part of the resuscitative thoracotomy, separate members should be designated for procedures and instructed where to be in the room such as airway management (head of the bead), vascular access/pelvic binder/tourniquet placement on the right lower end of the bed, assistant and team for thoracotomy on both sides of the patient's torso. Ensure the team is donned in personal protective equipment ideally before the patient arrives to reduce the incidence of pathogen exposure and remind individuals to practice closed-loop communication, particularly when passing instruments.

Equipment needed can be found in thoracotomy trays and should include these basic instruments:

#10 or #20 Scalpel.

Mayo and Metzenbaum Scissors.

Finochietto retractor.

Lebsche knife and mallet.

Atraumatic vascular clamp: a Satinsky and DeBakey Aortic Occlusion Clamp.

Procedure

Position the patient supine with the left arm extended above the head. Cover the entire chest in betadine.

Incision and Access to the Thoracic Cavity

Perform a left lateral anterolateral thoracotomy incision beginning from the *right* sternal border on the fifth intercostal space. Advance the incision to the left and once past the left nipple, progress the incision toward the left axilla along the rib cage.

This curvilinear incision follows the inferior border of the pectoralis muscle. In women, the landmark is the inframammary fold and the breast may need to be retracted superiorly. This incision is the best choice for the resuscitative thoracotomy as it allows for optimal access, increased retraction, and in certain instances, better opportunity for surgical closure.

Divide the skin, subcutaneous tissue, and chest wall musculature rapidly. This can be done with the scalpel or scissors.

Attempt to incise the intercostal muscles on the *superior* edge of the rib to avoid the intercostal neurovascular bundle. It is important to get into the thoracic cavity quickly yet be mindful to avoid injuring the heart or the lung.

Once in the thoracic cavity, place the Finochietto retractor with the handle toward the axilla and spread the ribs.

Use the Lebsche knife and mallet to cross the sternum transversely. If extending the resuscitative thoracotomy to a clamshell thoracotomy,[a] extend the incision through the right 5th intercostal space to the *right axilla* extending from a left anterolateral thoracotomy to a clamshell.

Pericardiotomy and Cardiac Repair

Perform the pericardiotomy with an incision from the apex of the heart to the base of the aortic root. The incision should be parallel and anterior to the phrenic nerve. If the pericardium is not tense, it may need to be picked up with a toothed forceps.

Pericardiotomy should be routinely performed as tamponade cannot be ruled out visually.

Deliver the heart once the pericardium is widened, and remove clots and blood to allow for evaluation of the heart for injuries.

For cardiac injuries, there are a number of techniques that can be used for hemostasis. Any bleeding initially should be controlled with digital pressure. Subsequent

---

[a] The clamshell incision allows for access to the right hemothorax, facilitates life-saving interventions, and does not increase mortality when compared with isolated lateral thoracotomies.[35]

temporizing or definitive repair can be done rapidly with staples or sutures. While suturing on the ventricle be mindful to not occlude the coronary vessels and induce myocardial ischemia. A Foley catheter may be useful as it can be inserted into the laceration, then inflated to tamponade any bleeding. This has the potential for worsening injury as it can be dislodged and further the laceration. Other options include using intestinal Allis clamps or partial side-biting vascular clamps.

If no injury is noted, you can begin a bimanual massage. Compared with the one-hand technique, the bimanual "hinged clamping" technique for cardiac massage is preferred.

Noncardiac Injury Interventions

Evaluate the great vessels including the ascending and descending aorta, vena cava, and subclavian vessels using trajectory to guide evaluation. Though best controlled in the operating room, digital pressure or nonocclusive side-biting vascular clamps can be used to temporize bleeding.

Inspect the lung parenchyma starting from the hilum then evaluate further laterally. Compared with peripheral parenchymal injuries, hilar injuries can lead to extensive hemorrhage and can be temporized with digital pressure, umbilical tape, a nonocclusive vascular clamp, or by twisting the lung parenchyma around the hilum.

Aortic Clamp

Accessing the aorta for occlusion can be difficult, particularly in a pulseless, hypovolemic patient. Mobilize the lung superolaterally, which may require dissecting the inferior pulmonary ligament which can be found at the inferior lateral portion of the left lung parenchyma. Identify the aorta anterior to the spine and posterior to the esophagus.

Under direct visualization, dissect the aorta from the esophagus and vertebrae. Then place a nonocclusive straight clamp perpendicular to the aorta.

Placing a nasogastric tube can help identify the esophagus. If the aorta cannot be separated from the esophagus, a clinician can apply direct digital pressure on the aorta against the spine.

Aortic occlusion can provide for control of inferodiaphragmatic vascular occlusion to assist in hemostasis as well as increase diastolic afterload for cerebral and coronary perfusion. The efficacy of this is debated and there is potential for ischemia and reperfusion injury calling this technique for routine resuscitation into question.

Post-Procedure

If return of spontaneous circulation is achieved and patient has achieved some resemblance of stability, the patient should be taken to the operating room for repair and continued damage control resuscitation. Though a lifesaving procedure, resuscitative thoracotomy is riddled with risks and complications. First and foremost is exposure to blood-borne pathogens or iatrogenic injury to a team member. If there is any concern, infection control should be contacted. Early complications for the patient include iatrogenic injury to the heart and other intrathoracic injuries. Particularly with the clamshell technique, return of circulation can lead to bleeding from the internal mammary arteries which will require ligation. Later complications include infection and post-cardiotomy syndrome. Though there is evidence of therapeutic hypothermia in medical cardiac arrest, with the ongoing goal of normalizing coagulopathy, optimizing acid-base status, and correcting hypothermia to achieve hemostasis, therapeutic hypothermia should be avoided.

Summary

Resuscitative thoracotomy is one of the most dramatic and controversial procedures in medicine—the objective of the clinician in this intervention is to make it the complete opposite. One must control themselves before one can control the room. Be purposeful with the indications and objectives of the procedure, efficient with incisions, and continue all other efforts for resuscitation simultaneously. The outcomes of resuscitative thoracotomy have been reviewed and evaluated for more than 50 years and have led to controversy including the indications and ethical issues yet the most current guidance suggests the best outcomes in penetrating trauma with signs of life and cardiac arrest in less than 15 min.

BURR HOLE CRANIOTOMY

Key points

- Burr hole craniotomy should be performed in patients with deteriorating neurologic status, a Glasgow Coma Scale < 8, lateralizing signs, and evidence of epidural or subdural hematoma when there is an absence of timely neurosurgical intervention.

- Most common location of hematoma is the temple though imaging can help guide location.

- There will be more bleeding than expected both during and after the procedure. Do not make attempts to control bleeding as this can injure vascular structures.

- Continue management of traumatic brain injury and DO NOT delay transfer to a location with neurosurgical intervention.

Introduction

Traumatic brain injury accounts for 2.5 million ED visits and over a quarter million hospital admissions. 1/3 of all traumatic deaths involve traumatic brain injury. A strategy to relieve pressure from the brain is burr hole craniotomy or trephination.

Craniotomy is not a new concept. As possibly the earliest form of surgery to be performed, archeological studies on ancient skulls around the world confirm that there was a purposeful procedure done that patients survived.[36-38] It has been practiced through history particularly in wartime, which has then been expanded and refined during the World Wars.[39,40] With the advent of computerized tomography, the indications of burr holes narrowed and its frequency decreased with the ability for non-invasive rapid diagnosis. This coupled with the development of trauma management systems and access to neurosurgery, burr hole craniotomy in the trauma bay or emergency department has become very rare. Though in austere locations or instances without access to a neurosurgeon, time to decompression is crucial and bedside burr hole craniotomy can be performed to improve survival.

Nature of the Problem

The physiology of death in traumatic brain injury begins initially with primary injury from immediate impact. This then leads to an evolving cellular response causing edema and a cyclic increase in intracranial pressure, a decrease in cerebral perfusion pressure, ischemia, and further edema. A strategy to emergently relieve this increase in intracranial pressure and stop the cycle is by trephination or more commonly known as burr hole craniotomy. This is defined by the Monroe-Kelly doctrine stated the skull has a finite amount of space and its components change in volume affect each other.

Bricolo and Pasut found that regardless of the Glasgow coma score (GCS) on presentation when the GCS at the time of surgery was >8, 100% had good recovery compared with 40% if the GCS was 3 to 4.[41] Seelig and colleagues[42] reported that a delay of >4 h before surgery in acute subdural hematoma changed the mortality from 30% to 90%. In instances where decompression is delayed due to location or resource availability, bedside burr hole craniotomy can be performed by a trauma surgeon or emergency medicine physician safely and effectively.

In a review of 116 patients who "talked and died" after head injury, the most common cause of preventable death was delay in evacuation of an intracranial hematoma.[43] The majority of extracerebral bleeds are accessible to standard burr holes with a low complication rate even if done at the bedside. Mahoney and colleagues[44] noted no complications in 51 burr holes made with a hand drill in the ED. A case series from austere hospitals in the Midwest showed five patients with epidural hematomas, who presented talking then deteriorated, and underwent cranial trephination before transfer. Time to pressure relief and improvement of symptoms was 1 h, there were zero complications and all patients survived hospital discharge with mild to no neurologic disability.[45,46]

Indications

1. No access to a neurosurgeon in a timely manner.
2. CT imaging showing—extradural hematoma with midline shift[b]
3. GCS 8 or less
4. Unequal pupils

Anatomy

It is important to identify landmarks for this procedure according to where the injury occurred (**Fig. 2**):

1. Temporal bone above the zygoma located 2 cm anterior and 2 cm superior to the tragus
2. Frontal bone approximately 10 cm behind the midpupillary line over the coronal suture
3. Parietal bone over the parietal eminence found 3 cm superior and 4 cm posterior to the external auditory meatus

Pre-procedure Planning

It is important to have early and frequent consultations with neurosurgery even if in a remote situation. Secure the patient's airway, administer peri-operative antibiotics, and if CT imaging is available, evaluate skull thickness to dura at the location of the anticipated burr hole. The patient should be placed supine and the end of the bed elevated to 30°. The head turned to the contralateral side of the injury.

Equipment needed includes:

Hair trimmer or shaving blade.

Skin preparation solution.

Scalpel.

Self-retaining scalp retractor.

Drill: these vary from manual hand drills and electronic drills.

---

[b] can be an exception if a computed tomography (CT) scan is unavailable and there is a high level of suspicion.

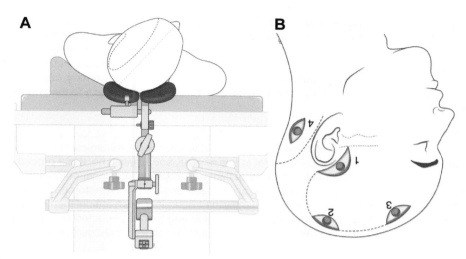

Fig. 2. Burr holes location. (https://www.clinicalkey.com/#!/content/book/3-s2.0-B97803236
61928003918?scrollTo=%23hl0001014.)

Procedure

Shave the patient's hair, clean the scalp, and then mark a 3 to 5 cm line for your incision. Make an incision straight down to the bone. Attempt to be anterior to the superficial temporal artery though if incised, do not worry about bleeding. This can be
controlled with direct pressure while continuing the procedure.

Use forceps to move the periosteum and place the self-retaining retractor.

Beginning trephination by pushing down firmly with the drill against the ostium and
keeping the drill perpendicular to the skull. Ensure an assistant is holding the head still
and ideally apply sterile saline wash as you drill.

Depending on the equipment available the technique here will vary though a manual
crank drill or an air drill will be used down to the dura and can be adjusted based on
skull depth seen on CT. A Hudson-brace crank first uses a perforator drill bit then
switches to the conical burr when the inner portion of the skull noted by jerking motion
with the crank.

Remove drill. Use the blunt hook to remove the remaining bone fragments. Extradural blood should now escape.

If the blood is subdural, very carefully open the dura using a sharp hook to tent the
dura up, and a new sharp knife to incise the dura with a cruciate cut. Subdural blood is
likely to be more clotted and difficult to remove. Manual removal of clot could be
considered, but avoid suctioning as this may disrupt bridging veins and may damage
brain tissue.

If no blood is found either extra or subdurally, stop, check the site of the burr hold to
ensure it was performed on the correct side and location of the head. This may need to
be done in another location, if performed without CT scan. Above all, transfer to a center with neurosurgical capabilities should *not* be delayed.

Post-Procedure

During and after burr hole craniotomy there will be more bleeding than expected. If
fresh blood is continuing to ooze from the wound, do not try to tamponade. Leaving

the self-retainer in place may stop the bleeding. Continue medical management of traumatic brain injury including head of the bed elevation, hyperosmolar therapy, blood pressure control, and optimizing acid/base status. Traumatic brain injury can induce coagulopathy with disruption of the blood–brain barrier and correcting this coagulopathy should be a continued focus of resuscitation. The primary objective above all else is transferred to neurosurgical capabilities and admission to the neurologic intensive care unit.

Summary

Performing a burr hole craniotomy in the trauma bay without neurosurgical is the definition of up a river without a paddle. Yet in this remote, and lonely time, it is a procedure that can potentially save the life of a patient and improve functional outcomes. If there are lateralizing signs, presence of an epidural or subdural hematoma, deteriorating clinical status, and absence of timely neurosurgical intervention then a burr hole should be performed. There will be more bleeding than is expected before and after the procedure. Do not delay transfer and continue medical management of traumatic brain injury.

THE RESUSCITATIVE HYSTEROTOMY

Key points

- Resuscitative hysterotomy should be considered in all women in the 3rd trimester of pregnancy who present in the extremis after traumatic injury
- Outcomes for both the fetus and mother improve the sooner the procedure is performed
- The adage of this to be performed within 4 min is driven by initial data, but survival has been seen up to 30 min of extremis
- Call for help early including the operating room, obstetrics, and neonatal team
- Utilize a large midline incision for the abdomen and uterus. Iatrogenic injury may happen but can be managed afterward
- Be sure to deliver the placenta and pack the uterus after delivery

---

Introduction

A pregnant trauma patient in the extremis may be the most challenging and stressful patient that a trauma surgeon or emergency physician encounters. Trauma is the leading cause of non-obstetric death in pregnant women with motor vehicle collisions and assault as the primary mechanisms. Physiology in pregnancy is altered depending on the trimester and can further complicate the diagnostic and therapeutic course. The resuscitative hysterotomy or perimortem cesarean section (C-section) is the most maximally invasive therapy that can be performed for a pregnant patient in the trauma bay as a lifesaving intervention. As it is one of the rarest procedures performed by a clinician primarily caring for trauma patients, it is riddled with stress, yet if done efficiently and effectively, has the potential to save more than one life.

Resuscitative hysterotomy refers to an emergent surgical fetal delivery before or after maternal death. Though the origins of this procedure can be fabled back to the description in Greek mythology, its historical origin is speculated from the birth of Julius Caesar and a law declared in his name that a fetus should be removed after mother's death for potential survival or a separate burial.[47,48] Modern medicine accounts come from the sixteenth to eighteenth centuries where this procedure was described with the survival of the mother.[47] The twentieth and twenty-first century began using the cesarean section for complicated pregnancies or difficult vaginal deliveries and the perimortem cesarean section became a variant from ancient times.[49]

Outcomes

Fetal salvage and perimortem C-section were first suggested to be beneficial in the seminal review in 1986 theorizing the procedure would relieve the effect of cavoatrial compression and optimize maternal circulation.[50] This led to 1992 American Heart Association guidelines supporting resuscitative hysterotomy in special situations and has been as part of their guidelines since.[51] Maternal survival ranges are quoted from 34% to 54%.[52,53] Fetal survival ranges from 0% to 89% in various studies with outcomes worsening with less than 24 weeks gestation for both mother and fetus.[54–57] With reports of no hemodynamic instability after perimortem C-section, it has been suggested to be the most important part of resuscitation in a pregnant woman in cardiac arrest.

Indications

Outcomes and importance of perimortem C-section are evidently important, yet the indications are debated. The follow-up landmark series in 2005 by Katz and colleagues[53] built from their initial study in 1986 and suggested performing a resuscitative hysterotomy in 4 min could improve neonatal outcomes. Further reports showed benefits to mothers with this timeframe applied leading to The American College of Obstetricians and Gynecologists endorsing this time frame.[58] There are reports of survival up to 15 min for the mother and 30 min for the fetus. With this in mind, survival is higher if performed within 4 min of maternal arrest and resuscitative hysterotomy should be considered in all moribund pregnant women in their 3rd trimester with less than 30 min of cardiac arrest.

Gestational age of 24 weeks is generally considered viable for a fetus though this may range from institutions.[59] A multi-center study showed improved survival in fetuses after 25 weeks gestation and that 60% of infant deaths resulted from delays in recognizing fetal distress.[57] This study also found maternal injury to be independent of fetal outcome. For maternal benefit, resuscitative hysterotomy is not considered beneficial before 24 weeks gestation as the uterine size and blood volume are unlikely to contribute to hemodynamic lability.[60] Thereby indicating 24 weeks or gestational age considered by the local institution as an indication for resuscitative hysterotomy recognizing this may be difficult to ascertain in the emergency department.[54]

A debated condition is the presence or absence of fetal heart tones. One study showed 0% survival in the absence of fetal heart tones yet another showed fetal survival despite the absence of fetal heart tones.[57,61] This underscores the importance or technology for assessing the fetal heart and the inherent limitations of technology in various clinical scenarios.

Pre-procedure Planning

Ensure your team has personal protective equipment. If able, set up suction, prepare the room for an endotracheal intubation, and initiate massive transfusion protocol. Though resuscitative hysterotomy will take the attention of most members of the team, it is important to remember other measures of traumatic and cardiac resuscitation. Important variations to traditional resuscitation in a pregnant woman include chest compressions 2 to 3 cm higher, manual displacement of the uterus to the left, and the avoidance of femoral lines if possible.

Equipment needed will mostly be found in a thoracotomy tray. The primary instruments needed include:

- #10 or 20 Scalpel
- Mayo and Metzenbaum scissors
- 2 Kelly clamps

Procedure

- (**Fig. 3**) Lay the patient in a supine position if possible, 30° toward the left lateral decubitus position. As time and stability allow, cover the abdomen with an anti-septic such as betadine. Stand on the side of your dominant hand with an assistant on the opposite side
- Begin with a vertical incision from the sternum at the xiphoid process to the pubic symphysis. This should be a big incision as time is of the essence and rapidly go through the skin, subcutaneous tissue, and musculature.
- Once in the peritoneum with the outer abdomen retracted, make a 1- to 2-cm incision (enough space for a finger and scissors) in the inferior portion of the uterus
- Using scissors, make a vertical cut up the uterus, protecting the fetus with your finger
- Deliver the baby through the incision. This may require your assistant giving fundal pressure
- Using the two Kelley clamps, attach them to the umbilical cord, cut the cord between them with scissors
- Hand the baby to the neonatal team
- Deliver the placenta with a sterile towel over your hand and gentle traction. Inspect to make sure it is intact
- Pack the uterus with sterile towels and briefly perform uterine massage then pack the abdomen further with sterile towels

PERIMORTEM C-SECTION

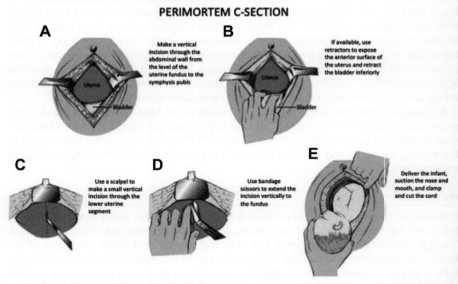

Fig. 3. Perimortem c-section. (https://www.clinicalkey.com/#!/content/journal/1-s2.0-S07338 62720300663?scrollTo=%23hl0000721.)

Post-Procedure

If the mother survives, she will need to go to the operative room at the least with the obstetrics and gynecology team for closure. As this is an infrequently performed procedure done emergently, there is potential for iatrogenic injury to the bladder or hollow viscus structures which warrants thorough inspection intra-operatively. Continued management of traumatic injuries with admission to the ICU for both the mother and baby is important.

Summary

The resuscitative hysterotomy is a stressful procedure as it defines the term "double jeopardy" as there are two lives on the line. A woman in extremis after trauma suspected to be greater than 24 weeks gestation identified crudely by womb above the umbilicus should be considered for a perimortem cesarean section. Time is of the essence for both the fetus and the mother to move quickly and efficiently. Call for help early and consider having three teams one for the trauma, one for the procedure, and one for neonatal resuscitation. Outcomes for both the mother and fetus are highest the sooner the procedure is performed. Take a deep breath, control yourself before controlling the room, and make that big cut.

LATERAL CANTHOTOMY

> **Key points**
>
> - Orbital compartment syndrome is defined by increasing intra-orbital pressure that can lead to blindness by ischemia
> - Elevated intraocular pressure either by palpation or measured greater than 40 mm Hg is considered an indication for lateral canthotomy if there is a concern for orbital compartment syndrome
> - If decompression is not successful with a complete dissection of the inferior crus, consider dissection of the superior crus.
> - The most common pitfall is an incomplete dissection of the inferior crus and should be interrogated if there is still a concern for incomplete decompression.

Introduction

Ocular trauma is a common cause of acquired blindness, particularly in developing countries and under resourced areas. As one of the most baneful consequences to craniomaxillofacial injury, blindness can lead to great financial strain and morbidity.[62] The primary mechanism for blindness after an injury is direct traumatic optic neuritis. Although spontaneous recovery is possible, it is rare.[63] Lateral canthotomy is a bedside procedure that can emergently decompress the orbital compartment and save a patient from progressing to blindness.

Lateral canthotomy was first described in 1950 and has refined over the years to a valuable tool used at the bedside tool to rescue vision in the trauma bay.[64] Surgical opening of the lateral canthus can reverse traumatic blindness within 90 to 120 min.[65–67] Though a lateral canthotomy has a straightforward technique, there are multiple suboptimal outcomes that have been attributed to a lack of knowledge and confidence by clinicians in the trauma bay performing this procedure.[68] With proper preparation and training, lateral canthotomy can be a sight-saving procedure.

Nature of the Problem

Orbital compartment syndrome is defined by increasing intra-orbital pressure that can lead to blindness by ischemia. Direct trauma to the eye can lead to orbital hemorrhage. As bleeding increases, pressure in the retrobulbar space increases, compressing the optic nerve. This coupled with edema from the response to injury leads to ischemia of the optic nerve. This direct traumatic optic neuritis progresses to blindness through the clinical presentation of proptosis, diminished extraocular movement, vision change, increase intraocular pressure, and pupillary defect or loss of reaction.

Anatomy

The orbital cavity is approximately 30 mL of space enclosed by multiple bones of the face and skull. Within this bony cavity rests the orbit along with the optic nerve, ophthalmic vasculature, and extraocular muscles. The eye is kept from displacing anteriorly by the confluence of tarsal places on either side of the orbit known as the medial and lateral canthal tendons. These canthi become natural junctions for the upper and lower lid while the skull bones provide support from posterior displacement and connection to nerves and vasculature. Owing to its superficial location and distance from other anatomic structures, the lateral canthal tendon is the recommended anatomic structure to decompress the orbital compartment.

Indications

The indications for lateral canthotomy have become refined in the second half of the twentieth century. I believe lateral canthotomy should be considered in any patient with direct craniomaxillofacial trauma and diminishing eyesight. The primary indication for lateral canthotomy is orbital compartment syndrome. Orbital compartment syndrome is ultimately a clinical diagnosis described as a constellation of symptoms including proptosis, elevated intraocular pressure, visual, afferent pupillary, or extraocular movement defect.[69] As the most common cause for orbital compartment syndrome is a retrobulbar hematoma, a CT scan can be helpful for identifying this associated injury. Elevated intraocular pressure either by palpation or measured greater than 40 mm Hg is considered an indication for lateral canthotomy if there is a concern for orbital compartment syndrome. Owing to the risk of rapid progression of vision loss, orbital compartment syndrome is a clinical diagnosis and lateral canthotomy should not be delayed for imaging or other measurements. The relative contraindication for lateral canthotomy is evidence of globe rupture due to the high risk of bleeding and infection.[70]

Pre-procedure Planning

It is important to notify the ophthalmology service when considering lateral canthotomy. If available, they may assist in diagnosis and intervention. When the patient arrives, position the head of the bed 10 to 15° and restrain the head with tape or an assistant. Patients with other injuries or altered states may require intubation and sedation.

Equipment Needed

- Lidocaine 1% to 2% with or without epinephrine in a syringe with a 25- to 27-gauge needle
- Normal saline for irrigation
- Straight hemostat
- Sterile scissors either iris or suture or curved Stevens scissors
- Forceps with $\geq$0.3-mm teeth

Procedure

- True sterile preparation is impractical with an emergent procedure, yet using normal saline to lavage the eye can help remove debris and foreign objects **(Fig. 4)**
- Infiltrate the skin of the lateral canthus with approximately 1 cc of lidocaine and epinephrine directing the needle to the lateral orbit and begin injecting when the needle hit bone. The addition of epinephrine can help with hemostasis as well

Lateral Canthotomy And Cantholysis

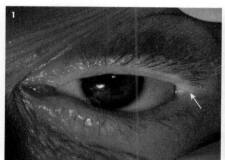

Identify the lateral canthus (arrow). Cleanse the area with antiseptic and anesthetize with 1% lidocaine with epinephrine. (The left eye is depicted in this image sequence.)

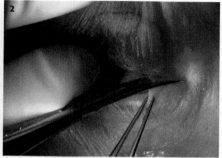

Crush the lateral canthus with a hemostat for 1 to 2 minutes to reduce incisional bleeding (not shown). Then, cut through the crushed tissue with iris scissors (as depicted above) to perform the canthotomy.

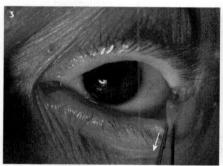

Pull the lower eyelid away from the globe with toothed forceps (arrow).

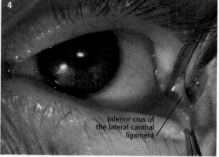

Inferior crus of the lateral canthal ligament

"Strum" the tissue under the canthotomy with the scissors to identify the inferior crus of the lateral canthal ligament. Cut through this ligament with scissors to perform the inferior cantholysis. Note that the scissors are directed inferiorly during this step, perpendicular to the canthotomy incision.

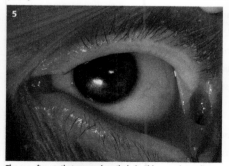

> NOTE:
> If intraocular pressure remains elevated after inferior cantholysis, the superior crus of the lateral canthal ligament may be released in a similar fashion.

The eye after canthotomy and cantholysis. This procedure relieves increased intraocular pressure by allowing the globe and orbital contents to move forward.

Fig. 4. Lateral canthotomy. (https://www.clinicalkey.com/#!/content/book/3-s2.0-B97803 23354783000622?scrollTo=%23hl0001528.)

- Apply the hemostat and clamp the canthus for approximately 60 s the crush and devascularize the skin. This also helps to mark the next incision
- Using the scissors, cut the skin laterally to the lateral border of the orbit of approximately 1 cm. This position minimizes iatrogenic injury to the orbit
- Apply traction to the lower lid to identify the inferior lateral crus. Cut this using scissors directed inferiorly and laterally with an incision that is approximately 1 cm
- The inferior lid will displace relieving pressure from the orbital compartment.
- If further intervention is still needed, divide the superior crus with a superolateral incision bring mindful of the lacrimal gland which is in close proximity
- This should improve the laxity of the upper lid, further relieving the orbital compartment

Post-Procedure

It is important to have a thorough evaluation by ophthalmology and reassess for other traumatic injuries. The most common pitfall is an incomplete dissection of the inferior crus and should be interrogated if there is still a concern for incomplete decompression. Immediate complications include iatrogenic injuries to the globe and surrounding structures as this is inherently a blind procedure. Delayed complications include infection, functional impairment, and cosmetic deformity. Hospital admission is not necessary if this is an isolated injury.

SUMMARY

Lateral canthotomy is a sight-saving procedure that should be considered in all patients with craniomaxillofacial trauma and concern for vision loss. Indication is orbital compartment syndrome, and as this has the potential for rapid irreversible vision loss, lateral canthotomy should not be delayed for diagnostic testing. While performing the procedure, consider the phrase "one is the number," 1 cm of injection, 1 min of compression, identify 1 tendon 1st, and incise 1 cm.

CLINICS CARE POINTS

- The biggest mistake in regard to a cricothyroidotomy is not performing the procedure soon enough.
- Key equipment: scalpel, bougie, and endotracheal tube.
- Laryngeal handshake will keep you midline and assist in maintaining landmarks.
- There will be more bleeding than you expect.
- Prepare the team, system, and yourself as soon as possible in the setting of thoracotomy.
- Deprioritize chest compressions during cardiac arrest in trauma
- Clamshell thoracotomy allows of greater access, assists in intervention, and does not increase mortality.
- Always perform the pericardiotomy.
- Detach the inferior pulmonary ligament to mobilize the left lung.
- Cross-clamping the aorta has variable benefits and can potentiate harm
- Burr hole craniotomy should be performed in patients with deteriorating neurologic status, a Glasgow Coma Scale < 8, lateralizing signs, and evidence of epidural or subdural hematoma when there is an absence of timely neurosurgical intervention.

- Most common location of hematoma is the temple though imaging can help guide location.
- There will be more bleeding than expected both during and after the procedure. Do not make attempts to control bleeding as this can injure vascular structures.
- Continue management of traumatic brain injury and DO NOT delay transfer to a location with neurosurgical intervention.
- Resuscitative hysterotomy should be considered in all women in the 3rd trimester of pregnancy who present in the extremis after traumatic injury
- Outcomes for both the fetus and mother improve the sooner the procedure is performed
- The adage of this to be performed within 4 min is driven by initial data, but survival has been seen up to 30 min of extremis
- Call for help early including the operating room, obstetrics, and neonatal team
- Utilize a large midline incision for the abdomen and uterus. Iatrogenic injury may happen but can be managed afterward
- Be sure to deliver the placenta and pack the uterus after delivery
- Orbital compartment syndrome is defined by increasing intra-orbital pressure that can lead to blindness by ischemia
- Elevated intraocular pressure either by palpation or measured greater than 40 mm Hg is considered an indication for lateral canthotomy if there is a concern for orbital compartment syndrome
- If decompression is not successful with a complete dissection of the inferior crus, consider dissection of the superior crus.
- The most common pitfall is an incomplete dissection of the inferior crus and should be interrogated if there is still a concern for incomplete decompression.

DISCLOSURE

The authors have nothing to disclose.

REFERENCES

1. Hussain L, Redmond A. Are pre-hospital deaths from accidental injury preventable? BMJ 1994;308:1077–80.
2. Talucci R, Shaikh K, Schwab C. Rapid sequence induction with oral endotracheal intubation in the multiple injured patient. AmSurg 1988;54:185–7.
3. Rotondo MF, McGonigal MD, Schwab CW, et al. Uregent paralysis and intubation of trauma patients: Is it safe? J Trauma 1993;34:242–6.
4. Zewdie A, Tagesse D, Alemayehu S, et al. The success rate of endotracheal intubation in the emergency department of tertiary care hospital in ethiopia, one-year retrospective study. Emerg Med Int 2021;2021:9590859.
5. Ollerton JE. NSW Institute of trauma and injury management. North Ryde: NSW; 2007. Adult trauma clinical practice guidelines: Emergency airway management in the trauma patients.
6. Stephens CT, Kahntroff S, Dutton RP. The success of emergency endotracheal intubation in trauma patients: a 10-year experience at a major adult trauma referral center. Anesth Analg 2009;109(3):866–72.
7. McGill J, Clinton JE, Ruiz E. Cricothyrotomy in the emergency department. Ann Emerg Med 1982;11(7):361–4.

8. Erlandson MJ, Clinton JE, Ruiz E, et al. Cricothyrotomy in the emergency department revisited. J Emerg Med 1989;7(2):115–8.

9. Chang RS, Hamilton RJ, Carter WA. Declining rate of cricothyrotomy in trauma patients with an emergency medicine residency: implications for skills training. Acad Emerg Med 1998;5(3):247–51.

10. Scrase I, Woollard M. Needle vs surgical cricothyroidotomy: a short cut to effective ventilation. Anaesthesia 2006;61(10):962–74.

11. Black AE, Flynn PE, Smith HL, et al. Development of a guideline for the management of the unanticipated difficult airway in pediatric practice. Paediatr Anaesth 2015;25:346–62.

12. Poole O, Vargo M, Zhang J, et al. A comparison of three techniques for cricothyrotomy on a manikin. Can J Respir Ther 2017;53(2):29–32.

13. Bair AE, Panacek EA, Wisner DH, et al. Cricothyrotomy: a 5-year experience at one institution. J Emerg Med 2003;24(2):151–6.

14. Wright MJ, Greenberg DE, Hunt JP, et al. Surgical cricothyroidotomy in trauma patients. South Med J 2003;96(5):465–7.

15. Hermreck AS. The history of cardiopulmonary resuscitation. Am J Surg 1988; 156(6):430–6.

16. Kouwenhoven WB, Jude JR, Knickerbocker GG. Closed-chest cardiac massage. JAMA 1960;173:1064–7.

17. Safar P. Initiation of closed-chest cardiopulmonary resuscitation basic life support. a personal history. Resuscitation 1989;18(1):7–20.

18. Zoll PM, Linenthal AJ, Norman LR, et al. Treatment of unexpected cardiac arrest by external electric stimulation of the heart. N Engl J Med 1956;254:541–6.

19. Beall AC Jr, Diethrich EB, Cooley DA, et al. Surgical management of penetrating cardiovascular trauma. South Med J 1967;60:698–704.

20. Graham JM, Mattox KL, Beall AC Jr. Penetrating trauma of the lung. J Trauma 1979;19(9):665–9.

21. Feliciano DV, Bitondo CG, Cruse PA, et al. Liberal use of emergency center thoracotomy. Am J Surg 1986;152(6):654–9.

22. Meshkinfamfard M, Narvestad JK, Wiik Larsen J, et al. Structured and systematic team and procedure training in severe trauma: going from 'zero to hero'for a time-critical, low-volume emergency procedure over three time periods. World J Surg 2021;45(5):1340–8.

23. Cogbill TH, Moore EE, Millikan JS, et al. Rationale for selective application of emergency department thoracotomy in trauma. J Trauma 1983;23:453–60.

24. Moore EE, Moore JB, Galloway AC, et al. Postinjury thoracotomy in the emergency department: a critical evaluation. Surgery 1979;86:590–8.

25. Rhee PM, Acosta J, Bridgeman A, et al. Survival after emergency department thoracotomy: review of published data from the past 25 years. J Am Coll Surg 2000;190:288–98.

26. Working Group. Ad Hoc subcommittee on outcomes, american college of surgeons. committee on trauma. practice management guidelines for emergency department thoracotomy. J Am Coll Surg 2001;193:303–9.

27. Modes ME, Engelberg RA, Downey L, et al. Toward understanding the relationship between prioritized values and preferences for cardiopulmonary resuscitation among seriously Ill adults. J Pain Symptom Manage 2019;58(4):567–77.e1.

28. Brouwer TF, Walker RG, Chapman FW, et al. Association between chest compression interruptions and clinical outcomes of ventricular fibrillation out-of-hospital cardiac arrest. Circulation 2015;132(11):1030–7.

29. Luna GK, Pavlin EG, Kirkman T, et al. Hemodynamic effects of external cardiac massage in trauma shock. J Trauma 1989;29(10):1430–3.
30. Cabrini L, Biondi-Zoccai G, Landoni G, et al. Bystander-initiated chest compression-only CPR is better than standard CPR in out-of-hospital cardiac arrest. HSR Proc Intensive Care Cardiovasc Anesth 2010;2(4):279–85.
31. Konesky KL, Guo WA. Revisiting traumatic cardiac arrest: should CPR be initiated? Eur J Trauma Emerg Surg 2018;44(6):903–8.
32. Seamon MJ, Haut ER, Van Arendonk K, et al. An evidence-based approach to patient selection for emergency department thoracotomy: a practice management guideline from the Eastern Association for the Surgery of Trauma. J Trauma Acute Care Surg 2015;79(1):159–73.
33. Burlew CC, Moore EE, Moore FA, et al. Western Trauma Association critical decisions in trauma: resuscitative thoracotomy. J Trauma Acute Care Surg 2012;73(6): 1359–63.
34. Hansen CK, Hosokawa PW, Mcintyre RC, et al. A National Study of Emergency Thoracotomy for Trauma. J Emerg Trauma Shock 2021;14(1):14–7.
35. DuBose JJ, Morrison J, Moore LJ, et al. Does clamshell thoracotomy better facilitate thoracic life-saving procedures without increased complication compared with an anterolateral approach to resuscitative thoracotomy? results from the american association for the surgery of trauma aortic occlusion for resuscitation in trauma and acute care surgery registry. J Am Coll Surg 2020;231(6):713–9.e1.
36. Breasted JH. The Edwin Smith surgical papyrus. In: Breasted JH, editor. Neurosurgical classics. Park Ridge (IL): American Association of Neurological Surgeons; 1992. p. 1–5.
37. Gurdjian ES. The treatment of penetrating wounds of the brain sustained in warfare. J Neurosurg 1974;39:157–67.
38. Velasco-Suarez M, Martinez JB, Oliveros RG, et al. Archaeological origins of cranial surgery: trephination in Mexico. Neurosurgery 1992;21:313–8.
39. Maltby GL. Penetrating craniocerebral injuries, evaluation of the late results in a group of 200 consecutive penetrating cranial war wounds. J Neurosurg 1946;3: 239–49.
40. Craig WM. Neurosurgery in World War II. U.S Armed Forces J 1952;3:1–13.
41. Bricolo AP, Pasut ML. Extradural hematoma: toward zero mortality: a prospective study. Neurosurg 1984;14:8–11.
42. Seelig JM, Becker DP, Miller JD, et al. Traumatic acute subdural hematoma: major mortality reduction in comatose patients treated within four hours. N Engl J Med 1981;304:1511–8.
43. Rose J, Valtonen S, Jennett B. Avoidable factors contributing to death after head injury. Br Med J 1977;2(6087):615–8.
44. Mahoney BD, Rockswold GL, Ruiz E, et al. Emergency twist drill trephination. Neurosurgery 1981;8(5):551–4.
45. Smith SW, Clark M, Nelson J, et al. Emergency department skull trephination for epidural hematoma in patients who are awake but deteriorate rapidly. J Emerg Med 2010;39(3):377–83.
46. Laroche M, Kutcher ME, Huang MC, et al. Coagulopathy after traumatic brain injury. Neurosurgery 2012;70(6):1334–45.
47. Todman D. A history of caesarean section: from ancient world to the modern era. Aust N Z J Obstet Gynaecol 2007;47(5):357–61.
48. Ellis H. The early days of caesarian section. J Perioper Pract 2010;20(5):183–4.
49. Lurie S. The changing motives of cesarean section: from the ancient world to the twenty-first century. Arch Gynecol Obstet 2005;271(4):281–5.

50. Katz VL, Dotters DJ, Droegemueller W. Perimortem cesarean delivery. Obstet Gynecol 1986;68(4):571–6.
51. Guidelines for cardiopulmonary resuscitation and emergency cardiac care. Emergency Cardiac Care Committee and Subcommittees, American Heart Association. Part IV. Special resuscitation situations. JAMA 1992;268(16):2242–50.
52. Einav S, Kaufman N, Sela HY. Maternal cardiac arrest and perimortem caesarean delivery: evidence or expert-based? Resuscitation 2012;83(10):1191–200.
53. Katz V, Balderston K, DeFreest M. Perimortem cesarean delivery: were our assumptions correct? Am J Obstet Gynecol 2005;192(6):1916–21.
54. Strong TH Jr, Lowe RA. Perimortem cesarean section. Am J Emerg Med 1989; 7(5):489–94.
55. Luppi CJ. Cardiopulmonary resuscitation: pregnant women are different. AACN Clin Issues 1997;8(4):574–85.
56. Selden BS, Burke TJ. Complete maternal and fetal recovery after prolonged cardiac arrest. Ann Emerg Med 1988;17(4):346–9.
57. Morris JA Jr, Rosenbower TJ, Jurkovich GJ, et al. Infant survival after cesarean section for trauma. Ann Surg 1996;223(5):481–91.
58. American College of Obstetricians and Gynecologists. ACOG Practice Bulletin No. 100: critical care in pregnancy. Obstet Gynecol 2009;113:443–50.
59. Allen MC, Donohue PK, Dusman AE. The limit of viability–neonatal outcome of infants born at 22 to 25 weeks' gestation. N Engl J Med 1993;329:1597–601.
60. Murphy N, Reed S. Maternal resuscitation and trauma. [book auth. In: Eisinger SH, Damos JR, editors. Advanced life support in obstetrics (ALSO) provider course syllabus. Leawood, KS: American Academy of Family Physicians; 2000. p. 1–25.
61. Ritter JW. Postmortem cesarean section. JAMA 1961;175:715–6.
62. Thylefors B. Epidemiological patterns of ocular trauma. Aust New Zealand J Ophthalmol 1992;20(2):95–8.
63. Atkins EJ, Newman NJ, Biousse V. Post-traumatic visual loss. Rev Neurol Dis 2008;5(2):73–81.
64. Nguyen MV. A Historical Perspective of Lateral Canthotomy and Its Adoption as an Emergency Medicine Procedure. J Emerg Med 2019;56(1):46–52.
65. Larsen M, Wieslander S. Acute orbital compartment syndrome after lateral blowout fracture effectively relieved by lateral cantholysis. Acta Ophthalmol Scand 1999;77(2):232–3.
66. Sun MT, Chan WO, Selva D. Traumatic orbital compartment syndrome: importance of the lateral canthomy and cantholysis. Emerg Med Australas 2014; 26(3):274–8.
67. Popat H, Doyle PT, Davies SJ. Blindness following retrobulbar haemorrhage–it can be prevented. Br J Oral Maxillofac Surg 2007;45(2):163–4.
68. Fox A, Janson B, Stiff H, et al. A multidisciplinary educational curriculum for the management of orbital compartment syndrome. Am J Emerg Med 2020;38(6): 1278–80.
69. McInnes G, Howes DW. Lateral canthotomy and cantholysis: a simple, vision-saving procedure. CJEM 2002;4(1):49–52.
70. Murali S, Davis C, McCrea MJ, et al. Orbital compartment syndrome: Pearls and pitfalls for the emergency physician. J Am Coll Emerg Physicians Open 2021; 2(2):e12372. Published 2021 Mar 6.

Trauma in the Aging Population

Geriatric Trauma Pearls

Lorraine Lau, MScA, MD, FRCPC[a],*, Henry Ajzenberg, MD[b],
Barbara Haas, MD, PhD, FRCSC[c], Camilla L. Wong, MHSc, MD, FRCPC[d]

KEYWORDS

- Geriatric trauma • Trauma • Older adults • Falls

KEY POINTS

- Approach to trauma among older adults should take into consideration the anatomic and physiologic differences in older adults.
- In older adults, medical comorbidities and pathologies as a precipitating factor to the traumatic mechanism should be considered early in the course of care.
- A proactive geriatric consultation service can improve outcomes in older adults with traumatic injury.
- Patients' goals of care, baseline functional status, and preinjury frailty are particularly important in the approach to geriatric trauma.

INTRODUCTION
Epidemiology

As global populations age, those who provide frontline care will continue to see a rapid increase in the number of geriatric trauma patients. Data from North America show that between 30% and 40% of trauma patients are now older than the age of 65, a number that has roughly doubled since 2006.[1–3] A national registry study of seriously ill trauma patients in the United Kingdom showed that the mean age of a trauma patient increased from 36 years in 1990 to 54 years in 2013. The same study showed that the proportion of trauma patients older than the age of 75 increased from 8% to 27%.[4]

[a] Department of Emergency Medicine, McGill University Health Centre, 1001 Decarie Boulevard, Montreal, Quebec H4A 3J1, Canada; [b] Division of Emergency Medicine, University of Toronto, 500 University Avenue Suite 602, Toronto, Ontario M5G 1V7, Canada; [c] Department of Surgery and Interdepartmental Division of Critical Care Medicine, University of Toronto, Sunnybrook Health Sciences Centre, 2075 Bayview Avenue, Toronto, Ontario M4N 3M5, Canada; [d] Division of Geriatric Medicine, St. Michael's Hospital, 30 Bond Street, Toronto, Ontario M5B 1W8, Canada
* Corresponding author.
E-mail address: lorraine.lau@mcgill.ca

Emerg Med Clin N Am 41 (2023) 183–203
https://doi.org/10.1016/j.emc.2022.09.006
0733-8627/23/© 2022 Elsevier Inc. All rights reserved.

A national registry study from Japan revealed that the percentage of patients older than 60 years increased from 32% to 60% between 2004 and 2015.[5] The resuscitation and management of patients who are older adults and present with severe injuries will be a common part of any trauma practice in the coming decades.

What Defines Geriatric Trauma?

There is no universally agreed on age cutoff that defines a geriatric trauma patient. A wide range of cutoffs has been used in defining and studying geriatric trauma patients.[6,7] Age 65 is commonly used in research and clinical settings, although this arbitrary number is likely based more on historical than physiologic factors. One cross-sectional study of more than 75,000 trauma patients showed that when stratified by Injury Severity Score, mortality increased significantly older than the age of 70.[6] The authors therefore argue that 70 would be a more appropriate age at which to define a geriatric trauma patient. Another retrospective study of more than 100,000 patients demonstrated a significant increase in mortality after the age of 57.[7] Rather than memorizing an age cutoff, it is important for the emergency physician to be aware that frailty, increasing comorbidities, decreased physiologic reserve, and other factors that contribute to worse outcomes in geriatric trauma patients can occur at different ages and must be assessed on an individualized basis. It is worthwhile to note that the preferred term for geriatric patients, endorsed by the *Journal of the American Geriatric Society*, is "older adults." We are increasingly aware of the importance of language in molding conscious and subconscious attitudes. The use of the terms "elderly," "elders," and "seniors" are associated with negative attitudes and may result in patients receiving substandard care.[8]

Mechanisms of Injury and Injury Patterns in Geriatric Trauma

Geriatric trauma patients have higher mortality than their younger counterparts, even when matched for illness severity.[5,9–11] They are more likely to require intensive care unit (ICU) admission and be discharged to a long-term care facility or nursing home than their younger counterparts.[12] A seemingly minor mechanism is capable of causing serious injury and complications.

Low-energy mechanisms cause most geriatric trauma,[13] with falls and motor-vehicle collisions making up the first and second most frequent causes, respectively.[14] Falls are exceptionally common among older adults; 27% of adults 65 years of age and older fall each year.[15] Even ground-level falls can cause significant injury, and are associated with a 1-year mortality rate of 33.2%. Risk factors for falls include a history of falls, cognitive impairment, visual impairment, polypharmacy, home hazards, orthostatic hypotension, and gait instability.[16] In addition, medical events related to underlying comorbidities are the precipitants of a traumatic injury. Falls and motor vehicle accidents, for example, can be caused by underlying orthostatic hypotension, cardiac syncope, or cerebrovascular accident.

ANATOMIC AND PHYSIOLOGIC CONSIDERATIONS IN GERIATRIC TRAUMA PATIENTS

Anatomic and physiologic changes related to aging can affect the clinical presentation and early management of geriatric trauma patients. **Table 1** summarizes age-related anatomic and physiologic changes and their clinical implications in trauma management.

Triage algorithms for injured patients often rely on the presence of abnormal vital signs to identify the presence of severe injury.[17] However, injured older adults often present atypically and can have "normal" vital signs even in the face of severe

Table 1
Age-related changes and clinical implications in trauma[24,25]

Organ System	Age-Related Changes	Clinical Implications
Neurologic	Brain atrophy Decreased cerebral blood flow Decreased autonomic neural responses	Increased risk of cerebral and vascular injuries Increased risk of delirium Blunted responses to stress
Respiratory	Decreased vital capacity Decreased inspiratory reserve volume Decreased alveolar quantity and size Decreased chest wall compliance	Decreased respiratory reserve Increased risk of desaturation during intubation Increased risk of respiratory complications
Cardiovascular	Decreased cardiac output Increased systemic vascular resistance Decreased response to adrenergic catecholamines	Decreased cardiac reserve Increased risk of fluid overload Vital signs not reflective of severity of shock and injury
Gastrointestinal	Decreased pain sensation Decreased abdominal musculature	Increased risk of intra-abdominal injury Unreliable physical examination (absent peritoneal signs despite injury)
Renal	Decreased glomerular filtration rate Decreased renal mass	Increased risk of kidney injury Increased risk of electrolyte and acid-base abnormalities Decreased clearance of certain medications
Hepatic	Decreased hepatic function	Decreased metabolism and clearance of certain medications
Musculoskeletal	Decreased muscle mass Decreased bone mineral density	Increased risk of fracture
Integumentary	Loss of collagen and elastin Thinning of epidermis Decreased subcutaneous fat and tissue	Increased risk of soft tissue injuries, skin tears Increased risk of pressure injuries

inury.[18–20] Multiple factors that may affect vital signs in the older adult include underlying cardiovascular comorbidities, medications (eg, β-blockers), and physiologic changes related to aging itself. Multiple groups have suggested modifications to triage algorithms to better identify severely injured older adults. For example, a heart rate greater than 90 beats per minute and systolic blood pressure less than 110 mm Hg as a cutoff value has been associated with increased mortality in the geriatric trauma patient, and have been suggested as a criteria for trauma team activation.[21] The Shock Index, defined as heart rate divided by systolic blood pressure, is a tool used as a predictor of mortality, critical bleeding, and need for massive transfusion in trauma patients.[22] Given the unreliability of vital signs in older adults, the Age-Adjusted Shock Index (AASI) (**Box 1**) has been proposed as a more sensitive alternative.[23] In older adults, an AASI of greater than 50 was associated with a mortality of approximately 10% and seemed to be a predictor of early mortality and the need for blood products.[23] Although the AASI is an important tool for clinicians, used alone it is not sensitive enough to rule out critical injuries.

> **Box 1**
> **Age-adjusted shock index**
>
> $$\frac{Heart\ Rate\ (bpm)}{Systolic\ Blood\ Pressure\ (mm\ Hg)} \times Age\ (years)$$
>
> AASI greater than 50 = concerns for shock.

In addition to vital signs, other aspects of the trauma assessment may be confounded by older adults' underlying comorbidities. For example, it may be difficult to assess neurocognitive status, and identify a treatable head injury, in a patient with dementia. Patients with neurocognitive disorders likely have more difficulty providing a history or localizing pain. The presence of osteoporosis and frailty may cause a minor mechanism (eg, ground level fall) to result in severe multisystem injuries. Overall, the clinician assessing an older adult after a traumatic mechanism of injury must maintain a high level of suspicion that severe injury may be present and should not rely exclusively on vital signs and other physiologic measure to exclude the presence of severe injury.

FRAILTY

The term frailty describes a dynamic state of decreased reserves in multiple domains including physical, cognitive, psychological, and social, which can lead to vulnerability and increased risk of adverse health outcomes.[26] There is no consensus definition and there are multiple validated instruments that are used to measure an individual's level of frailty.[27] For example, the Canadian Study of Health and Aging Clinical Frailty Scale is a commonly used and easily interpretable frailty scale (**Fig. 1**, **Table 2**).

Preinjury frailty is strongly associated with adverse outcomes following injury including mortality, in-hospital complications, and adverse discharge disposition (ie, long-term care facility).[28–31] Frailty is likely a stronger predictor of outcome than age or comorbidities.[32] The association between frailty and adverse outcomes in geriatric trauma patients has been demonstrated consistently by multiple frailty measures use in various clinical contexts.[33] As such, an assessment of preinjury frailty can identify those at highest risk of adverse outcomes; early identification of these patients may allow for the mobilization of specialized resources (eg, lower threshold for ICU admission, early assessment by an interdisciplinary team). Frailty screening for all geriatric trauma patients and development of an institutional frailty standardized care pathway is recommended by the American College of Surgeons.[34]

TRAUMA SYSTEMS AND TRAUMA IN OLDER ADULTS

Undertriage of older adults with severe injury is a systemic issue across multiple jurisdictions.[35,36] A multitude of studies have shown that older adults with severe traumatic injuries are less likely to be transported to a trauma center and to have trauma team activation, compared with younger patients.[35–40] In the prehospital setting, standard adult physiologic parameters have poor sensitivity for severe injury in older adults and may lead to missed severe injuries in geriatric patients.[35] As a result, multiple prehospital trauma triage guidelines emphasize advanced age as a special consideration for the triage of injured patients, with lower threshold for trauma center transport for older adults.[17,34,41,42] In addition to different field triage, multiple guidelines also support a lower threshold for trauma team activation for older adults treated at trauma

CLINICAL FRAILTY SCALE

	1	**VERY FIT**	People who are robust, active, energetic and motivated. They tend to exercise regularly and are among the fittest for their age.
	2	**FIT**	People who have **no active disease** symptoms but are less fit than category 1. Often, they exercise or are very **active** occasionally, e.g., seasonally.
	3	**MANAGING WELL**	People whose **medical problems are well controlled**, even if occasionally symptomatic, but often are **not regularly active** beyond routine walking.
	4	**LIVING WITH VERY MILD FRAILTY**	Previously "vulnerable," this category marks early transition from complete independence. While **not dependent on** others for daily help, often **symptoms limit activities**. A common complaint is being "slowed up" and/or being tired during the day.
	5	**LIVING WITH MILD FRAILTY**	People who often have **more evident slowing**, and need help with **high order instrumental activities of daily living** (finances, transportation, heavy housework). Typically, mild frailty progressively impairs shopping and walking outside alone, meal preparation, medications and begins to restrict light housework.
	6	**LIVING WITH MODERATE FRAILTY**	People who need help with **all outside activities** and with keeping house. Inside, they often have problems with stairs and need **help with bathing** and might need minimal assistance (cuing, standby) with dressing.
	7	**LIVING WITH SEVERE FRAILTY**	**Completely dependent for personal care**, from whatever cause (physical or cognitive). Even so, they seem stable and not at high risk of dying (within ~6 months).
	8	**LIVING WITH VERY SEVERE FRAILTY**	Completely dependent for personal care and approaching end of life. Typically, they could not recover even from a minor illness.
	9	**TERMINALLY ILL**	Approaching the end of life. This category applies to people with a **life expectancy <6 months**, who are not otherwise living with severe frailty. (Many terminally ill people can still exercise until very close to death.)

SCORING FRAILTY IN PEOPLE WITH DEMENTIA

The degree of frailty generally corresponds to the degree of dementia. Common **symptoms in mild dementia** include forgetting the details of a recent event, though still remembering the event itself, repeating the same question/story and social withdrawal.

In **moderate dementia**, recent memory is very impaired, even though they seemingly can remember their past life events well. They can do personal care with prompting.

In **severe dementia**, they cannot do personal care without help.

In **very severe dementia** they are often bedfast. Many are virtually mute.

DALHOUSIE UNIVERSITY

Fig. 1. Clinical frailty scale.

center.[34,42] Nevertheless, although these modifications increase the sensitivity of triage criteria, their specificity is lowered.[43]

Although there is a concern that system resources might be overwhelmed if triage criteria are further modified and more older adults are triaged to trauma centers, prevailing evidence suggests that undertriage, rather than overtriage, remains the prevalent issue affecting severely injured older adults. Even among adults meeting EMS field trauma triage criteria, a large proportion are undertriaged, with older adults being overrepresented among those that are transported to a nontrauma center.[44] Although triage criteria suggest older adults at higher risk of adverse outcomes should have lower thresholds for trauma center transfer, such risk factors as frailty and advance age are paradoxically associated with a lower likelihood of transfer to trauma center care.[44,45] We propose that addressing systemic undertriage of older adults with severe injury is one of the most pressing issues in trauma care in the next two decades.

Trauma Center Performance

Older adults who are treated at a trauma center have lower morbidity and mortality when compared with those treated at a nontrauma center.[46] Despite this, there exists significant variation in outcomes across different trauma centers.[47] The reasons for this variation are multifactorial. Volume is one predictor of outcomes, where a higher volume of geriatric trauma at a given trauma center is associated with decreased mortality.[48,49] The proportion of geriatric trauma patients that a trauma center treats is independently associated with lower mortality, and may play a larger role than absolute volume.[50] However, the factors accounting for significant survival variation across trauma centers are poorly understood.

Table 2 Clinical frailty scale[26]		
1	Very fit	People who are robust, active, energetic, and motivated. They tend to exercise regularly and are among the fittest for their age.
2	Fit	People have **no active disease symptoms** but are less fit than category 1. Often, they exercise or are very **active occasionally**, such as seasonally.
3	Managing well	People whose **medical problems are well controlled**, even if occasionally symptomatic, but often are **not regularly active** beyond routine walking.
4	Living with very mild frailty	Previously "vulnerable," this category marks early transition from complete independence. Although **not dependent** on others for daily help, often **symptoms limit activities**. A common complaint is being "slowed up" and/or being tired during the day.
5	Living with mild frailty	People who often have **more evident slowing**, and need help with **high order instrumental activities of daily living** (finances, transportation, heavy housework). Typically, mild frailty progressively impairs shopping and walking outside alone, meal preparation, medications, and begins to restrict light housework.
6	Living with moderate frailty	People who need help with **all outside activities** and with **keeping house**. Inside, they often have problems with stairs and need **help with bathing** and might need minimal assistance (cuing, standby) with dressing.
7	Living with severe frailty	**Completely dependent for personal care**, from whatever cause (physical or cognitive). Even so, they seem stable and not at high risk of dying (within ~6 mo).
8	Living with very severe frailty	Completely dependent for personal care and approaching end of life. Typically, they could not recover from even a minor illness.
9	Terminally ill	Approaching the end of life. This category applies to people with a **life expectancy <6 mo**, who are **not otherwise living with severe frailty**. (Many terminally ill people can still exercise until very close to death).

INITIAL RESUSCITATION OF THE GERIATRIC TRAUMA PATIENT
Airway Considerations

Anatomic and physiologic changes of normal aging can complicate airway management.[51] Lips are often dry, thin, and more prone to laceration with minimal manipulation from laryngoscopy. Teeth may be absent or loose. Dentures are common and should be removed before intubation. Saliva production is generally reduced among older adults and this may make laryngoscope blade insertion difficult.[51] Despite the classic teaching that being edentulous makes bag-mask ventilation more difficult, multiple large studies have failed to consistently find this to be true.[52–54] Decreased neck mobility is common among older adults and can lead to difficulty with laryngoscopy.[55] Additionally, multiple studies have shown that manual inline stabilization makes laryngoscopy more difficult.[56–58] Therefore, videolaryngoscopy should be first line, because it is associated with an improved first pass success rate and may be especially useful in a trauma patient where cervical immobilization is required.[59,60]

Cardiovascular and respiratory changes in older adults occur because of normal aging, the increased prevalence of disease, and polypharmacy. The end result is an increased sensitivity to medications and decreased physiologic reserve.[61] Preexisting coronary artery disease, valvular disease, and diastolic or systolic dysfunction can limit cardiac output in older adults with hemorrhagic shock or medication-induced vasodilation.[62,63] Underlying hypertension is common, and what is an apparently normal blood pressure may represent significant hypotension for the older patient.[19] Caution must be used when administering sedative medications as a part of induction for rapid sequence intubation. Although no induction medication is hemodynamically neutral, such agents as ketamine or etomidate have generally been preferred because they cause less peri-intubation hypotension.[64,65] Given concerns for adrenal suppression and recent data showing increased mortality with etomidate, ketamine is likely the safest option for all trauma patients. Regardless of which induction medication is used, doses should generally be reduced by 40% to 50% for older adults to avoid hypotension.[63,66]

Aging causes numerous mechanical and physiologic changes that lead to decreased global pulmonary reserve, predisposing patients to hypoxemia. Increased lung parenchymal compliance and increased closing volume leads to the collapse of small airways. Decreased compliance of the chest wall leads to increased work of breathing.[61] Oxygen diffusion capacity is reduced.[51] Older adults are more susceptible to aspiration because of decreased protective cough and swallowing reflexes. Short periods of altered breathing may be less well tolerated because of decreased compensatory ventilatory responses to hypoxemia or hypercarbia.[61]

Investigations

Elevated lactate and base deficit are associated with significantly increased mortality in normotensive geriatric trauma patients and should be part of the initial bloodwork drawn. Older trauma patients with a lactate greater than 4 mmol/L or base deficit less than -6 mEq/L have an approximately 40% mortality rate.[67,68] Several studies have found that lactate greater than or equal to 2.5 mmol/L is independently associated with increased mortality.[69,70] These elevated markers are associated with a high probability of severe injury and mortality in all trauma patients, and may be particularly concerning in older patients despite normal vital signs.

Cardiac troponin should also be considered as part of the initial trauma panel for the older patient. With increased prevalence of cardiovascular comorbidities among older adults, the clinician must consider cardiac pathology as a cause of the trauma and/or a secondary complication caused by the stress of traumatic injuries (eg, type II myocardial infarction). An elevated troponin is an independent prognostic factor predicting all-cause morbidity and mortality in geriatric patients without acute coronary syndrome and should therefore be measured in the context of trauma.[71]

Anticoagulation Reversal

Many older adults are on anticoagulants for various indications. Prompt assessment of the severity of injury and extent of bleeding, along with laboratory testing (eg, coagulation studies) and appropriate diagnostic imaging are required to determine if immediate anticoagulation reversal is required. For urgent surgical interventions, presence of hemorrhagic shock, need for transfusion, and major traumatic injuries, reversal should be immediately initiated. Intracranial hemorrhage is also an indication for anticoagulation reversal because it reduces hemorrhage progression and mortality.[72]

TRAUMATIC BRAIN INJURY

With physiologic changes related to aging, white matter and cerebral vasculature become more susceptible to injury.[73] Geriatric patients with traumatic brain injury (TBI) experience higher morbidity and mortality, slower recovery, and worse outcomes.[74–77] Falls from standing height or from low height are the leading cause of TBI in older adults.[78]

The Glasgow Coma Scale (GCS) is not a reliable tool to assess TBI in a geriatric trauma patient because of higher prevalence of preexisting comorbidities and conditions, such as neurocognitive disorders, cognitive impairment, delirium, and polypharmacy.[79,80] Other factors, such as age-related cerebral atrophy, can also lead to delayed clinical findings because it provides more space for an intracranial hemorrhage to expand. Furthermore, older adults were found to have worse outcomes despite better GCS scores than younger patients with more severe or comparable injuries.[81,82] As such, clinicians should be cautious and not be falsely reassured by the clinical assessment and GCS score in a geriatric trauma patient.

There is currently no validated geriatric TBI neuroimaging guideline. There are multiple validated clinical decision rules to assist clinicians with making the decision to investigate with computed tomography (CT) head imaging in the context of adult blunt head trauma, including the Canadian CT Head Rule, New Orleans Criteria, and the National Emergency X-Ray Utilization Study (NEXUS) II Head CT Rule.[83,84] However, older age is listed as a high-risk factor for intracranial trauma for these rules and therefore generally support the routine use of CT head for all older adults. Canadian CT Head Rule and Nexus II identified patients greater than or equal to the age of 65 as a high-risk factor requiring imaging, whereas New Orleans Criteria listed greater than the age of 60. The mild TBI clinical policy from the American College of Emergency Physician also supports these recommendations.[85] The decision to pursue diagnostic imaging should also take into consideration the patient's goals of care and incorporate shared decision making.

SPINE INJURIES

Decreased bone mineral density and degenerative changes predispose older adults to increased risk of spinal injuries. Older adults are also more likely to have baseline comorbidities, such as osteoarthritis, osteoporosis, disk disease, rheumatic disorders, and spinal stenosis. Older patients are therefore at risk for severe spinal injury despite seemingly minor trauma, such as falling from standing height.[86] In this population, midline cervical spine (c-spine) tenderness is often absent, and is an unreliable indicator of fracture.[87,88] Because of degenerative changes and decreased lower c-spine mobility, geriatric patients have an increased incidence of injuries at the craniocervical junction and upper c-spine, especially at the level of C2 and the odontoid.[89] Type II odontoid fractures are one of the most common c-spine fractures among older adults.[86]

As with TBI, there is a lack of high-quality evidence currently to support the use of clinical decision rules in the older adult population. The Canadian C-Spine Rule considers patients older than 65 years of age as a high-risk criterion and therefore recommends imaging for all older adults.[90] For the NEXUS criteria, studies have shown variable sensitivity in older adults, ranging from 65.9% to 100%.[91–93] Multiple studies have questioned the validity of this tool to rule out the need for imaging for older adults.[91,93]

Given the high risk of c-spine fractures despite low-energy mechanisms and atypical clinical presentations, there should be a low threshold to order diagnostic imaging in older patients. Plain radiographs for c-spine injuries have a false-negative rate of 15% to 40% and are also particularly poor at diagnosing dense fractures.[89,94] CT, not plain radiographs, should therefore be performed.[95] For geriatric trauma patients who require a CT head, a concurrent CT of the c-spine should be strongly considered because there is a 5% likelihood of fracture, regardless of intracranial injury.[94]

Timely spinal precaution clearance is particularly critical among injured older adults. Prolonged immobilization is particularly detrimental to older adults, potentially leading to loss of muscle mass, venous thromboembolism, aspiration, respiratory complications, delirium, and pressure ulcers.[96] Prolonged use of a cervical collar can also lead to significant skin breakdown.[97] Within institutional limitations, prompt radiologic reporting of diagnostic imaging and early evaluation by surgical spine service if available and indicated should be advocated. In obtunded adult blunt trauma patients, EAST guidelines currently conditionally recommend c-spine collar removal and clearance after a negative high-quality c-spine CT scan.[98] However, this recommendation is based on low-quality evidence, is not specific to older adults, and there is a pending update in progress. Of note, standard cervical collar immobilization with a patient supine on a flat surface may not adequately put the spine in a neutral position in older adults. Age-related thoracic kyphosis and cervical hyperlordosis means that lying flat without occipital cushioning can place the cervical spine in hyperextension.[99]

RIB FRACTURES

Rib fractures are diagnosed in approximately 35% of patients with blunt thoracic trauma and are present in 10% of all patients presenting to a trauma center.[100,101] Among older adults, rib fractures are associated with significant morbidity and mortality.[102–108] In this patient population, each additional broken rib is associated with a 19% relative increase in mortality.[109] Several studies have sought to identify a threshold number of rib fractures over which mortality significantly increases. Although this number varies based on the study, what is clear is that the frequency of complications and mortality increases proportionally to the number of ribs fractured.[105,110,111]

Given the implications on patient morbidity and mortality and hospital length of stay, appropriate investigation and management of rib fractures in older adults are critical. Imaging is particularly important for diagnosis and prognosis in patients with blunt chest trauma. Because plain radiographs miss up to 50% of rib fractures, CT scans should be considered given the higher incidence of intrathoracic injuries in older adults.[112]

Optimized analgesia is the cornerstone of rib fracture management. Inadequate analgesia from rib fractures contributes to patient morbidity including splinting, hypoventilation, and pneumonia; therefore, early pain management is crucial in older patients. Multiple guidelines recommend the use of a multimodal analgesic approach using opioid and nonopioid adjuncts, including nerve blocks, to improve pain management and patient outcomes in patients with blunt thoracic trauma.[34,113,114] Multiple observational studies also demonstrate the utility of spirometry (typically forced vital capacity) to risk-stratify patients, and identify those that may benefit from closer observation in the ICU.[115–117] Formalizing the approach to rib fracture management, including early assessment, risk stratification for ICU care, analgesia, and other aspects of care in a clinical pathway or protocol has also been associated with decreased morbidity and mortality in geriatric trauma patients.[114,118–120] One key aspect of this approach is the involvement of multidisciplinary teams, such as a pain service, respiratory therapy, and physical and occupational therapy.[121] Several risk stratification and management pathways exist. The Western Trauma Association rib fracture algorithm suggests that any patient with two or more rib fractures older than the age of 65 be admitted to an ICU or step-down unit.

HIP AND PELVIC FRACTURES

Hip and pelvic fractures are one of the most common traumatic injuries among older adults.[122] Plain radiographs have an estimated sensitivity of 90% to 98% for hip fractures and should reveal most fractures.[123] However, if there is persistent clinical suspicion despite normal radiographs (eg, pain, inability to ambulate), then further imaging should be pursued to rule out occult fracture.

Among patients with hip fractures, preoperative wait times greater than 24 hours are associated with increased complications and mortality.[124,125] A recent randomized trial demonstrated that surgery within 6 hours of diagnosis resulted in a lower risk of delirium, better pain management, earlier mobilization, and earlier hospital discharge.[126] These data suggest there should be prompt consultation or transfer to a facility with orthopedic surgery to help expedite surgical intervention if indicated. As with rib fractures, aggressive pain management is the mainstay of treatment while awaiting more definitive care or admission. The literature also supports the implementation of a comprehensive, interdisciplinary approach in geriatric hip fracture care.[127–129] Interdisciplinary teams could include geriatricians, physical and occupational therapists, and social workers. Studies have shown that this team-based approach decreases morbidity and mortality, and optimizes discharge planning.[129–134]

For pelvic fractures, older adults are more likely to sustain lateral compression fractures and are at higher risk for bleeding and mortality, and therefore more likely to require transfusion and angiographic embolization.[135,136] With potential previous comorbidities and anticoagulation therapy, clinicians should consider anticoagulation reversal and early interventional radiology consultation for consideration of angiographic embolization.[137] There are no widely accepted criteria for angioembolization but the threshold should be lower in older adults.[89] General indications include hemodynamic instability, CT showing pelvic hematoma or active contrast extravasation, and requirement for massive transfusion.[89]

SOFT TISSUE INJURIES

With age, skin loses elastin and collagen, the epidermis becomes thin, and there is decreased subcutaneous support.[138] Older adults are therefore more prone to soft tissue injury and the wound healing process is prolonged. In the context of geriatric trauma, there are certain particular considerations.

Prolonged Immobilization

Early trauma care is often associated with immobilization, including backboards, spine precautions, and cervical collars. Patients can be immobilized for a prolonged period of time while they await evaluation, investigations, and diagnostic imaging.[139] Prolonged immobilization can lead to skin breakdown and development of pressure ulcers, which may develop in 4 to 6 hours.[140] Clinicians should be even more mindful of minimizing immobilization to prevent iatrogenic soft tissue injuries, especially in older adults, and consider using reactive gel surface mattresses to reduce pressure ulcer risk.[141,142]

Management of Skin Tears

Among older adults, skin tears have a significant risk of evolving into complex chronic wounds. The International Skin Tear Advisory Panel classifies skin tears into three types: type 1 has no skin loss, with a flap that can be repositioned; type 2 has partial skin loss, where the wound cannot be completed covered; and type 3 has total flap loss, where the entire wound bed is exposed.[143] Depending on the type and extent of injury, the involvement of a wound care nurse or even plastic surgeon may be advisable. Best practice recommendations include cleansing with saline or clear tap water at a low pressure to remove clots and dried blood, debridement of nonviable tissue, and reapposition of any skin flap over the wound bed.[144] Given the fragility of the skin flaps, suturing and staples are not recommended.[145] Skin glue or adhesive strips (Steri-Strips) may be used to approximate the wound edges if the wound bed is appropriately covered by the flap.

ELDER ABUSE

Elder abuse includes physical, psychological, sexual, and financial abuse, and neglect. Although few studies have accurately captured the prevalence of elder abuse and neglect, a 2016 scoping review of international literature on elder abuse found a worldwide mean prevalence of 7%.[146] Another review of studies across 28 countries found that one in six older adults older than the age of 60 were subjected to some form of abuse.[147]

Emergency physicians frequently miss and underreport elder abuse.[148–150] In the context of geriatric trauma, clinicians should always maintain a high level of suspicion of elder abuse, especially if there is a delayed presentation, inconsistent history, and atypical injury patterns. Risk factors for abuse include: problems with physical health; mental illness; substance use; functional, financial, social or emotional dependency; problems with stress and coping; previous abuse; interpersonal conflicts; and social isolation.[151] Although these risk factors are broad, the key takeaway is to be cognizant of potential nonaccidental trauma in older adult patients and to intervene as needed.

The legal duty to report elder abuse and neglect depends on multiple factors, such as geographic location of residence, the patient's place of residence (ie, care facility), and if a criminal act has occurred. Health care providers should therefore inform themselves about their local laws relevant to elder abuse and legal obligations to report to the authorities.

Given the challenges in identifying elder abuse, adopting a team-based approach involving interdisciplinary health care professionals, including geriatric emergency nurses and social workers, is useful.[152] There are also multiple screening tools that are available that could be used to help detect elder abuse, although there is no single tool that is considered to be the gold standard.[153] The American College of Surgeons Best Practice Guideline suggests that providers consider screening older adults for elder abuse, and lays out the approach to doing so.[154] Overall, it is essential to maintain high suspicion for elder abuse in the context of geriatric trauma and to involve an interdisciplinary team for support if there are concerns.

GOALS OF CARE

With increased morbidity and mortality in geriatric trauma, clinicians should promptly engage in goals of care discussions with the patient, their substitute decision maker, and their family. Previous directives need to be noted by the treatment team and approach to management must reflect the patient's values and preferences for care at the end of life. The clinician needs to avoid ageism and also appreciate the patient's preinjury functional status. Goals of care discussions should be approached with empathy and clarity.[155]

TRANSITIONS TO INPATIENT CARE
Delirium Prevention

Delirium is an acute neuropsychiatric syndrome that is distressing to patients and is associated with serious adverse outcomes. It is essential to incorporate multicomponent nonpharmacologic delirium prevention strategies, such as optimizing the older patient's environment (eg, having a clock and calendar, room with windows, placing familiar objects or pictures in hospital room) and addressing basic needs (eg, correct sensory impairments with glasses, hearing aids, addressing hunger and thirst). Nonpharmacologic strategies have clearly been shown to reduce incidence of delirium compared with usual care (relative risk, 0.57; 95% confidence interval, 0.46–0.71).[156] These interventions to prevent delirium must be implemented as soon as possible, starting in the emergency department.

Medication: Right Medication, Right Dose, Right Time

Careful management of medication is imperative in the care of older adults. Accurately represcribing and adjusting medication is crucial to avoid potential adverse effects and withdrawal. For example, patients with Parkinson disease require their medication to be administered on time to prevent freezing and hypokinesia. Older adults are also more susceptible to adverse effects of opioid analgesics. Clinicians need to approach medication prescription for geriatric trauma patients cautiously, considering their medical comorbidities and adjusting dosing as needed (eg, adjusted for age, kidney failure). The Beers Criteria is a published list of medications that highlight those that may not be the safest or most appropriate options for older adults and is a useful resource to review.[157]

Geriatric Consultation Service

Providing optimal management of hospitalized geriatric trauma patients is often complex, and needs to balance the care of acute injuries with preinjury comorbidities, frailty, fall risk, postinjury complications, and social and functional issues. Current guidelines support the implementation of a proactive geriatric consultation service, consisting of geriatric specialists who evaluate patients early in their admission, before the development of complications. Assessment and management by a dedicated geriatric service is associated with decreases in the incidence of delirium, length of stay, discharge to long-term care facilities, and hospital-acquired complications (eg, functional decline and falls).[158–160]

SUMMARY

Older adults who experience trauma have unique needs compared with their younger counterparts. There are several specific considerations that a provider must take into account when involved in their care. Recognition of illness severity based on different physiologic parameters, avoiding undertriage of patients, liberal use of diagnostic imaging, and involving multidisciplinary teams to optimize outcomes are all crucial. On an institutional level, leaders must ensure that care pathways are standardized and that trauma teams have specific training in geriatric trauma.

CLINICS CARE POINTS

- Use the Clinical Frailty Scale to ascertain frailty as frailty is strongly associated with adverse outcomes.
- Older adults with traumatic injurt who require a CT head should have a concurrent CT of the c-spine as there is a high likelihood of fracture, regardless of intracranial injury.
- Plain radiographs often miss rib fractures.
- Delirium prevention should not be an afterthought to trauma care as non-pharmacology strategies can reduce the incidence of delirium (relative risk 0.57, 95% confidence interval, 0.46–0.71)

DISCLOSURE

All authors certify that they have no affiliations with or involvement in any organization or entity with any financial interest or nonfinancial interest in the subject matter or materials discussed in this article.

REFERENCES

1. Hill AD, Pinto R, Nathens AB, et al. Age-related trends in severe injury hospitalization in Canada. J Trauma Acute Care Surg 2014;77(4):608–13.
2. Cioffi WG, Connolly MD, Adams CA, et al. The National Trauma Data Bank Annual Report. Encycl Intensive Care Med 2012;2206.
3. Clark D, Fantus R. National Trauma Data Bank Annual Report 2007. Am Coll Surg 2007.
4. Kehoe A, Smith JE, Edwards A, et al. The changing face of major trauma in the UK. Emerg Med J 2015;32(12):911–5.
5. Kojima M, Endo A, Shiraishi A, et al. Age-related characteristics and outcomes for patients with severe trauma: analysis of Japan's Nationwide Trauma Registry. Ann Emerg Med 2019;73(3):281–90.
6. Caterino JM, Valasek T, Werman HA. Identification of an age cutoff for increased mortality in patients with elderly trauma. Am J Emerg Med 2010;28(2):151–8.
7. Goodmanson NW, Rosengart MR, Barnato AE, et al. Defining geriatric trauma: when does age make a difference? Surg (United States) 2012;152(4):668–75.
8. Lundebjerg NE, Trucil DE, Hammond EC, et al. When it comes to older adults, language matters: Journal of the American Geriatrics Society Adopts Modified American Medical Association Style. J Am Geriatr Soc 2017;65(7):1386–8.
9. Sammy I, Lecky F, Sutton A, et al. Factors affecting mortality in older trauma patients: a systematic review and meta-analysis. Injury 2016;47(6):1170–83.
10. Savioli G, Ceresa IF, Macedonio S, et al. Major trauma in elderly patients: worse mortality and outcomes in an Italian trauma center. J Emerg Trauma Shock 2021; 14(2):98–103.
11. Perdue PW, Watts DD, Kaufmann CR, et al. Differences in mortality between elderly and younger adult trauma patients: geriatric status increases risk of delayed death. J Trauma 1998;45(4):805–10.
12. Aitken LM, Burmeister E, Lang J, et al. Characteristics and outcomes of injured older adults after hospital admission. J Am Geriatr Soc 2010;58(3):442–9.
13. Konda SR, Lott A, Mandel J, et al. Who is the geriatric trauma patient? An analysis of patient characteristics, hospital quality measures, and inpatient cost. Geriatr Orthop Surg Rehabil 2020;11:1–8.

14. Labib N, Nouh T, Winocour S, et al. Severely injured geriatric population: morbidity, mortality, and risk factors. J Trauma 2011;71(6):1908–14.
15. Ganz DA, Bao Y, Shekelle PG, et al. Will my patient fall? JAMA 2007;297(1): 77–86.
16. Kwan E, Straus SE, Kwan E. Mayores 2 2014;186(16).
17. Newgard CD, Fischer PE, Gestring M, et al. National guideline for the field triage of injured patients: recommendations of the national expert panel on field triage, 2021. J Trauma Acute Care Surg 2022;(2). https://doi.org/10.1097/ta.0000000000003627.
18. Heffernan DS, Thakkar RK, Monaghan SF, et al. Normal presenting vital signs are unreliable in geriatric blunt trauma victims. J Trauma 2010;69(4):813–20.
19. Martin JT, Alkhoury F, O'Connor JA, et al. Normal" vital signs belie occult hypoperfusion in geriatric trauma patients. Am Surg 2010;76(1):65–9. http://www.ncbi.nlm.nih.gov/pubmed/20135942.
20. Demetriades D, Sava J, Alo K, et al. Old age as a criterion for trauma team activation. J Trauma 2001;51(4):754–6 [discussion: 756–7].
21. Brown JB, Gestring ML, Forsythe RM, et al. Systolic blood pressure criteria in the National Trauma Triage Protocol for geriatric trauma: 110 is the new 90. J Trauma Acute Care Surg 2015;78(2):352–9.
22. Mutschler M, Nienaber U, Münzberg M, et al. The Shock Index revisited: a fast guide to transfusion requirement? A retrospective analysis on 21,853 patients derived from the TraumaRegister DGU. Crit Care 2013;17(4):R172.
23. Zarzaur BL, Croce MA, Fischer PE, et al. New vitals after injury: shock index for the young and age x shock index for the old. J Surg Res 2008;147(2):229–36.
24. Navaratnarajah A, Jackson SHD. The physiology of ageing. Medicine (Baltimore) 2013;41(1):5–8.
25. Aalami OO, Fang TD, Song HM, et al. Physiological features of aging persons. Arch Surg 2003;138(10):1068–76.
26. Rockwood K. A global clinical measure of fitness and frailty in elderly people. Can Med Assoc J 2005;173(5):489–95.
27. Faller JW, Pereira D do N, de Souza S, et al. Instruments for the detection of frailty syndrome in older adults: a systematic review. PLoS One 2019;14(4): e0216166.
28. Cheung A, Haas B, Ringer TJ, et al. Canadian Study of Health and Aging Clinical Frailty Scale: does it predict adverse outcomes among geriatric trauma patients? J Am Coll Surg 2017;225(5):658–65.e3.
29. Joseph B, Orouji Jokar T, Hassan A, et al. Redefining the association between old age and poor outcomes after trauma: the impact of frailty syndrome. J Trauma Acute Care Surg 2017;82(3):575–81.
30. Joseph B, Pandit V, Zangbar B, et al. Superiority of frailty over age in predicting outcomes among geriatric trauma patients: a prospective analysis. JAMA Surg 2014;149(8):766–72.
31. Poulton A, Shaw JF, Nguyen F, et al. The association of frailty with adverse outcomes after multisystem trauma: a systematic review and meta-analysis. Anesth Analg 2020;130(6):1482–92.
32. Haas B, Wunsch H. How does prior health status (age, comorbidities and frailty) determine critical illness and outcome? Curr Opin Crit Care 2016;22(5):500–5.
33. Cubitt M, Downie E, Shakerian R, et al. Timing and methods of frailty assessments in geriatric trauma patients: a systematic review. Injury 2019;50(11): 1795–808.

34. ACS Committee on Trauma. ACS TQIP Geriatric Trauma Management Guidelines. Am Coll Surg 2013;1–31. Available at: https://www.facs.org/~/media/files/quality programs/trauma/tqip/geriatric guide tqip.ashx.

35. Alshibani A, Alharbi M, Conroy S. Under-triage of older trauma patients in pre-hospital care: a systematic review. Eur Geriatr Med 2021;12(5):903–19.

36. Chang DC, Bass RR, Cornwell EE, et al. Undertriage of elderly trauma patients to state-designated trauma centers. Arch Surg 2008;143(8):776–81 [discussion:.782].

37. Nordgarden T, Odland P, Guttormsen AB, et al. Undertriage of major trauma patients at a university hospital: a retrospective cohort study. Scand J Trauma Resusc Emerg Med 2018;26(1):64.

38. Anantha RV, Painter MD, Diaz-Garelli F, et al. undertriage despite use of geriatric-specific trauma team activation guidelines : who are we missing? Am Surg 2021;87(3):419–26.

39. Xiang H, Wheeler KK, Groner JI, et al. Undertriage of major trauma patients in the US emergency departments. Am J Emerg Med 2014;32(9):997–1004.

40. Ichwan B, Darbha S, Shah MN, et al. Geriatric-specific triage criteria are more sensitive than standard adult criteria in identifying need for trauma center care in injured older adults. Ann Emerg Med 2015;65(1):92–100.e3.

41. Field Trauma Triage and Air Ambulance Utilization Standards. Emergency Health Services Branch, Ministry of Health and Long-Term Care. https://www.health.gov.on.ca/en/pro/programs/emergency_health/docs/ehs_training_blltn113_en.pdf. [Accessed 30 October 2022].

42. Barraco R, Chiu W, Bard M, et al. Practice management guidelines for the appropriate triage of the victim of trauma. 2010. Available at: https://www.east.org/Content/documents/practicemanagementguidelines/TraumaTriage.pdf.

43. Boulton AJ, Peel D, Rahman U, et al. Evaluation of elderly specific pre-hospital trauma triage criteria: a systematic review. Scand J Trauma Resusc Emerg Med 2021;29(1). https://doi.org/10.1186/s13049-021-00940-z.

44. Gomez D, Haas B, Doumouras AG, et al. A population-based analysis of the discrepancy between potential and realized access to trauma center care. Ann Surg 2013;257(1):160–5.

45. Tillmann BW, Nathens AB, Guttman MP, et al. Hospital resources do not predict accuracy of secondary trauma triage: a population-based analysis. J Trauma Acute Care Surg 2020;88(2):230–41.

46. MacKenzie EJ, Rivara FP, Jurkovich GJ, et al. A national evaluation of the effect of trauma-center care on mortality. N Engl J Med 2006;354(4):366–78.

47. Haas B, Gomez D, Xiong W, et al. External benchmarking of trauma center performance: have we forgotten our elders? Ann Surg 2011;253(1):144–50.

48. Pandya SR, Yelon JA, Sullivan TS, et al. Geriatric motor vehicle collision survival: the role of institutional trauma volume. J Trauma 2011;70(6):1326–30.

49. Zafar SN, Obirieze A, Schneider EB, et al. Outcomes of trauma care at centers treating a higher proportion of older patients: the case for geriatric trauma centers. J Trauma Acute Care Surg 2015;78(4):852–9.

50. Olufajo OA, Metcalfe D, Rios-Diaz A, et al. Does hospital experience rather than volume improve outcomes in geriatric trauma patients? J Am Coll Surg 2016;223(1):32–40.e1.

51. Bryan Y, Johnson K, Botros D, et al. Anatomic and physiopathologic changes affecting the airway of the elderly patient: implications for geriatric-focused airway management. Clin Interv Aging 2015;1925. https://doi.org/10.2147/CIA.S93796.

52. Langeron O, Masso E, Huraux C, et al. Prediction of difficult mask ventilation. Anesthesiology 2000;92(5):1229–36.

53. Kheterpal S, Han R, Tremper KK, et al. Incidence and predictors of difficult and impossible mask ventilation. Anesthesiology 2006;105(5):885–91.

54. Kheterpal S, Martin L, Shanks AM, et al. Prediction and outcomes of impossible mask ventilation: a review of 50,000 anesthetics. Anesthesiology 2009;110(4): 891–7.

55. Detsky ME, Jivraj N, Adhikari NK, et al. Will this patient be difficult to intubate? JAMA 2019;321(5):493.

56. Goutcher CM, Lochhead V. Reduction in mouth opening with semi-rigid cervical collars † †Presented as a poster at the Difficult Airway Society Annual Scientific Meeting, Leicester, UK, November 25–26, 2004. Br J Anaesth 2005;95(3):344–8.

57. Yuk M, Yeo W, Lee K, et al. Cervical collar makes difficult airway: a simulation study using the LEMON criteria. Clin Exp Emerg Med 2018;5(1):22–8.

58. Thiboutot F, Nicole PC, Trépanier CA, et al. Effect of manual in-line stabilization of the cervical spine in adults on the rate of difficult orotracheal intubation by direct laryngoscopy: a randomized controlled trial. Can J Anesth Can D'anesthésie 2009;56(6):412–8.

59. Lewis SR, Butler AR, Parker J, et al. Videolaryngoscopy versus direct laryngoscopy for adult patients requiring tracheal intubation: a Cochrane Systematic Review. Br J Anaesth 2017;119(3):369–83.

60. Singleton BN, Morris FK, Yet B, et al. Effectiveness of intubation devices in patients with cervical spine immobilisation: a systematic review and network meta-analysis. Br J Anaesth 2021;126(5):1055–66.

61. Sprung J, Gajic O, Warner DO. Review article: age related alterations in respiratory function:- anesthetic considerations. Can J Anaesth 2006;53(12): 1244–57.

62. Dimitriou R, Calori GM, Giannoudis PV. Polytrauma in the elderly: specific considerations and current concepts of management. Eur J Trauma Emerg Surg 2011;37(6):539–48.

63. Rivera R, Antognini JF, Riou B. Perioperative drug therapy in elderly patients. Anesthesiology 2009;110(5):1176–81.

64. Upchurch CP, Grijalva CG, Russ S, et al. Comparison of etomidate and ketamine for induction during rapid sequence intubation of adult trauma patients. Ann Emerg Med 2017;69(1):24–33.e2.

65. Kovacs G, Sowers N. Airway management in trauma. Emerg Med Clin North Am 2018;36(1):61–84.

66. Matchett G, Gasanova I, Riccio CA, et al. Etomidate versus ketamine for emergency endotracheal intubation: a randomized clinical trial. Intensive Care Med 2022;48(1):78–91.

67. Callaway DW, Shapiro NI, Donnino MW, et al. Serum lactate and base deficit as predictors of mortality in normotensive elderly blunt trauma patients. J Trauma 2009;66(4):1040–4.

68. Davis JW, Kaups KL. Base deficit in the elderly: a marker of severe injury and death. J Trauma 1998;45(5):873–7.

69. Salottolo KM, Mains CW, Offner PJ, et al. A retrospective analysis of geriatric trauma patients: venous lactate is a better predictor of mortality than traditional vital signs. Scand J Trauma Resusc Emerg Med 2013;21:7.

70. Neville AL, Nemtsev D, Manasrah R, et al. Mortality risk stratification in elderly trauma patients based on initial arterial lactate and base deficit levels. Am

Surg 2011;77(10):1337–41. Available at: http://www.ncbi.nlm.nih.gov/pubmed/22127083.

71. Sedighi SM, Nguyen M, Khalil A, et al. The impact of cardiac troponin in elderly patients in the absence of acute coronary syndrome: a systematic review. Int J Cardiol Hear Vasc 2020;31:100629.

72. Ivascu FA, Howells GA, Junn FS, et al. Rapid warfarin reversal in anticoagulated patients with traumatic intracranial hemorrhage reduces hemorrhage progression and mortality. J Trauma 2005;59(5):1131–7 [discussion: 1137–9].

73. Liu H, Yang Y, Xia Y, et al. Aging of cerebral white matter. Ageing Res Rev 2017;34:64–76.

74. Mosenthal AC, Livingston DH, Lavery RF, et al. The effect of age on functional outcome in mild traumatic brain injury: 6-month report of a prospective multicenter trial. J Trauma 2004;56(5):1042–8.

75. McIntyre A, Mehta S, Aubut J, et al. Mortality among older adults after a traumatic brain injury: a meta-analysis. Brain Inj 2013;27(1):31–40.

76. Thompson HJ, Dikmen S, Temkin N. Prevalence of comorbidity and its association with traumatic brain injury and outcomes in older adults. Res Gerontol Nurs 2012;5(1):17–24.

77. Coronado VG, Thomas KE, Sattin RW, et al. The CDC traumatic brain injury surveillance system: characteristics of persons aged 65 years and older hospitalized with a TBI. J Head Trauma Rehabil 2005;20(3):215–28.

78. Harvey LA, Close JCT. Traumatic brain injury in older adults: characteristics, causes and consequences. Injury 2012;43(11):1821–6.

79. Kehoe A, Rennie S, Smith JE. Glasgow Coma Scale is unreliable for the prediction of severe head injury in elderly trauma patients. Emerg Med J 2015;32(8):613–5.

80. Salottolo K, Levy AS, Slone DS, et al. The effect of age on Glasgow Coma Scale score in patients with traumatic brain injury. JAMA Surg 2014;149(7):727–34.

81. Susman M, DiRusso SM, Sullivan T, et al. Traumatic brain injury in the elderly: increased mortality and worse functional outcome at discharge despite lower injury severity. J Trauma 2002;53(2):219–23 [discussion: 223–4].

82. Demetriades D, Kuncir E, Murray J, et al. Mortality prediction of head Abbreviated Injury Score and Glasgow Coma Scale: analysis of 7,764 head injuries. J Am Coll Surg 2004;199(2):216–22.

83. Mower WR, Hoffman JR, Herbert M, et al. Developing a decision instrument to guide computed tomographic imaging of blunt head injury patients. J Trauma 2005;59(4):954–9.

84. Stiell IG, Clement CM, Rowe BH, et al. Comparison of the Canadian CT Head Rule and the New Orleans Criteria in patients with minor head injury. JAMA 2005;294(12):1511–8.

85. Jagoda AS, Bazarian JJ, Bruns JJ, et al. Clinical policy: neuroimaging and decisionmaking in adult mild traumatic brain injury in the acute setting. J Emerg Nurs 2009;35(2):e5–40.

86. Lomoschitz FM, Blackmore CC, Mirza SK, et al. Cervical spine injuries in patients 65 years old and older: epidemiologic analysis regarding the effects of age and injury mechanism on distribution, type, and stability of injuries. AJR Am J Roentgenol 2002;178(3):573–7.

87. Healey CD, Spilman SK, King BD, et al. Asymptomatic cervical spine fractures: current guidelines can fail older patients. J Trauma Acute Care Surg 2017;83(1):119–25.

88. Schrag SP, Toedter LJ, McQuay N. Cervical spine fractures in geriatric blunt trauma patients with low-energy mechanism: are clinical predictors adequate? Am J Surg 2008;195(2):170–3.

89. Sadro CT, Sandstrom CK, Verma N, et al. Geriatric trauma: a radiologist's guide to imaging trauma patients aged 65 years and older. Radiographics 2015;35(4): 1263–85.

90. Stiell IG, Wells GA, Vandemheen KL, et al. The Canadian C-spine rule for radiography in alert and stable trauma patients. JAMA 2001;286(15):1841–8.

91. Goode T, Young A, Wilson SP, et al. Evaluation of cervical spine fracture in the elderly: can we trust our physical examination? Am Surg 2014;80(2):182–4.

92. Touger M, Gennis P, Nathanson N, et al. Validity of a decision rule to reduce cervical spine radiography in elderly patients with blunt trauma. Ann Emerg Med 2002;40(3):287–93.

93. Denver D, Shetty A, Unwin D. Falls and Implementation of NEXUS in the Elderly (The FINE Study). J Emerg Med 2015;49(3):294–300.

94. Bub LD, Blackmore CC, Mann FA, et al. Cervical spine fractures in patients 65 years and older: a clinical prediction rule for blunt trauma. Radiology 2005; 234(1):143–9.

95. Como JJ, Diaz JJ, Dunham CM, et al. Practice management guidelines for identification of cervical spine injuries following trauma: update from the eastern association for the surgery of trauma practice management guidelines committee. J Trauma 2009;67(3):651–9.

96. Laksmi PW, Harimurti K, Setiati S, et al. Management of immobilization and its complication for elderly. Acta Med Indones 2008;40(4):233–40. Available at: http://www.ncbi.nlm.nih.gov/pubmed/19151453.

97. Powers J, Daniels D, McGuire C, et al. The incidence of skin breakdown associated with use of cervical collars. J Trauma Nurs 2006;13(4):198–200.

98. Patel MB, Humble SS, Cullinane DC, et al. Cervical spine collar clearance in the obtunded adult blunt trauma patient: a systematic review and practice management guideline from the Eastern Association for the Surgery of Trauma. J Trauma Acute Care Surg 2015;78(2):430–41.

99. Rao PJ, Phan K, Mobbs RJ, et al. Cervical spine immobilization in the elderly population. J Spine Surg (Hong Kong) 2016;2(1):41–6.

100. Ziegler DW, Agarwal NN. The morbidity and mortality of rib fractures. J Trauma 1994;37(6):975–9.

101. Liman ST, Kuzucu A, Tastepe AI, et al. Chest injury due to blunt trauma. Eur J Cardiothorac Surg 2003;23(3):374–8.

102. Marini CP, Petrone P, Soto-Sánchez A, et al. Predictors of mortality in patients with rib fractures. Eur J Trauma Emerg Surg 2021;47(5):1527–34.

103. Stawicki SP, Grossman MD, Hoey BA, et al. Rib fractures in the elderly: a marker of injury severity. J Am Geriatr Soc 2004;52(5):805–8.

104. Shi HH, Esquivel M, Staudenmayer KL, et al. Effects of mechanism of injury and patient age on outcomes in geriatric rib fracture patients. Trauma Surg Acute Care Open 2017;2(1):e000074.

105. Battle CE, Hutchings H, Evans PA. Risk factors that predict mortality in patients with blunt chest wall trauma: a systematic review and meta-analysis. Injury 2012;43(1):8–17.

106. Barnea Y, Kashtan H, Skornick Y, et al. Isolated rib fractures in elderly patients: mortality and morbidity. Can J Surg 2002;45(1):43–6. Available at: http://www.ncbi.nlm.nih.gov/pubmed/11837920.

107. Meyer DE, Vincent LE, Fox EE, et al. Every minute counts: time to delivery of initial massive transfusion cooler and its impact on mortality. J Trauma Acute Care Surg 2017. https://doi.org/10.1097/TA.0000000000001531.

108. Bergeron E, Lavoie A, Clas D, et al. Elderly trauma patients with rib fractures are at greater risk of death and pneumonia. J Trauma 2003;54(3):478–85.

109. Bulger EM, Arneson MA, Mock CN, et al. Rib fractures in the elderly. J Trauma 2000;48(6):1040–6 [discussion: 1046–7].

110. Sirmali M, Türüt H, Topçu S, et al. A comprehensive analysis of traumatic rib fractures: morbidity, mortality and management. Eur J Cardiothorac Surg 2003;24(1):133–8.

111. Shulzhenko NO, Zens TJ, Beems MV, et al. Number of rib fractures thresholds independently predict worse outcomes in older patients with blunt trauma. Surgery 2017;161(4):1083–9.

112. Livingston DH, Shogan B, John P, et al. CT diagnosis of rib fractures and the prediction of acute respiratory failure. J Trauma 2008;64(4):905–11.

113. Galvagno SM, Smith CE, Varon AJ, et al. Pain management for blunt thoracic trauma: a joint practice management guideline from the Eastern Association for the Surgery of Trauma and Trauma Anesthesiology Society. J Trauma Acute Care Surg 2016;81(5):936–51.

114. Brasel KJ, Moore EE, Albrecht RA, et al. Western Trauma Association critical decisions in trauma: management of rib fractures. J Trauma Acute Care Surg 2017; 82(1):200–3.

115. Billings JD, Khan AD, Clement LP, et al. A clinical practice guideline using percentage of predicted forced vital capacity improves resource allocation for rib fracture patients. J Trauma Acute Care Surg 2021;90(5):769–75.

116. Carver TW, Milia DJ, Somberg C, et al. Vital capacity helps predict pulmonary complications after rib fractures. J Trauma Acute Care Surg 2015;79(3):413–6.

117. Warner R, Knollinger P, Hobbs G, et al. Forced vital capacity less than 1: a mark for high-risk patients. J Trauma Acute Care Surg 2018;85(2):271–4.

118. Sahr SM, Webb ML, Renner CH, et al. Implementation of a rib fracture triage protocol in elderly trauma patients. J Trauma Nurs 2013;20(4):172–5 [quiz: 176–7].

119. Hamilton C, Barnett L, Trop A, et al. Emergency department management of patients with rib fracture based on a clinical practice guideline. Trauma Surg Acute Care Open 2017;2(1):e000133.

120. Flarity K, Rhodes WC, Berson AJ, et al. Guideline-driven care improves outcomes in patients with traumatic rib fractures. Am Surg 2017;83(9):1012–7. Available at: http://www.ncbi.nlm.nih.gov/pubmed/28958283.

121. Todd SR, McNally MM, Holcomb JB, et al. A multidisciplinary clinical pathway decreases rib fracture-associated infectious morbidity and mortality in high-risk trauma patients. Am J Surg 2006;192(6):806–11.

122. Veronese N, Maggi S. Epidemiology and social costs of hip fracture. Injury 2018; 49(8):1458–60.

123. Cannon J, Silvestri S, Munro M. Imaging choices in occult hip fracture. J Emerg Med 2009;37(2):144–52.

124. Uzoigwe CE, Burnand HGF, Cheesman CL, et al. Early and ultra-early surgery in hip fracture patients improves survival. Injury 2013;44(6):726–9.

125. Simunovic N, Devereaux PJ, Sprague S, et al. Effect of early surgery after hip fracture on mortality and complications: systematic review and meta-analysis. CMAJ 2010;182(15):1609–16.

126. HIP ATTACK Investigators. Accelerated surgery versus standard care in hip fracture (HIP ATTACK): an international, randomised, controlled trial. Lancet (London, England) 2020;395(10225):698–708.

127. Patel JN, Klein DS, Sreekumar S, et al. Outcomes in multidisciplinary team-based approach in geriatric hip fracture care: a systematic review. J Am Acad Orthop Surg 2020;28(3):128–33.

128. Zuckerman JD, Sakales SR, Fabian DR, et al. Hip fractures in geriatric patients. Results of an interdisciplinary hospital care program. Clin Orthop Relat Res 1992;274:213–25. Available at: http://www.ncbi.nlm.nih.gov/pubmed/1729006.

129. Lau TW, Leung F, Siu D, et al. Geriatric hip fracture clinical pathway: the Hong Kong experience. Osteoporos Int 2010;21(Suppl 4):S627–36.

130. Adunsky A, Lerner-Geva L, Blumstein T, et al. Improved survival of hip fracture patients treated within a comprehensive geriatric hip fracture unit, compared with standard of care treatment. J Am Med Dir Assoc 2011;12(6):439–44.

131. Schnell S, Friedman SM, Mendelson DA, et al. The 1-year mortality of patients treated in a hip fracture program for elders. Geriatr Orthop Surg Rehabil 2010;1(1):6–14.

132. Giannoulis D, Calori GM, Giannoudis PV. Thirty-day mortality after hip fractures: has anything changed? Eur J Orthop Surg Traumatol 2016;26(4):365–70.

133. Lau T-W, Fang C, Leung F. The effectiveness of a geriatric hip fracture clinical pathway in reducing hospital and rehabilitation length of stay and improving short-term mortality rates. Geriatr Orthop Surg Rehabil 2013;4(1):3–9.

134. Moyet J, Deschasse G, Marquant B, et al. Which is the optimal orthogeriatric care model to prevent mortality of elderly subjects post hip fractures? A systematic review and meta-analysis based on current clinical practice. Int Orthop 2019;43(6):1449–54.

135. Henry SM, Pollak AN, Jones AL, et al. Pelvic fracture in geriatric patients: a distinct clinical entity. J Trauma 2002;53(1):15–20.

136. Kanezaki S, Miyazaki M, Notani N, et al. Clinical presentation of geriatric polytrauma patients with severe pelvic fractures: comparison with younger adult patients. Eur J Orthop Surg Traumatol 2016;26(8):885–90.

137. Kimbrell BJ, Velmahos GC, Chan LS, et al. Angiographic embolization for pelvic fractures in older patients. Arch Surg 2004;139(7):728–32 [discussion: 732–3].

138. Farage MA, Miller KW, Elsner P, et al. Characteristics of the aging skin. Adv Wound Care 2013;2(1):5–10.

139. Stagg MJ, Lovell ME. A repeat audit of spinal board usage in the emergency department. Injury 2008;39(3):323–6.

140. Gefen A. How much time does it take to get a pressure ulcer? Integrated evidence from human, animal, and in vitro studies. Ostomy Wound Manage 2008;54(10):26–8, 30-35. http://www.ncbi.nlm.nih.gov/pubmed/18927481.

141. Kwan I, Bunn F, Roberts I. Spinal immobilisation for trauma patients. Cochrane Database Syst Rev 2001;(2):CD002803.

142. Shi C, Dumville JC, Cullum N, et al. Beds, overlays and mattresses for preventing and treating pressure ulcers: an overview of Cochrane Reviews and network meta-analysis. Cochrane Database Syst Rev 2021;(8):2021. https://doi.org/10.1002/14651858.CD013761.pub2.

143. Van Tiggelen H, LeBlanc K, Campbell K, et al. Standardizing the classification of skin tears: validity and reliability testing of the International Skin Tear Advisory Panel Classification System in 44 countries. Br J Dermatol 2020;183(1):146–54.

144. LeBlanc K, Campbell KE, Wood E, et al. Best practice recommendations for prevention and management of skin tears in aged skin: an overview. J Wound Ostomy Cont Nurs 2018;45(6):540–2.

145. LeBlanc K, Baranoski S. Skin Tear Consensus Panel Members. Skin tears: state of the science: consensus statements for the prevention, prediction, assessment, and treatment of skin tears. Adv Skin Wound Care 2011;24(9 Suppl):2–15.

146. Pillemer K, Burnes D, Riffin C, et al. Elder abuse: global situation, risk factors, and prevention strategies. Gerontologist 2016;56(Suppl 2):S194–205.

147. Yon Y, Mikton CR, Gassoumis ZD, et al. Elder abuse prevalence in community settings: a systematic review and meta-analysis. Lancet Glob Heal 2017;5(2): e147–56.

148. Dong X, Simon MA. Association between elder abuse and use of ED: findings from the Chicago Health and Aging Project. Am J Emerg Med 2013;31(4): 693–8.

149. Mercier É, Nadeau A, Brousseau A-A, et al. Elder abuse in the out-of-hospital and emergency department settings: a scoping review. Ann Emerg Med 2020;75(2):181–91.

150. Mandiracioglu A, Govsa F, Celikli S, et al. Emergency health care personnel's knowledge and experience of elder abuse in Izmir. Arch Gerontol Geriatr 2006;43(2):267–76.

151. Storey JE. Risk factors for elder abuse and neglect: a review of the literature. Aggress Violent Behav 2020;50:101339.

152. Rosen T, Hargarten S, Flomenbaum NE, et al. Identifying elder abuse in the emergency department: toward a multidisciplinary team-based approach. Ann Emerg Med 2016;68(3):378–82.

153. Gallione C, Dal Molin A, Cristina FVB, et al. Screening tools for identification of elder abuse: a systematic review. J Clin Nurs 2017;26(15–16):2154–76.

154. Abuse C, Abuse E, Violence IP, et al. Best practices guidelines for trauma center recognition of child abuse, elder abuse. Am Coll Surg 2019;52–3.

155. Palliative Care Best Practices Guidelines. American College of Surgeons. 2017. Available at: https://www.facs.org/media/g3rfegcn/palliative_guidelines.pdf. Accessed August 20, 2022.

156. Burton JK, Craig LE, Yong SQ, et al. Non-pharmacological interventions for preventing delirium in hospitalised non-ICU patients. Cochrane Database Syst Rev 2021;2021(7). https://doi.org/10.1002/14651858.CD013307.pub2.

157. By the 2019 American Geriatrics Society Beers Criteria® Update Expert Panel. American Geriatrics Society 2019 Updated AGS Beers Criteria® for potentially inappropriate medication use in older adults. J Am Geriatr Soc 2019;67(4): 674–94.

158. Fallon WF, Rader E, Zyzanski S, et al. Geriatric outcomes are improved by a geriatric trauma consultation service. J Trauma 2006;61(5):1040–6.

159. Lenartowicz M, Parkovnick M, McFarlan A, et al. An evaluation of a proactive geriatric trauma consultation service. Ann Surg 2012;256(6):1098–101.

160. Eagles D, Godwin B, Cheng W, et al. A systematic review and meta-analysis evaluating geriatric consultation on older trauma patients. J Trauma Acute Care Surg 2020;88(3):446–53.

Pediatric Trauma

Jennifer Guyther, MD[a,b,*], Rachel Wiltjer, DO[c]

KEYWORDS

- Pediatric trauma • Penetrating • Blunt • TXA • TEG • Blood transfusion • Arrest

KEY POINTS

- In major pediatric trauma, start with the ABCDE evaluation, keeping in mind the anatomical differences, age-appropriate vital signs, and developmental milestones.
- Use weight-based medication dosing and appropriately sized equipment on all pediatric patients.
- Although the guidelines currently recommend crystalloid first in hemorrhagic shock, pediatric studies are promising in the use of whole blood, blood components, and tranexamic acid.
- Penetrating trauma in young children is more often the result of non-missile weapons or other common objects.
- Use a stepwise approach to laboratories and imaging in the hemodynamically stable blunt trauma patient.

INITIAL TRAUMA EVALUATION

The saying "kids aren't just little adults" holds true when discussing the evaluation and management of a critically ill pediatric trauma patient. There are a variety of anatomic and physiologic differences that impact the impressions taken from the examination and objective data and can affect the decisions made in care. Broadly, normal ranges for vital signs change as a child grows, and it is important to interpret vital signs as well as examination findings within the context of age. In addition, hemodynamic compensation is enhanced in children, leading to hypotension as a very late sign of shock. Weight and size become important for both the dosing of medication and the size of the equipment used. References and tools such as the Broselow tape exist to help with estimation of weight as well as dosing of critical medications. Communication can also be difficult, even with children who are verbal. Having a parent at bedside, especially if there is staff available to explain to the parent what is happening, can be helpful for both parent and child. The core of the trauma examination remains

[a] Department of Emergency Medicine, University of Maryland School of Medicine, 110 South Paca Street, 6th Floor, Suite 200, Baltimore, MD 21201, USA; [b] Department of Pediatrics, University of Maryland School of Medicine, 110 South Paca Street, 6th Floor, Suite 200, Baltimore, MD 21201, USA; [c] University of Maryland Medical Center, 22 South Greene Street, Baltimore, MD 21201, USA
* Corresponding author.
E-mail address: jguyther@som.umaryland.edu

Emerg Med Clin N Am 41 (2023) 205–222
https://doi.org/10.1016/j.emc.2022.09.002
0733-8627/23/© 2022 Elsevier Inc. All rights reserved.

emed.theclinics.com

the same—ABCDE—but each portion of the examination will require subtle adjustments from adult algorithms.

THE CRITICAL TRAUMA
Airway

The pediatric airway develops throughout childhood and adolescence. Infants and young children have an anterior, narrow, and shorter airway, which can lead to difficulties in airway management. The pediatric airway is also easily occluded, either by foreign body or obstruction by the tongue.[1] As children become hypoxic easily and hypoxia can lead to significant hemodynamic effects, knowledge of effective airway management—both intubation and more simple supportive maneuvers—is paramount. Preoxygenation is more important the smaller a child is for these reasons as well.

If airway assessment indicates a need for intervention, consider positioning as well as adjuncts. For younger children, the head is often large, and placement of a shoulder roll can help bring the airway into alignment. For older children and adolescents, especially those who are obese, more standard positioning and even ramping is likely appropriate. The trachea is more compressible in younger patients, so use laryngeal manipulation with caution, as there is a risk of iatrogenic obstruction of the airway. Placement of an airway adjunct—either a nasopharyngeal airway in children with a gag or oropharyngeal airway in those without—may assist in effective oxygenation and ventilation before placement of an advanced airway. Consider using a bedside resource to assist in determination of correct sizing of equipment. The use of cuffed endotracheal tubes in pediatrics has been evolving over the past several years, with the American Heart Association now stating that cuffed tubes are a reasonable option over uncuffed endotracheal tubes in children under 8 years. Much of the recent literature demonstrates safety and improved outcomes with cuffed endotracheal tubes down to the neonatal period.[2,3,4] Video assistive technology is available in pediatric sizes; however, this is not available in many facilities and should not be depended on. First-pass success rate is lower in pediatric patients than in adult patients, and approximately one-third of pediatric patients will have a desaturation event with intubation, so set yourself up for success from the start.[4,5]

Airway obstruction is a rare but serious event with a high mortality rate. The pediatric airway is smaller and the tracheal rings are less calcified than the adult. Because of this traditional cricothyroidotomy is impractical in smaller children. Classically, the teaching has been that a cricothyroidotomy can first be performed between the ages of 10 and 12 years; however, this should also be based on the size of the child.[6] The procedure may be inappropriate in a child who is small for his age. A needle cricothyroidotomy is an alternate procedure that can be used as a temporary means of oxygenation (not ventilation) until either a surgical tracheostomy can be placed or the airway obstruction resolves.[7] If there is complete airway obstruction, the respiratory rate given through needle cricothyroidotomy should be lower than the typical rate to decrease the risk of barotrauma.

Breathing

Respiratory rate slows as an individual grows, with normal respiratory rates in an infant being as high as 60 breaths per minute. If ventilatory assistance is required, it is important to approximate physiologic rates and volumes. There are alternative ventilator setups (namely high-frequency oscillatory ventilation) for infants and young children who are difficult to ventilate. However, the use of these alternatives in the acute trauma setting is unlikely to be appropriate and would best be managed by pediatric critical care.

Circulation

Hemodynamic assessment of the pediatric patient is nuanced secondary to robust compensatory mechanisms. Blood pressure is often maintained after injury even with up to 30% blood loss, leading to hypotension being a late sign of shock.[8] Tachycardia presents before hypotension but can take longer to develop as well. Capillary refill can be used as a marker of impending shock, although this can be misleading due to temperature differences, individual range of response to hypovolemia, and potential variability in interobserver reliability.[9] The pediatric total blood volume can be as small as 250 to 300 mL in a term newborn. This is an important consideration both in the drawing of laboratories as well as in fluid and blood resuscitation. For resuscitation, it may be more effective to hand push fluids or blood as opposed to using a pressure bag. The hand push fluids use a stopcock to perform the "push-pull" method where a bolus is drawn into a syringe from a larger bag and then pushed manually into the patient. Many of the commercial products for massive transfusion and blood warming will be inappropriate for the pediatric patient due to minimum volume and flow requirements, although some products make inserts and/or adaptors to allow for pediatric and neonatal volume needs.[10] Children are particularly susceptible to hypothermia, and even warmed blood at lower flow rates can lose heat in intravenous (IV) tubing. Warming equipment and insulated IV tubing for pediatric transfusion exists but may not be available in all centers.[11] If warming blood is not situationally possible, monitor for hypothermia and use other forms of warming to attempt to maintain normothermia.

Massive transfusions are a rare event and associated with high morbidity and mortality.[12] Evidence to guide the timing of use and the choice between crystalloid fluids and blood products is not robust, and controversy exists. Some pediatric protocols may still advocate for isotonic fluid resuscitation up to 60 mL/kg (in aliquots of 20 mL/kg) before initiation of blood; however, newer literature suggests a benefit to earlier blood administration.[13] The most recent edition of Advanced Trauma Life Support also takes note of this research, recommending only one 20 mL/kg bolus of isotonic fluid before initiating blood transfusion.[14] Blood products should be transfused in aliquots of 10 mL/kg. Early research into whole blood administration in children also shows promise with a potential to decrease transfusion requirements and also decrease time to resolution of shock.[15] The definition of "massive transfusion" is also not consistent throughout the literature, and ranges from transfusion of 50% of blood volume (or about 40 mL/kg) to 100% of blood volume in 24 hours. Studies have shown that up to half of children who receive blood volumes that constitute a massive transfusion do not receive any platelets or fresh frozen plasma (FFP).[16] Ideal product ratios have yet to be definitively determined for the pediatric population, although newer studies lean toward a 1:1 ratio of packed red blood cells and FFP.[17–19] Coagulopathy is of particular concern in neonatal populations, as the hemostatic system is not fully developed until approximately 6 months of age.[16]

Given the difficulty in predicting which pediatric patients will require a massive transfusion, potential triggers have been assessed. Tools to help determine the need for massive transfusion are currently limited; one possible upcoming method is the base deficit, INR, and GCS (BIS) score which includes base deficit, International normalized ratio (INR), and a pediatric shock index (shock index, pediatric age adjusted [SIPA]) (Phillips).[19] The BIS score has not yet undergone prospective external validation. In the adult population, thromboelastography (TEG) has been shown to reduce mortality when guiding massive transfusion resuscitation (Philips 21, WIKKEL).[20,21] A retrospective analysis of 117 patients 18 years and younger compared patients who received greater than 40 cc/kg of blood to those who did not. This study showed that patients who required greater than 40 cc/kg of blood had a lower alpha angle, maximal amplitude (MA) value, and platelet count. The investigators concluded that TEG could help identify patients who may benefit from transfusion of cryoprecipitate or platelets.[20]

IV access can be difficult to establish in smaller children or children with depleted blood volumes. Intraosseous (IO) access is generally the preferred method for initial resuscitation if IV is unable to be established (within 2–3 attempts or 90 seconds) or is insufficient for resuscitation. Potential sites for IO access in a young child include the distal femur in addition to both proximal and distal tibia. The humeral head can be used once the greater tuberosity can be palpated, at approximately 6 years of age.[22] Central venous access is an option, but can be technically difficult in younger children, requires appropriately sized equipment, and has a higher risk of complications. Surgical cut down should remain a last resort.[23] Code drugs can be given endotracheally for the patient in arrest; however, this is a suboptimal means of delivery due to variable absorption and does not allow for volume resuscitation.

Disability

The Glasgow Coma Scale (GCS) has a validated pediatric format with verbal subscores broken down by more specific age ranges to allow for comparison to an age-appropriate norm. The pediatric GCS also incorporates minor changes to the motor and eye-opening scoring to allow for scoring of children who are too young to understand commands. A GCS score of 8 or lower is concerning for severe brain injury and may necessitate intubation as in adults, although assessment of the individual clinical scenario is important as well as the performance of controlled intubation when possible. Neurologic examination may be more challenging in younger populations; however, many movements and responses may be able to be elicited by drawing the child's attention in various directions with assistance from a parent if available. A basic understanding of developmental milestones may also help in interpreting examination findings as normal or abnormal.

Cervical spine immobilization also can present challenges in children of all ages—from finding an appropriately sized cervical collar to encouraging a child to leave it on. Sizing is particularly important as an incorrectly sized collar can create excessive flexion or extension and rates of pediatric cervical spine injuries tend to be higher in the areas where movement may occur. If a correctly sized cervical collar is unavailable or conventional collars are inappropriately shaped for a child (which can occur with some dysmorphia), roll towels and tape them in place for stabilization. The majority of spinal injuries in the pediatric population occur in the cervical spine, so appropriate immobilization is important.[24]

The routine use of backboards is not recommended. Studies show no change in rates of spinal cord injury with routine use. There are concerns for increased time to definitive care, pressure injuries, pain secondary to the backboard, and risk of respiratory compromise.[25–28] Much of the literature on prehospital backboard use is in adult patients, but the results can be extrapolated to the pediatric population, who face the same challenges. Although backboards may be necessary for extrication in the prehospital setting, patients should be removed from backboards as soon as is feasible. Patients should be logrolled for placement and removal from the backboard, at which time it is appropriate to assess for risk of spinal injury to determine need for continued logrolling. It is common and appropriate for Emergency Medical Service (EMS) to bring a child to the hospital in the car seat if the child is stable and without apparent neurologic deficits and the car seat has no visible damage.[29] When removing a child from the car seat, manual in-line stabilization should be used, even if a cervical collar is in place. After the child is unbuckled and in-line stabilization is held, the back of the car seat should be placed parallel to the ground and the child slid out the superior portion of the car seat onto the stretcher to maintain spinal alignment.

Exposure

Just as in adult patients, injuries must be uncovered to be visualized. The removal of all coverings for thorough examination is important, including the diaper. Younger children will become hypothermic more quickly and easily than adults, however, and this carries with it the usual trend toward coagulopathy. Aggressively cover children with warm blankets or use noninvasive warming devices as necessary to maintain normothermia.

WORKUP AND INITIAL MANAGEMENT OF THE CRITICAL TRAUMA PATIENT

As noted, the ABCDE algorithm should be addressed. Another important initial step is estimation of weight and size. Most medications are dosed in a weight-based fashion and equipment varies based on the size and weight of the child. The most used tool for estimation of weight in the pediatric population is the Broselow tape. This is found in many pediatric code carts and is the tool that many physicians are familiar with. Although there are concerns that it may underestimate weight in obese children, it provides a starting point and many initial medications, such as pain control, anesthetics, and vasoactive, can be titrated to effect.[30]

Numerous trauma mortality assessment tools can be applied to pediatrics with the Injury Severity Score being the most widely used and outperforms other pediatric trauma scores (pediatric trauma score, BIG score, and the revised trauma score) when predicting mortality.[31–33] This score is not intended to be a bedside emergency tool, but can be used in the research setting and may allow for prognostication after initial stabilization.[31,34,35] Knowledge of the mortality risk may help counsel families and facilitate communication between facilities during transfer.[31]

Internal Trauma Activation

Trauma centers have their own internal systems for activating hospital resources and trauma teams. Gutierrez and colleagues[36] showed that the use of physiologic criteria for activating internal trauma systems is a more accurate predictor of significant injury compared with both physician discretion and mechanism of injury. Although the majority of internal trauma activations are due to EMS prehospital alerts, Rubens and colleagues[37] found that 15% of pediatric patients arriving outside of EMS required immediate operative intervention or ICU-level care, but these patients represented only 1.8% of the trauma activations. This could delay definitive care and subspecialty consults and lead to unnecessary testing or worse outcomes.[38] Internal trauma activation systems should be based on objective data and be applied irrespective of mode of arrival.

Laboratory Testing

Laboratory work will be similar for pediatric and adult patients with clear multisystem injuries. Laboratories including a complete blood count, comprehensive metabolic panel, lipase, type and screen, coagulation factors, and urinalysis should be obtained. Lactate and base deficit have both been studied for their applicability in the pediatric population. Base deficit has some evidence to show that it may assist in prediction of the need for blood product transfusion.[38] The evidence is not robust enough to state that obtaining a Venous Blood Gas (VBG) for base deficit should be standard of care, but it is reasonable to obtain as an adjunct in determining the full picture. Elevated lactate levels (with cutoffs varying from 2.9 up to 5.1 mmol/L) have been associated in multiple studies with an increase in mortality; however, exact utilization in practice and changes in management are still unclear.[38] This again is a reasonable value to obtain. Troponin and Electrocardiogram (EKG) are indicated if concern for blunt cardiac injury exists. Toxicologic screening and pregnancy tests should be obtained as indicated by the clinical scenario.

Imaging

Imaging in critical trauma is also similar in pediatric and adult patients. Computerized tomography (CT) scan use should be considered more judiciously given the risk of radiation, but with concern for significant multisystem trauma it can still be appropriate to use scans of the head, neck, chest, and abdomen with the addition of x-rays as clinically indicated. Hemodynamically unstable patients who are not stable enough for CT should be considered for Operating Room (OR). Focused Assessment with Sonography for Trauma Evaluation (FAST) is used less commonly in pediatric trauma than in adult trauma but has been studied. The negative predictive value of FAST is lower in pediatric patients with between 26% and 35% of patients with hemoperitoneum on CT not being detected on FAST. A positive FAST in an unstable pediatric trauma patient, however, is helpful evidence of the need for emergent operative management.[8] Chest x-ray is a useful screening before chest CT even in an ill child, as a normal chest x-ray in the pediatric population is a good rule-out test for thoracic injury that will require intervention. Chest CT should be reserved for patients with physical examination findings to suggest major thoracic trauma, abnormal x-ray, or a suspected tracheo-bronchial injury.[39] Pelvic x-ray has a role for the hemodynamically unstable patient in whom a pelvic fracture is suspected, but sensitivity for pelvic fracture in the pediatric population is as low as 50%, making it inappropriate as a basis for ruling out pelvic fracture.[40]

Pain Management

Depending on the age of the child, communication may be limited or difficult. Infants experience pain and have physiologic stress responses as a result of pain. Pain control should be given just as freely in adults. Sedation of the pediatric patient should be considered if stable enough, before painful procedures such as fracture reduction or burn debridement.

Tranexamic Acid

The CRASH-2 trial showed decreased mortality and bleeding deaths in patients who received tranexamic acid (TXA).[41] In pediatric patients, the correlation between hemorrhage and mortality has not been as strong as in the adult population, possibly related to pediatric patients having a much lower rate of penetrating trauma.[42] Early coagulopathy, however, is linked to pediatric mortality, raising the possibility that TXA may have some benefit in this population.[42] Routine surgical procedures in pediatric cardiac, spine, and craniofacial surgeries have shown a decrease in intraoperative blood loss and transfusion needs with an acceptable safety profile when TXA was used.[41,43] Given the lack of large studies, there is significant variability in usage and dosing of TXA.[43] A survey of centers caring for victims of pediatric trauma showed that 35% are using TXA in these patients with the most common initial dose being 15 mg/kg and many giving a subsequent infusion of 2 mg/kg/h for 8 h.[43]

The PED-TRAX study was one of the first trials to examine TXA administration in the pediatric trauma population specifically.[41] Ten percent of the 766 patients 18 years and younger in this study received TXA. In this combat zone population, the investigators found that TXA use was independently associated with decreased mortality without any difference in thromboembolic or cardiovascular complications.[41] A standard dose of 1 gram IV within 3 hours of injury was used with redosing decided by the treating team.[41] Another study looked at 48 patients 16 years and younger who received blood products under the institutions massive transfusion protocol.[42] TXA (15 mg/kg to a maximum of 1 gram over 10 minutes with an infusion of 2 mg/kg/h over 8 hours) was used in 60% of these patients with no difference in mortality or thrombus.[42] A different study also looked at patients who received massive transfusions and TXA and showed that patients who received TXA were less likely to die (with an odds ratio of 0.35) in the hospital compared with those who did not receive TXA.[44] The TIC-TOC study is a multicenter study looking at the benefits of TXA in the pediatric trauma patient with hemorrhage involving the torso or brain. This study is an ongoing look at placebo versus two different weight-based dosing therapies.[45] The limited data currently available from this study do not seem to show an increase in thromboembolic events and there may be an improvement in mortality among those patients who require massive transfusion. The results of the TIC-TOC study will help to confirm these thoughts and provide guidance on proper dosing.

PEDIATRIC TRAUMATIC ARREST

Patterns in pediatric traumatic arrest are similar to adult traumatic arrest, with penetrating trauma and drowning most likely to have the best outcomes. Blunt trauma and strangulation/hanging have dismal outcomes. The incidence of pediatric traumatic arrest is low, and literature on the topic is sparse, but some small studies have attempted to describe the epidemiology and use of interventions.

Epinephrine has been a topic of study and debate in adult cardiac arrest and has been de-emphasized in adult traumatic cardiac arrest, but the pediatric data are quite limited. Once recent study found an association between early epinephrine administration and increased mortality in cardiac arrest due to hemorrhagic shock, however this is not yet definitive and more data are required before drawing actionable conclusions.[46–48] This serves as a reminder of the importance of other priorities in traumatic arrest such as hemorrhage control, fluid resuscitation, and high-quality Cardiopulmonary Resuscitation (CPR).[46]

There are not clear, widely accepted guidelines for when performance of resuscitative thoracotomy is appropriate in the pediatric population. Most case studies are small and report poor outcomes. Several studies involve patient ages ranging up to 18 years, with a trend toward older patients, which limits their applicability to younger populations. What has been established is that patients most likely to have a good outcome are those with penetrating injury, specifically cardiac injury.[43] It has also been demonstrated that patients presenting with signs of life (organized electrocardiographic activity, pupillary response, attempt at spontaneous respiration or movements, or an unassisted blood pressure) have better outcomes, and it has been proposed that the presence of signs of life should be a strong criterion in the decision to perform a resuscitative thoracotomy.[49]

Resuscitative endovascular balloon occlusion of the aorta (REBOA) is becoming more commonplace in adult traumatic resuscitation, but the translation to pediatrics is unclear. The balloon manufacturer does not recommend its use in aortas less than 15 mm in diameter which has been correlated with approximately 12 years of age although case reports exist of other balloon catheters being used off label.[50,51] The lowest documented age of successful REBOA use is 9 years old. Concerns also exist over the size of the femoral sheath versus the femoral artery in smaller children, although a 7 Fr option now exists as opposed to the original 12 Fr sheath.[50] Although there may be situations in which use is appropriate, these would be in larger children/adolescents, and care must be taken not to overinflate the balloon. REBOA is not a standard practice and should be generally reserved for extraordinary or investigative scenarios for smaller children.

PEDIATRIC PENETRATING TRAUMA

Penetrating injuries occur less often in the pediatric population compared with the adult population. Although there is scant literature and consensus on how to approach these patients, some key differences in the initial management of the pediatric penetrating trauma patient can be outlined here.

Head Injuries

Pediatric penetrating head injuries are rare and carry a mortality of up to 40%.[52] When assessing the pediatric patient, the examination should include a GCS and age-appropriate neurologic examination. Admission GCS score has been shown to be a reliable prognostic indicator in the pediatric population.[52] The mechanism of head injuries is also different in children. Although adolescents may be more prone to GSW or intentional self-inflicted head trauma, younger patients tend to suffer from accidental injuries. In accidental injuries, objects tend to enter the thinner roof of the orbit or the squamous part of the temporal bone.[52] Children are also more prone to infectious complications in penetrating head injury compared with their adult counterparts, with infections seen in up to 50% of pediatric patients. Risk factors for infections include cerebrospinal fluid (CSF) leak, sinus involvement, and injury materials such as graphite or wood.[52] Antibiotics to cover *Staphylococcus*, gram-negative bacteria, and *Clostridium* should be routinely administered in the emergency department (ED).[52] Data for seizure prophylaxis in younger children are lacking, but practice patterns suggest the prophylactic use of anticonvulsant medications initially and deferring to the treating neurosurgery team on the long-term prophylactic anticonvulsant therapy.[52]

Vascular Injuries

Vascular injuries are typically the result of gunshot wounds but are seen with non-missile projectiles that can be as innocuous as woodchips.[53] If vascular injury to the head or neck is suspected, the initial study of choice is CTA of the brain/neck as it can provide additional information such as trajectory, retained foreign body, and associated injuries not seen with digital subtraction angiography (DSA).[52] DSA remains the gold standard for the diagnosis of cerebrovascular injuries as CTA has a sensitivity of 73% for detecting these injuries.[53] DSA should be used for diagnosis and treatment planning.[53]

Neck injuries

Pediatric penetrating neck trauma is exceedingly rare, with hypotension on ED presentation or vascular injury being associated with death.[54] Injury pattern differs by age. In patients 0 to 5 years, there is a higher likelihood of injury to the aerodigestive tract. Patients aged 5 to 14 years more commonly injure the vasculature, nerves, or spinal cord in comparison with the younger age group.[55] Evaluation and surgical management decisions align with the management of the adult patient. Hard signs, such as active hemorrhage, expanding or pulsatile hematoma, pulse deficit, significant subcutaneous emphysema, respiratory distress, shock, or airway compromise mandate surgical exploration.[56] In the absence of these hard signs, a CTA of the neck is recommended before any surgical intervention.[55]

Palate injuries

Penetrating palate injuries are fairly unique to the pediatric population and typically result from a fall with an object in the mouth. Complications include retropharyngeal abscess, phlegmon, mediastinitis, internal jugular (IJ) thrombosis, and retained foreign body.[57] Prophylactic antibiotics are not recommended unless the associated laceration is larger than 1 to 2 cm or the wound is grossly contaminated.[57,58] Although most patients do well without intervention, a rare complication (occurring in <1% of these patients) is injury to the internal carotid artery, which could present as a delayed stroke.[57,58] The initial carotid injury would require a CTA.[57,59] Unfortunately, the location, appearance, or severity of the wound has not been correlated with the likelihood of neurological sequalae.[57,60] Outside of multiple case series and reports, the most recent retrospective study done in 2010 by Hennelly and colleagues[60] showed that the morbidity from penetrating palate trauma in the well-appearing patient was very low, with no cases of stroke seen in 122 patients. The decision to obtain a CTA in these patients is still not clear-cut. Decision-making should be shared with the parents while weighing the risks and benefits of imaging and definitive diagnosis with radiation and potential sedation.[57,59,60] One study has found promising results with a reduced-dose-targeted CT protocol specifically for penetrating palate injuries which includes images from the skull base to the hyoid bone. This technique would help to reduce radiation while maintaining diagnostic accuracy.[59]

Thorax injuries

With penetrating thorax trauma, there should be a high suspicion for multiple injuries and potential decompensation.[61] In pediatric penetrating thoracic trauma, mortality is inversely proportional to patient age, and death occurs in up to 14% of cases.[62,63] Hemothorax and concomitant head injury are independently associated with mortality. Compared with the adult population, pediatric patients have a lower risk of rib or sternal fractures, flail chest, and hemothorax.[62] Pediatric patients with penetrating thoracic trauma have also been shown to need a greater amount of blood products per kilogram compared with their adult counterparts.[62] Up to 35% of these patients will require operative intervention, and approximately one-third of these injuries will be able to be managed with tube thoracotomy alone.[63]

Abdominal injuries

In penetrating abdominal injuries, the small bowel is injured more often than the large bowel, which is injured more often than the liver. The risk of complications can be predicted by clinical shock, the number of organs injured, the mL/kg of blood transfusions needed, and concomitant thoracic trauma.[64] In a study looking at solid organ injuries related to penetrating stab wounds, the kidneys were the most commonly injured organ, followed by the liver and the spleen. Hollow viscus injuries were also found in a substantial portion of these patients.[65]

Exploratory laparotomy has been considered the gold standard for management of pediatric patients with penetrating abdominal trauma, but recent studies are show that minimally invasive laparoscopic surgery, or observation, can be used in the hemodynamically stable patient.[65,66] This approach may decrease morbidity and mortality associated with exploratory laparotomy.[67] In one study with 102 cases of penetrating pediatric trauma, minimally invasive surgery identified all of the injured organs.[66] Butler and colleagues[68] conducted a study in which surgeons were asked how they would manage a 9-year-old with a stab wound to the abdomen. The surgeons were asked to choose between observation, diagnostic laparoscopy, exploratory laparotomy, and local wound exploration.[68] The largest percentage (39.1%) of surgeons chose observation, 31.5% chose laparoscopy, and 29.5% chose local wound exploration; no respondent chose the laparotomy. Pediatric surgeons were more likely to choose laparoscopy over observation.[68]

PEDIATRIC BLUNT TRAUMA
Head Injuries

Head injury is particularly common, especially in infants and young children, due to their proportionally large heads and weak cervical muscles. The widely used PECARN criteria were studied and implemented in an attempt to decrease unnecessary CT scans in the pediatric population. This objective has had variable success nationwide, but it has been demonstrated that usage can decrease rates of CT scan, so PECARN criteria should be evaluated when deciding on brain imaging for a stable child with a GCS of 14 or greater.[69–71] For patients with a recommendation of observation versus imaging, there is not a definitive rule in which patients may benefit from imaging, but take into consideration ease and likelihood of return to care if patient worsens on discharge as well as family and provider comfort. Patients with GCS of less than 14 or concern for basilar skull fracture should have imaging. Although CT has been the imaging modality of choice, fast MRI protocols have been becoming more available, represent a reasonable alternative for stable patients, and do not involve radiation.[72] MRI can also be used to monitor progression of injuries.

Similar injury patterns can be seen in children and adults—including epidural, subdural, subarachnoid, and intraparenchymal hemorrhages as well as cerebral contusions and diffuse axonal injury.[73] The etiology of epidural hematomas is often different in children, with bleeding from the edges of fracture sites, often venous in nature, being the predominant cause.[74] Subdural hematomas may be associated with more severe injury to various structures in children in comparison with epidural hematomas.[74] A pathology unique to the neonate is the subgaleal hemorrhage. Subgaleal hemorrhages originate from the emissary veins which connect the scalp veins to the dural sinuses, although most cases are associated with birth trauma, cases have also been attributed to traumatic causes including nonaccidental trauma (NAT) and bleeding disorders.[75–77] The subgaleal space can expand enough to accommodate blood loss of up to 70% of an infant's circulating volume. Although subgaleal hematomas can occur in older individuals, they are unlikely to represent a source of significant blood loss. Intracranial bleeding without a developmentally appropriate traumatic etiology should prompt workup for NAT. Either concurrently or, if the workup for NAT is negative, consider evaluating for bleeding disorders.

Intracranial bleeding should be managed in conjunction with neurosurgical consultation. If concern for herniation is present, hyperosmolar therapy with either mannitol or hypertonic saline is appropriate. Evidence for hypertonic saline is more robust and mannitol has less high-quality evidence but is still commonly used.[78] A recent study suggests possible superiority of hypertonic saline due to both a decrease in intracranial pressure and an increase in cerebral perfusion pressure (CPP) versus an isolated increase in CPP with mannitol.[79] At this time, the decision should be driven by availability of agents and consultant or institutional preference, but should lean toward hypertonic saline if available. The Guidelines for the Management of Pediatric Severe Brain Injury give a level II recommendation for an initial bolus dose of 3% hypertonic saline at 2 to 5 mL/kg given over 10 to 20 minutes.[78]

Skull fractures are not uncommon and can be seen either in conjunction with intracranial hemorrhage or as an isolated injury. Simple linear skull fractures are often appropriate for supportive care, but depressed or comminuted fractures require neurosurgical input and potential intervention.[80] Concussions are also common in the pediatric population; they can range from mild symptoms that resolve quickly to near debilitating symptoms that can take months to resolve. Pediatric patients can take longer to recover than adults. For the athlete, evaluations such as the CHILD SCAT5 can be used to help guide return to play. Consider referring the patient for neurology or concussion specific follow-up, especially if symptoms do not resolve after 2 to 4 weeks.[81]

Neck Injuries

Cervical spine trauma, though uncommon, is the most common form of spine trauma in pediatrics and can carry with it significant morbidity and mortality. Injuries are more common in the lower cervical spine in older children. Under 8 years, common injuries are in the upper cervical spine secondary to this being the area of maximal mobility.[24] Specifically, atlantooccipital dislocation is the most common injury under 2 years of age, whereas from ages 2 to 7 atlantoaxial rotatory subluxation becomes common as well. X-rays are the initial test of choice for cervical spine injury, with an initial lateral view being used often for screening. Sensitivity in pediatric patients has been demonstrated to be as high as 90% in the setting of blunt trauma.[82] It is important to note that there are several normal findings on pediatric cervical spine x-ray that can mimic pathology, so films should be read with the pediatric normal in mind. CT should be considered in the case of injury seen on x-ray that needs to be characterized, high clinical suspicion that requires the diagnosis be made quickly, or inability to perform adequate x-rays. MRI should also be considered when feasible when the cervical collar is unable to be cleared clinically and the patient is stable, especially given the risk for ligamentous injury in pediatrics.[24]

Clearance of the cervical collar is not as clear an issue in pediatric patients as it is in adults. The Canadian Cervical Spine Rule was studied in patients 16 and older, which limits the generalizability, although the NEXUS trial included pediatric patients, the numbers were small. NEXUS guidelines can reasonably be applied to developmentally normal children 8 year of age and older, whereas caution should be used with younger children. Other proposed guidelines have similar criteria as NEXUS.[82] It is helpful to have a written protocol for cervical spine clearance for pediatric patients as there is not a definitive standard of care and there is a wide variability in practice.[83] Blunt cerebrovascular injury (BCVI) is rare in pediatrics. Out of over 69,000 blunt pediatric trauma patients, less than 0.2% had BCVI. Factors that were independently associated with BCVI included skull base fracture, cervical spine fracture, intracranial hemorrhage, GCS of eight or less, and a mandibular fracture.[84] Motor vehicle accidents were not independently associated with BCVI in this study.[84] Multiple screening tools have been proposed, but to date none have external validation showing appropriate sensitivity and specificity.[84,85] Treatment of BCVI in pediatrics is not standardized; a recent study showed no difference in rates of complications between antiplatelet and anticoagulation therapy. The study found a nonsignificant trend toward better rates of healing with use of antiplatelet therapy, but the numbers were small.[86]

Thoracic Trauma

Pediatric thoracic trauma is uncommon but carries with it a proportionally high morbidity and mortality. The rib cage is more flexible due to non-ossification of the costal cartilage, allowing higher forces to be transmitted to the underlying organs but decreasing the rates of rib fractures. The mediastinal structures also have increased mobility, leading more commonly to tension physiology.[87] Pulmonary contusions, pneumothorax, and hemothorax are all common. Mediastinal injuries are rare but can cause mortality rates of up to 32% in the first hour.[87] Chest x-ray is the most appropriate screening tool for thoracic injury.[34] Otherwise, diagnosis and treatment of these injuries is similar to that of adult patients.

Abdominal Trauma

Abdominal organs in pediatric patients are proportionally larger than in adults as well as less protected by the rib cage, secondary to the flexibility noted above. Workup should start with physical examination, with generalized abdominal pain and tenderness being a sensitive marker for intra-abdominal injury in a neurologically intact patient. Abdominal distention and bruising (including seatbelt signs) are also concerning markers.[8] Laboratory work can be used as a screening tool for intra-abdominal injury in the hemodynamically stable patient. Elevated transaminases with an AST above 200 U/L or ALT above 125 U/L in known blunt abdominal trauma or an elevation above 80 U/L of either in the setting of NAT should prompt CT imaging. If microscopic hematuria is present, renal imaging should be considered.[8] Amylase and lipase levels have been classically part of the screening evaluation, although they will not be elevated at initial presentation even in the setting of pancreatic injury. Handlebar injuries in particular can cause delayed presentation and commonly involve pancreas and hollow viscus injuries.[9] These injuries are frequently missed and misdiagnosed, so have a high index of suspicion for this type of injury based on historical features. Solid organ injuries (spleen, liver, and kidney) are common and often can be managed nonoperatively. Multicenter studies show failure rates of nonoperative management less than 5% for hemodynamically stable patients.[9]

CT has classically been the test of choice in evaluation for intra-abdominal injury; however, given concerns about ionizing radiation, alternative evaluation tools have been studied. Contrast-enhanced ultrasound (CEUS) has shown promise. A 2021 systematic review from Italy showed a range of sensitivity of 85.7% to 100% and specificity of 89% to 100% for solid organ injury.[88] CEUS may represent a reasonable alternative to CT for screening tests, but it is not yet widely available and in use. MRI may be useful in the follow-up imaging of some conditions but does not currently have a role in imaging acute abdominal trauma.

Extremity Trauma

Extremity trauma is exceedingly common in pediatrics, and there are a few important considerations to note. The Salter–Harris classification is used for fractures involving the growth plate, which comprise up to 20% of pediatric fractures. Salter–Harris I fractures involve only the physis and may not be apparent on x-ray because of this.[89] If there is a clinical suspicion based on history and there is bony point tenderness on examination, these patients should be immobilized. Other important fractures to be aware of are those in a nonmobile infant, injuries that do not match the description of events or do not have a clear story, and multiple injuries at an early age. Some fracture patterns such as classical metaphyseal lesions (corner or bucket handle fracture) are more common in NAT; however, many fractures are nonspecific. Emergency physicians should be vigilant about accounting for the circumstances of all injuries.[90]

Peripheral vascular injury is uncommon but occurs in pediatrics and management practices have variability. CT is used frequently although Doppler ultrasound may also be effective in diagnosis. A significant proportion requires operative management with subsequent anticoagulant or antiplatelet therapy. There is little dedicated pediatric literature to inform practice on either management or optimal imaging.[91]

PEDIATRIC VERSUS ADULT TRAUMA CENTERS

Pediatric patients are better served at pediatric trauma centers (PTCs) with the advantage shown the clearest in younger and more severely injured children.[92] A study conducted by Kahil and colleagues, looked at just over 10,000 children in the National Trauma Data Bank. Patients were divided into two age groups: 0 to 14 years and 15 to 18 years. Primary outcomes were ED and inpatient mortality depending on whether they were taken to a PTC or an adult trauma center (ACT). Secondary outcomes included hospital length of stay, complication rate, ICU length of stay, and ventilator days.[93] Children in the 0 to 14 year age group had lower ED and inpatient mortality when treated at PTCs. This age group was also more likely to be discharged home and have fewer ICU and ventilator days when treated at PTCs. There was no difference in ED mortality or inpatient mortality in the 15- to18-year age group between PTCs and Adult Trauma Center (ATCs). There were no differences in complication rates in either age group between PTCs and ATCs.[93] In the case of penetrating injuries, there were equivalent survival outcomes between ATCs and PTCs in the Kahil and colleagues study, but Miyata and colleagues showed that younger penetrating trauma patients may have better functional outcomes when treated at PTCs.[93,94] The literature suggests that children aged 0 to 14 should ideally be evaluated primarily at PTCs, this may not always be feasible.[93] ATCs should therefore remain prepared to resuscitate critically ill pediatric trauma patients and may elect to transfer these patients to a PTC after stabilization.

SUMMARY

Emergency response to the pediatric trauma patient starts with the basics—ABCDE. Certain important differences in pediatric patients, such as airway physiology and drug dosing, must be considered, but standardized resources are available. Pediatric blunt and penetrating trauma evaluation and treatment also have mechanisms and nuances that distinguish them from adult cases. Much of the current treatment literature has its foundation in the adult literature, so future additions to the literature of pediatric trauma may establish evidence for important distinctions in testing or treatment between adult and pediatric trauma patients.

CLINICS CARE POINTS

- Use a systematic method for evaluation (ABCDE) to avoid missed data or being distracted by visible injury.
- Be aware of age appropriate vital signs and try to normalize vital signs to these values when resuscitating.
- Volume resuscitation begins with crystalloids for pediatric patients, but consider switching to blood products at 20 mL/kg of volume resuscitation and transfuse in 10 mL/kg aliquots.
- Utilize intraosseous access early if there are difficulties in peripheral intravenous access. Consider age appropriate development in interpretation of the neurologic exam.
- Children become hypothermic easily, cover and provide warming measures as soon as feasible to prevent this.
- Ionizing radiation should be used judiciously in pediatrics - for stable patients consider starting workup with focused physical exam and laboratory studies.
- FAST can provide helpful insight in the hemodynamically unstable patient, but can be falsely reassuring in the hemodynamically stable patient.

- Remember to evaluate for and treat pain, even in patients too young to verbalize their symptoms. Consider sedation for painful procedures.
- Think about non-accidental trauma when the injury is suspicious or the mechanism does not suggest the injury seen.

DISCLOSURE

The authors have nothing to disclose.

REFERENCES

1. Sulton C, Taylor T. The Pediatric Airway and Rapid Sequence Intubation in Trauma. Trauma Rep 2017;18:1–11.
2. Shi F, Xiao Y, Xiong W, et al. Cuffed versus uncuffed endotracheal tubes in children: a meta-analysis. J Anesth 2016 Feb;30(1):3–11.
3. Topjian AA, Raymond TT, Atkins D, et al. Part 4: pediatric basic and advanced life support 2020 american heart association guidelines for cardiopulmonary resuscitation and emergency cardiovascular care. Pediatrics 2021;147(Suppl 1):S88–159.
4. Kerrey BT, Rinderknecht AS, Geis GL, et al. Rapid sequence intubation for pediatric emergency patients: higher frequency of failed attempts and adverse effects found by video review. Ann Emerg Med 2012;60(3):251–9.
5. Sakles JC. Improving the Safety of Rapid Sequence Intubation in the Emergency Department. Ann Emerg Med 2017;69(1):7–9.
6. Roberts JR, Custalow CB, Thomsen TW. Roberts and Hedges' clinical procedures in emergency medicine and acute care. 7th edition. Philadelphia, PA: Elsevier; 2019. p. 127–41.
7. Morrison S, Aerts S, Saldien V. The ventrain device: a future role in difficult airway algorithms? A A Pract 2019;13(9):362–5.
8. Guyther J. Advances in pediatric abdominal trauma: what's new is assessment and management. Trauma Rep 2016;17:1–15.
9. Schacherer N, Miller J, Petronis K. Pediatric blunt abdominal trauma in the emergency department: evidence-based management techniques. Pediatr Emerg Med Pract 2014;11(10):1–23 [quiz 23-4]. Update in: Pediatr Emerg Med Pract. 2020 Jan 15;17(Suppl 1):1-59.
10. Barcelona SL, Thompson AA, Coté CJ. Intraoperative pediatric blood transfusion therapy: a review of common issues. Part I: hematologic and physiologic differences from adults; metabolic and infectious risks. Pediatr Anesth 2005;15(9):716–26.
11. Blain S. Paterson. Paediatric massive transfusion. BJA Education 2016;16(8):269–75.
12. Skelton T, Beno S. Massive transfusion in pediatric trauma: we need to focus more on "how. J Trauma Acute Care Surg 2017;82(1):211–5.
13. Shirek G, Phillips R, Shahi N, et al. To give or not to give? Blood for pediatric trauma patients prior to pediatric trauma center arrival. Pediatr Surg Int 2022;38(2):285–93.
14. American College of Surgeons. Committee on Trauma. Advanced trauma life support: student course manual. 10th edition. Chicago, IL: American College of Surgeons; 2018.
15. Anand T, Obaid O, Nelson A, et al. Whole blood hemostatic resuscitation in pediatric trauma: a nationwide propensity-matched analysis. J Trauma Acute Care Surg 2021;91(4):573–8.

16. Maw G, Furyk C. Pediatric massive transfusion: a systematic review. Pediatr Emerg Care 2018;34(8):594–8.

17. Evangelista ME, Gaffley M, Neff LP. Massive transfusion protocols for pediatric patients: current perspectives. J Blood Med 2020;11:163–72.

18. Noland DK, Apelt N, Greenwell C, et al. Massive transfusion in pediatric trauma: an ATOMAC perspective. J Pediatr Surg 2019;54(2):345–9.

19. Phillips R, Shahi N, Acker SN, et al. Not as simple as ABC: tools to trigger massive transfusion in pediatric trauma. J Trauma Acute Care Surg 2022;92(2): 422–7.

20. Phillips R, Moore H, Bensard D, et al. It is time for TEG in pediatric trauma: unveiling meaningful alterations in children who undergo massive transfusion. Pediatr Surg Int 2021;37(11):1613–20.

21. Wikkelsø A, Wetterslev J, Møller AM, et al. Thromboelastography (TEG) or thromboelastometry (ROTEM) to monitor haemostatic treatment versus usual care in adults or children with bleeding. Cochrane Database Syst Rev 2016;2016(8): CD007871.

22. Hoey G. and Keane O., Intraosseous access, Don't Forget the Bubbles, 2020. Available at: https://doi.org/10.31440/DFTB.31005.

23. Greene N, Bhananker S, Ramaiah R. Vascular access, fluid resuscitation, and blood transfusion in pediatric trauma. Int J Crit Illn Inj Sci 2012;2(3):135–42.

24. Li Y, Glotzbecker M, Hedequist D, et al. Pediatric spinal trauma. Trauma 2012;14: 82–96.

25. Abram S, Bulstrode C. Routine spinal immobilization in trauma patients: what are the advantages and disadvantages? Surgeon 2010;8(4):218–22.

26. Nolte PC, Liao S, Kuch M, et al. Development of a new emergency medicine spinal immobilization protocol for pediatric trauma patients and first applicability test on emergency medicine personnel. Pediatr Emerg Care 2022;38(1):e75–84.

27. Schafermeyer RW, Ribbeck BM, Gaskins J, et al. Respiratory effects of spinal immobilization in children. Ann Emerg Med 1991;20(9):1017–9.

28. Velopulos CG, Shihab HM, Lottenberg L, et al. Prehospital spine immobilization/ spinal motion restriction in penetrating trauma: a practice management guideline from the Eastern Association for the Surgery of Trauma (EAST). J Trauma Acute Care Surg 2018;84:736.

29. DeBoer SL, Seaver M. Pediatric spinal immobilization: C-spines, car seats, and color-coded collars. J Emerg Nurs 2004;30(5):481–4.

30. Tanner D, Negaard A, Huang R, et al. A prospective evaluation of the accuracy of weight estimation using the broselow tape in overweight and obese pediatric patients in the emergency department. Pediatr Emerg Care 2017;33(10):675–8.

31. Davis AL, Wales PW, Malik T, et al. The BIG score and prediction of mortality in pediatric blunt trauma. J Pediatr 2015;167(3):593–8.e1.

32. Hatchimonji J, Luks V, Swendiman R, et al. Settling the score. Pediatr Emerg Care 2022;38(2):e828–32.

33. Huang YT, Huang YH, Hsieh CH, et al. Comparison of injury severity score, glasgow coma scale, and revised trauma score in predicting the mortality and prolonged ICU stay of traumatic young children: a cross-sectional retrospective study. Emerg Med Int 2019;2019:5453624.

34. Berger M, Ortego A. Calculated decisions: injury severity score (ISS). Pediatr Emerg Med Pract 2019;16(5):CD1–2.

35. Lecuyer M. Calculated decisions: pediatric trauma score (PTS). Pediatr Emerg Med Pract 2019;16(5):CD3–4.

36. Gutierrez P, Travers C, Geng Z, et al. Centralization of prehospital triage improves triage of prehospital pediatric trauma patients. Pediatr Emer Care 2021;37:11–6.

37. Rubens J, Ahmed O, Yenokyan G, et al. Mode of transport and trauma activation status in admitted pediatric trauma patients. J Surg Res 2020;246:153–9.

38. Huh Y, Ko Y, Hwang K, et al. Admission lactate and base deficit in predicting outcomes of pediatric trauma. Shock 2021;55(4):495–500.

39. Moore MA, Wallace EC, Westra SJ. The imaging of paediatric thoracic trauma. Pediatr Radiol 2009;39(5):485–96.

40. Guillamondegui O, Mahboubi S, Stafford P, et al. The utility of the pelvic radiograph in the assessment of pediatric pelvic fractures. J Trauma 2003;55:236–40.

41. Eckert MJ, Wertin TM, Tyner SD, et al. Tranexamic acid administration to pediatric trauma patients in a combat setting: the pediatric trauma and tranexamic acid study (PED-TRAX). J Trauma Acute Care Surg 2014;77(6):852–8.

42. Thomson JM, Huynh HH, Drone HM, et al. Experience in an urban level 1 trauma center with tranexamic acid in pediatric trauma: a retrospective chart review. J Intensive Care Med 2021;36(4):413–8.

43. Cornelius B, Cummings Q, Assercq M, et al. Current practices in tranexamic acid administration for pediatric trauma patients in the United States. J Trauma Nurs 2021;28(1):21–5.

44. Hamele M, Aden JK, Borgman MA. Tranexamic acid in pediatric combat trauma requiring massive transfusions and mortality. J Trauma Acute Care Surg 2020; 89(2S Suppl 2):S242–5.

45. Nishijima DK, VanBuren J, Hewes HA, et al. Traumatic injury clinical trial evaluating tranexamic acid in children (TIC-TOC): study protocol for a pilot randomized controlled trial. Trials 2018;19(1):593.

46. Lin YR, Wu MH, Chen TY, et al. Time to epinephrine treatment is associated with the risk of mortality in children who achieve sustained ROSC after traumatic out-of-hospital cardiac arrest. Crit Care 2019;23(1):101.

47. Post B, Nielsen DPD, Visram A. Comment upon "Time to epinephrine treatment is associated with the risk of mortality in children who achieve sustained ROSC after traumatic out-of-hospital cardiac arrest. Crit Care 2019;23(1):336.

48. Easter JS, Vinton DT, Haukoos JS. Emergent pediatric thoracotomy following traumatic arrest. Resuscitation 2012;83(12):1521–4.

49. Prieto JM, Van Gent JM, Calvo RY, et al. Nationwide analysis of resuscitative thoracotomy in pediatric trauma: time to differentiate from adult guidelines? J Trauma Acute Care Surg 2020;89(4):686–90.

50. Campagna GA, Cunningham ME, Hernandez JA, et al. The utility and promise of Resuscitative Endovascular Balloon Occlusion of the Aorta (REBOA) in the pediatric population: An evidence-based review. J Pediatr Surg 2020;55(10):2128–33.

51. Carrillo L, Skibber M, Kumar A, et al. Morphometric and physiologic modeling study for endovascular occlusion in pediatric trauma patients. ASAIO J 2020; 66(1):97–104.

52. Drosos E, Giakoumettis D, Blionas A, et al. Pediatric nonmissile penetrating head injury: case series and literature review. World Neurosurg 2018;110:193–205.

53. Ravindra V, Dewan M, Akbari H, et al. Management of penetrating cerebrovascular injuries in pediatric trauma: a retrospective multicenter study. Neurosurgery 2017;81:473–80.

54. Stone M, Farber B, Olorunfemi O, et al. Penetrating neck trauma in children: an uncommon entity described using the National Trauma Data Bank. J Trauma Acute Care Surg 2016;80:604–9.

55. Adbelmasih M, Kayssi A, Roche-Nagle G. Penetrating paediatric neck trauma. BMJ Case Rep 2019;12:e226436.

56. Tessler R, Nguyen H, Newton C, et al. Pediatric penetrating neck trauma: hard signs of injury and selective neck exploration. J Trauma Acute Care Surg 2017; 82:989–94.

57. Rose E, Sherwin T. Carotid dissection and cerebral infarction from posterior oropharyngeal trauma. Pediatr Emerg Care 2019;35(1):e17–21.

58. McCullum N, Guse S. Neck Trauma. Cervical spine, seatbelt sign, and penetrating palate injuries. Emerg Men Clin N Am 2021;39:573–88.

59. Choi J, Burton C, Danehy A, et al. Neck CT angiography examinations for pediatric oropharyngeal trauma: diagnostic yield and proposal of a new targeted technique. Pediatr Radiol 2020;50:1602–9.

60. Hennelly K, Kimia A, Lee L, et al. Incidence of morbidity from penetrating palate trauma. Pediatrics 2010;126:e1578–84.

61. Elkbuli A, Meneses E, Kinslow K, et al. Successful management of gunshot wound to the chest resulting in multiple intra-abdominal and thoracic injuries in a pediatric trauma patient: a case report and literature review. Int J Surg Care Rep 2020;76:372–6.

62. Keneally R, Shields C, Hsu A, et al. Pediatric thoracic trauma in Iraq and Afghanistan. Mil Med 2018;183:e596–602.

63. Mollberg N, Tabachnick D, Lin F, et al. Age-associated impact on presentation and outcome for penetrating thoracic trauma in the adult and pediatric populations. J Trauma Acute Care Surg 2013;76:273–8.

64. Iflazoglu N, Ureyen O, Oner OZ, et al. Complications and risk factors for mortality in penetrating abdominal firearm injuries: analysis of 120 cases. Int J Clin Exp Med 2015;8(4):6154–62.

65. Sakamoto R, Matsushima K, de Roulet A, et al. Nonoperative management of penetrating abdominal solid organ injuries in children. J Surg Res 2018;228: 188–93.

66. Mahmoud M, Daboos M, Bayoumi A, et al. Role of minimally invasive surgery in management of penetrating abdominal trauma in children. Eur J Pediatr Surg 2021;31:353–61.

67. Donati-Bourne J, Mohammad BI, Parikh D, et al. Paediatric penetrating thoraco-abdominal injury: role of minimally invasive surgery. Afr J Paediatr Surg 2014; 11(2):189–90.

68. Butler E, Groner J, Vavilala M, et al. Surgeon choice in management of pediatric abdominal trauma. J Pediatr Surg 2021;56:146–52.

69. Burstein B, Upton JEM, Terra HF, et al. Use of CT for Head Trauma: 2007-2015. Pediatrics 2018;142(4):e20180814.

70. Nigrovic LE, Kuppermann N. Children with minor blunt head trauma presenting to the emergency department. Pediatrics 2019;144(6):e20191495.

71. Ukwuoma OI, Allareddy V, Allareddy V, et al. Trends in head computed tomography utilization in children presenting to emergency departments after traumatic head injury. Pediatr Emerg Care 2021;37(7):e384–90.

72. Shope C, Alshareef M, Larrew T, et al. Utility of a pediatric fast magnetic resonance imaging protocol as surveillance scanning for traumatic brain injury. J Neurosurg Pediatr 2021;27(4):475–81.

73. Gelineau-Morel RN, Zinkus TP, Le Pichon JB. Pediatric head trauma: a review and update. Pediatr Rev 2019;40(9):468–81.

74. Figaji AA. Anatomical and physiological differences between children and adults relevant to traumatic brain injury and the implications for clinical assessment and care. Front Neurol 2017;8:685.

75. Bowens JP, Liker K. Subgaleal hemorrhage secondary to child physical abuse in a 4-year-old boy. Pediatr Emerg Care 2021;37(12):e1738–40.

76. Hepner MK, Hikmet F, Soe T. G296(P) A case of unexplained subgaleal bleed in an infant. Arch Dis Child 2016;101:A166.

77. Wetzel EA, Kingma PS. Subgaleal hemorrhage in a neonate with factor X deficiency following a non-traumatic cesarean section. J Perinatol 2012;32(4):304–5.

78. Kochanek PM, Tasker RC, Carney N, et al. Guidelines for the management of pediatric severe traumatic brain injury, third edition: update of the brain trauma foundation guidelines, executive summary. Neurosurgery 2019;84(6):1169–78.

79. Kochanek PM, Adelson PD, Rosario BL, et al. Comparison of intracranial pressure measurements before and after hypertonic saline or mannitol treatment in children with severe traumatic brain injury. JAMA Netw Open 2022;5(3):e220891.

80. Lyons TW, Stack AM, Monuteaux MC, et al. A QI initiative to reduce hospitalization for children with isolated skull fractures. Pediatrics 2016;137(6):e20153370.

81. Silverberg ND, Iaccarino MA, Panenka WJ, et al. Management of concussion and mild traumatic brain injury: a synthesis of practice guidelines. Arch Phys Med Rehabil 2020;101(2):382–93.

82. Guyther J. Advances in pediatric neck trauma: what's new is assessment and management. Trauma Rep 2020;21:1–13.

83. Pannu GS, Shah MP, Herman MJ. Cervical spine clearance in pediatric trauma centers: the need for standardization and an evidence-based protocol. J Pediatr Orthop 2017;37(3):e145–9.

84. Grigorian A, Dolich M, Lekawa M, et al. Analysis of blunt cerebrovascular injury in pediatric trauma. J Trauma Acute Care Surg 2019;87(6):1354–9.

85. Herbert JP, Venkataraman SS, Turkmani AH, et al. Pediatric blunt cerebrovascular injury: the McGovern screening score. J Neurosurg Pediatr 2018;21(6):639–49.

86. Ravindra VM, Bollo RJ, Dewan MC, et al. Comparison of anticoagulation and antiplatelet therapy for treatment of blunt cerebrovascular injury in children <10 years of age: a multicenter retrospective cohort study. Childs Nerv Syst 2021; 37(1):47–54.

87. Minervini F, Scarci M, Kocher G, et al. Pediatric chest trauma: a unique challenge. J Visualized Surg 2020;6:8.

88. Pegoraro F, Giusti G, Giacalone M, et al. Contrast-enhanced ultrasound in pediatric blunt abdominal trauma: a systematic review. J Ultrasound 2022;25(3): 419–27, published online ahead of print, 2022 Jan 18.

89. Kim HHR, Menashe SJ, Ngo AV, et al. Uniquely pediatric upper extremity injuries. Clin Imaging 2021;80:249–61.

90. Sink EL, Hyman JE, Matheny T, et al. Child abuse: the role of the orthopaedic surgeon in nonaccidental trauma. Clin Orthop Relat Res 2011;469(3):790–7.

91. Shahi N, Phillips R, Meier M, et al. Anti-coagulation management in pediatric traumatic vascular injuries. J Pediatr Surg 2020;55(2):324–30.

92. Sathya C, Alali A, Wales P, et al. Mortality among injured children treated at different trauma center types. JAMA Surg 2015;50:874–81.

93. Khalil M, Alawwa G, Pinto F, et al. Pediatric mortality at pediatric versus adult trauma centers. J Emerg Trauma Shock 2021;14:128–35.

94. Miyata S, Cho J, Lebedevskiy O. Trauma experts versus pediatric experts: comparison of outcomes in pediatric penetrating injuries. J Surg Res 2017;208:173–9.

Moving?

Make sure your subscription moves with you!

To notify us of your new address, find your **Clinics Account Number** (located on your mailing label above your name), and contact customer service at:

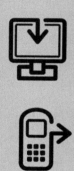

Email: journalscustomerservice-usa@elsevier.com

800-654-2452 (subscribers in the U.S. & Canada)
314-447-8871 (subscribers outside of the U.S. & Canada)

Fax number: 314-447-8029

Elsevier Health Sciences Division
Subscription Customer Service
3251 Riverport Lane
Maryland Heights, MO 63043

*To ensure uninterrupted delivery of your subscription, please notify us at least 4 weeks in advance of move.

Printed and bound by CPI Group (UK) Ltd, Croydon, CR0 4YY

08/05/2025

01864717-0002